MRCS... **PM**

500 SBAs and EMQs

SECOND EDITION

D1350483

MRCOG Part 2

500 SBAs and EMQs

SECOND EDITION

Rekha Wuntakal MBBS MD(O&G) DNB DFFP MRCOG
Consultant in Gynaecology and Gynaecological Oncology
Queen's Hospital, Romford, UK

Ziena Abdullah MBBS BSc MRCOG
Specialty Registrar in Obstetrics and Gynaecology
Newham General Hospital, London, UK

Edited by

Tony Hollingworth MBChB PhD MBA FRCS(Ed) FRCOG
Consultant in Obstetrics and Gynaecology
Whipps Cross University Hospital,
Barts Health NHS Trust, London, UK

David Redford MB FRCS FRCOG
Consultant in Obstetrics and Gynaecology
Royal Shrewsbury Hospital, Shrewsbury, UK

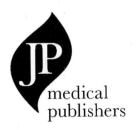

JP
medical
publishers

London • New Delhi • Panama City

© 2018 JP Medical Ltd.
Published by JP Medical Ltd
83 Victoria Street, London, SW1H 0HW, UK
Tel: +44 (0)20 3170 8910   Fax: +44 (0)20 3008 6180
Email: info@jpmedpub.com   Web: www.jpmedpub.com

ISBN: 978-1-909836-63-1

British Library Cataloguing in Publication Data
A catalogue record for this book is available from the British Library

Library of Congress Cataloging in Publication Data
A catalog record for this book is available from the Library of Congress

Commissioning Editor:	Steffan Clements
Editorial Assistant:	Adam Rajah
Design:	Designers Collective Ltd

Preface

The MRCOG examination is designed to set a standard of competent, safe practice for any doctor wanting to pursue a career in obstetrics and gynaecology. The exam has recently been divided into three parts. The Part 1 exam remains largely unchanged, while the Part 2 exam has been divided into two. The new Part 2 exam forms the theoretical element of the MRCOG, consisting of extended matching questions (EMQs) and single best answer questions (SBAs) instead of multiple choice questions (MCQs) and short answer questions (SAQs). The new Part 3 forms the clinical element of the MRCOG.

This book provides a revision aid for the Part 2 exam; accordingly, in this edition we have replaced MCQs and SAQs with 250 newly written SBAs. At the same time, we have replaced some of the 250 EMQs and updated those that have not been rewritten. The scenario-based questions are structured in the same way as the exam, which will enable trainees to identify areas of strength and weakness. It is important to keep up-to-date with guidelines in obstetrics and gynaecology, and to be familiar with the most recent studies in the field; the explanatory notes accompanying the answers will assist with this.

We hope that this book will prove useful in your revision for the MRCOG Part 2 exam.

Rekha Wuntakal
Ziena Abdullah
Tony Hollingworth
David Redford
September 2017

Dedication

Dedicated to my mother Akkamma, my brothers Sateesh, Nagu and Manjunath,
my sister Neelu and all my teachers in the UK.

Rekha Wuntakal

Dedicated to my mother Sajida, my sister Ayat and my husband Hasan.
Thank you for your support.

Ziena Abdullah

Acknowledgements

The authors wish to thank Miss Deepa Janga for her contribution to the chapter *Antenatal care*.

Contents

Preface   v
Dedication   vi
Acknowledgements   vi
Exam revision advice   viii

Chapter 1   Clinical skills   1

Chapter 2   Teaching, appraisal and assessment   17

Chapter 3   Information technology, clinical
            governance and research   27

Chapter 4   Core surgical skills   45

Chapter 5   Postoperative care   61

Chapter 6   Surgical procedures   71

Chapter 7   Antenatal care   81

Chapter 8   Maternal medicine   125

Chapter 9   Management of labour   155

Chapter 10 Management of delivery   173

Chapter 11 Postpartum problems (the puerperium)   189

Chapter 12 Gynaecological problems   205

Chapter 13 Subfertility   225

Chapter 14 Sexual and reproductive health   245

Chapter 15 Early pregnancy care   259

Chapter 16 Gynaecological oncology   279

Chapter 17 Urogynaecology and pelvic floor problems   321

Exam revision advice

Introduction and syllabus

The aim of the MRCOG exam is to set a standard for the competent and safe practice of obstetrics and gynaecology. The exam is made up of three parts:

- The MRCOG Part 1 deals with the basic sciences, and must be passed before taking the MRCOG Part 2.
- The MRCOG Part 2 is a written exam and aims to test the theory.
- The MRCOG Part 3 exam is an objective structured clinical examination (OSCE), which tests clinical knowledge.

The MRCOG Part 2 and 3 exams are aimed at the level of an ST5 trainee in obstetrics and gynaecology, and is 'blueprinted' to ensure that all of the syllabus is covered in both the written and OSCE components. The syllabus covers teaching and appraisal, information and technology, clinical governance and research, core surgical skills, postoperative care, surgical procedures, antenatal care, maternal medicine, fetal medicine, puerperium, management of labour and delivery, gynaecological problems, subfertility, early pregnancy care, women's sexual and reproductive health, gynaecology oncology and urogynaecology. A thorough description of the topics covered in each of these modules is available on the Royal College of Obstetricians and Gynaecologists' (RCOG) website (http://www.rcog.org.uk).

Format of the paper

The MRCOG Part 2 written exam is held twice a year, in March and September. It comprises single best answers (SBAs) and extended matching questions (EMQs). Only candidates who pass the written exam can proceed to the MRCOG Part 3 exam.

MRCOG Part 2 written exam consists of two papers. Marks are equally divided between these papers (50% for paper 1 and 50% for paper 2). Each paper is composed of single best answers (SBAs) and extended matching questions (EMQs). Paper 1 comprises 50 SBAs and 50 EMQs and is to be answered within 180 minutes. This is followed by a 60 minute lunch break. After lunch, paper 2 begins, which comprises 50 SBAs and 50 EMQs which must be answered within 180 minutes. For each paper, the RCOG suggests that candidates spend 70 minutes on SBA questions and 110 minutes on the EMQ questions. SBAs make up 40% of the total marks, and EMQs make up 60%.

The RCOG website provides details about the written exam format, with set examples of SBAs and EMQs. We have matched the RCOG format in this book.

How to prepare for the exam

The best time to sit the MRCOG Part 2 is while working at the level of an ST4 or ST5 trainee in obstetrics and gynaecology. Without realising it, the necessary knowledge should have been gathered by discussing cases with senior colleagues (senior registrars and consultants), attending consultant ward rounds, seeing obstetrics and gynaecology outpatients, and attending organised departmental and regional teaching sessions. However, a theoretical base is important to ensure that trainees understand why they are practicing the way they are when undertaking a particular task. The role of textbooks is essential to acquire this knowledge and to succeed in the exam.

Start planning for the exam at least 12 months before the exam date, especially if your clinical experience (post-registration training) has to be assessed for approval to sit for the exam (the application for assessment of training for entry to the MRCOG Part 2 exam is available via the RCOG website). Applications must reach the RCOG examination department by the preceding 1 October for the March exam or the preceding 1 April for the September exam. Doctors in training posts can sit the MRCOG Part 2 two years after passing the MRCOG Part 1, while doctors in Trust posts (clinical fellows) can sit the exam following four years of experience in obstetrics and gynaecology (MRCOG Part 2 regulations are also available on the RCOG website).

Start preparing and reading for the exam at least 6 months before the exam date and use the first month or two to build momentum to study faster. By this stage, you should have gathered all the necessary revision aids, including relevant textbooks, guidelines (RCOG, NICE, family planning) and exam revision books. Sign up to recommended exam revision websites and work through as many questions as many times as possible, in order to learn and memorise the topics. When doing this, you will be surprised at the amount of information you process and remember.

An effective method for exam study is to ensure that information is quickly and readily accessible. Organise yourself and take the time to learn about the exam: the format and the type of questions likely to be encountered. Make a list of common topics and repeated themes from the syllabus and past papers. Then three months before the exam, attend an MRCOG Part 2 theory course to speed up revision and develop knowledge further. Write down the important topic-based points in a small notebook or make revision cards. These can be used to revise topics in a short period of time several times over when the exam is approaching.

Plan ahead, make notes and revise common topics and themes. Practise answering a wealth of questions before the exam to acquire the necessary knowledge and identify any gaps in learning. The main emphasis is on reading the question and answering each one carefully. A week of study leave before the exam is ideal for revision purposes, and make sure you are not on call the day before the exam. Take note of the time and place of your exam, and arrive on time to avoid the added pressure of running late (remember you will not be allowed to sit for the exam if you arrive late).

To ensure success in the exam, it is important to develop and expand knowledge beyond the basics of the syllabus. A brief list of RCOG recommended guidelines and textbooks is given below:

MRCOG and Beyond series: http://www.rcog.org.uk/catalog/rcog-press/mrcog-and-beyond

RCOG Green-top Guidelines (all): http://www.rcog.org.uk/guidelines

Non-RCOG guidelines:

- The Faculty of Sexual & Reproductive Healthcare: www.fsrh.ord

- StratOG: https://stratog.rcog.org.uk/

- NICE guidelines in obstetrics and gynaecology: http://www.nice.org.uk

SIGN: www.sign.ac.uk

The Obstetrician & Gynaecologist (the MRCOG Part 2 questions are set 6 months prior to the set date for the exam, therefore read the issues covering at least three years prior to this period)

Luesley DM and Baker PN. Obstetrics and gynaecology: an evidence-based text for MRCOG (2nd edn). London: Hodder Arnold, 2010.

To help save time when preparing for the MRCOG exam, and to help you to broaden your knowledge on each topic, we have provided further reading (current key textbooks and journal articles) after many of the answers.

Extended matching questions (EMQs) and single best answers (SBAs)

The exam is a test of the knowledge and clinical experience expected of a ST5 or Year 3 specialist registrar. Your choice of answers should be based on the following criteria: which one provides the best care to patients, with the best available evidence after considering the resources and setting? If you are not certain about an answer, consider a patient you have discussed with a senior colleague or have managed in the past, in order to answer the question.

EMQs

Papers 1 and 2 consist of 100 EMQs. Each EMQ presents up to five stems with 10–14 options. To answer the EMQ, match the stem (typically a statement or clinical scenario) with one of the options available. The options are presented in alphabetical order and not all the options may be used. However, a single option may be used more than once. The questions are of a more practical nature than scientific, and the main focus is on the MRCOG Part 2 syllabus. Therefore you are likely to fail if you do not have the necessary knowledge or clinical experience before sitting the exam.

When answering EMQs, formulate an answer in your head before going through the 10–14 answer options. This may save time and avoid confusion. Sometimes you may not be sure between two similar options. In this case, choose the most likely option. If you do not know the answer, start eliminating the options one by one until you get a suitable option which seems like a close fit. Occasionally, you may not have any clue about the answer, or lack appropriate knowledge on the topic. If this is the case, relax and take a logical approach to make an educated guess. There is no negative marking for EMQs.

Finally, remember to read each question carefully. The question may seem familiar but it may not be exactly the question you read before, for instance the framing of the question may be different.

SBAs

A single best answer is a question where you choose one option out of five provided for that particular question. This type of question requires thorough knowledge of the subject in question. Therefore theoretical preparation of all topics in the RCOG curriculum is necessary.

Taking the exam

This question-and-answer book will help with preparation for the MRCOG Part 2 exams because it is written in line with the RCOG curriculum modules; there is a chapter for each module, and each chapter contains both SBAs and EMQs. An answer and explanation is provided for every question, and most answers have references for future reading. The references will help you to refer to further theory relevant to that topic and avoid wasting time.

Make sure you do not leave any questions unanswered because time constraints make it difficult to come back later. If you have time at the end, it is worth going back and reading through the difficult questions to check they are answered correctly. It is important not to get any answers out of sync.

Finally, remember this is your exam. Take a calm and collected approach, and be positive.

Ability is what you're capable of doing. Motivation determines what you do. Attitude determines how well you do it.

Lou Holtz

Good luck for the exam!

Chapter 1

Clinical skills

Questions: SBAs

For each question, select the single best answer from the five options listed.

1. You are doing a busy clinic with the consultant, assisted by a nurse. You have just taken a history from a woman who is complaining of menorrhagia and are about to examine her. You are waiting for the nurse but she is busy with the consultant. The patient is insisting that you examine her without a nurse because she is in a hurry to pick up her son up from school.

   Which of the following is the best course of action?

   A Explain that you are required to have a chaperone and will wait for the nurse
   B Examine the patient without a chaperone
   C Start the examination; the nurse will join you when she is free
   D Ask the patient's husband to chaperone
   E Refer the patient to a consultant who does not mind examining the patient without a chaperone

2. Non-technical skills are essential in obstetrics and gynaecology because they underpin technical ability.

   Which one of the following non-technical skills enables you to gather information, understand it and anticipate possible future developments?

   A Decision-making
   B Communication
   C Leadership
   D Situational awareness
   E Teamwork

3. Non-technical skills are extremely important in obstetrics and gynaecology because the various scenarios and emergencies on the labour ward often demand multitasking.

   Which non-technical skill leads to a good rapport with team members, provides the ability to delegate tasks appropriately and modifies behaviour according to the situation?

   A Decision-making
   B Communication
   C Leadership
   D Situation awareness
   E Teamworking

4. You are the on-call registrar for the gynaecology team and have been asked to go to theatre because the general surgeon wants your assistance with a 23-year-old woman with suspected appendicitis. On diagnostic laparoscopy, the appendix appeared normal but there is an ovarian cyst on the right ovary that measures 5 cm × 6 cm. There is no torsion. The surgeon thinks this is the cause of the woman's pain, and asks you to remove it. She is consented for 'appendectomy and proceed'.

    What is the appropriate management?

    A   Leave the cyst, close the abdomen and discharge the patient
    B   Leave the cyst and arrange follow-up in the gynaecology clinic
    C   Remove the cyst
    D   Take consent for cyst removal from the next of kin
    E   Wake the patient up, obtain consent and then perform a cystectomy

5. You are the on-call registrar for the labour ward and are in theatre with a primiparous woman. She had a prolonged labour but did not progress beyond 7 cm cervical dilatation despite 10 hours of syntocinon augmentation. She then developed clinical signs of chorioamnionitis, and a cardiotocograph trace showed fetal tachycardia of 200 bpm. You are therefore performing an emergency Caesarean section. Once the placenta has been delivered, the uterus is felt to be atonic. Uterotonics are administered in accordance with labour ward protocol. The blood loss is 2000 mL so you call the consultant in. The consultant places a B-Lynch suture but there is bleeding each time the needle is inserted into the myometrium. The anaesthetist is resuscitating the woman with blood products and gives her a general anaesthetic. The blood pressure is low and she becomes tachycardic. Her blood loss is now 4000 mL and the anaesthetist is worried she is going to have a cardiac arrest. The consultant wants to perform a hysterectomy, but you inform him that you have not consented her for hysterectomy. Another consultant is available but is 2 hours away.

    What is your next step in the management of this patient?

    A   Call the haematologist for advice
    B   Continue resuscitation until the bleeding stops
    C   Perform a hysterectomy
    D   Perform a hysterectomy and bilateral sapingo-oophrecotmy
    E   Wait for a second opinion from another consultant

6. Hospital staff have a right to work without fear of abuse or harassment. Conflict and aggression from patients and relatives is complex and often multifactorial. Clinicians therefore have to be aware of the signs that a patient or the partner are about to become aggressive.

    Which one of the following is a sign that a patient is about to become aggressive?

    A   Decreased respiratory rate
    B   Delusions or hallucinations (with violent content)
    C   Decreased restlessness
    D   Decreased volume of speech
    E   No eye contact

7. You are the on-call registrar for the gynaecology team. You have been asked to
    review a woman who is para 0 and has just had a pelvic ultrasound scan at 12
    weeks' gestation. This shows a fetal pole with a crown–rump length of 15 mm but
    no fetal heartbeat. The patient has a history of two previous ectopic pregnancies
    and laparoscopic bilateral salpingectomies. The current pregnancy resulted from
    in vitro fertilisation. The sonographers told her that the doctor will speak to her
    soon. You now have to break the bad news.

    Which one of the following will influence her reaction to the news?

    A   Culture
    B   Obstetric history
    C   Perception of the loss
    D   Religion
    E   All of the above

8. The UK's Department of Health defines clinical governance as 'A framework
    through which ... [health service] ... organisations are accountable for continuously
    improving the quality of their services and safeguarding high standards of care
    by creating an environment in which excellence in clinical care will flourish'. The
    framework is made up of seven elements.

    Which element of clinical governance is described as the right person, doing the
    right thing, at the right time, in the right place, with the right results?

    A   Audit
    B   Clinical effectiveness
    C   Education, training and continued professional development
    D   Information management and communication
    E   Risk management

9. Clinical governance is a framework within which health care systems can
    continually improve their services and make sure their standards are high. It
    consists of seven elements.

    Which element of clinical governance is described as a quality improvement
    process that aims to improve care by comparing current care with a standard in
    order to see if the standard has been achieved?

    A   Audit
    B   Clinical effectiveness
    C   Education, training and continued professional development
    D   Information management and communication
    E   Risk management

10. As the on-call registrar, you go to the postnatal ward to review a patient on whom you performed a Caesarean section the previous day. It was an uncomplicated Caesarean section with an estimated blood loss of 300 mL. When you see the woman, she appears upset and distressed. When you explore the reasons, she tells you that the midwifery staff on the postnatal ward have been rude and aggressive towards her and have not given her medication on time.

What is your advice to her?

A   To contact her lawyer
B   To complete an incident form
C   To think of the positive things on the ward
D   To contact the local advocacy and advisory service for hospital patients
E   Not to worry and that you will investigate further by speaking to the midwives on the postnatal ward

Questions: EMQs

Questions 11–15

Options for Questions 11–15

A	Autoimmune ovarian failure	I	Laurence–Moon–Bardet–Biedl syndrome
B	Constitutional delay		
C	Craniopharyngioma	J	Langerhans cell histiocytosis
D	Etoposide	K	McCune–Albright syndrome
E	Galactosaemia	L	Noonan's syndrome
F	Iatrogenic	M	Rubella
G	Irradiation	N	Turner's syndrome
H	Kallmann's syndrome	O	Tuberculosis

Instructions: For each clinical scenario described below, choose the single most appropriate diagnosis from the list of options above. Each option may be used once, more than once, or not at all.

11. A 16-year-old girl attends her local GP centre with her mother because she has not attained menarche. Clinical examination reveals short stature, cubitus valgus and coarctation of the aorta. Ultrasound scan shows streak gonads.

12. A 15-year-old girl attends the paediatric emergency department after a fall. Clinical examination reveals short stature, hypertelorism, downward slanting of the eyes and a right-sided heart murmur.

13. A 14-year-old girl attends her local GP centre with her mother because she has not attained menarche. She has a history of an unknown cancer at the age of 10 years, for which she received chemotherapy in Pakistan.

14. A 7-year-old girl attends the paediatric emergency department with her mother because she started to have monthly vaginal bleeding. Clinical examination reveals incomplete sexual precocity and café-au-lait spots with irregular borders.

15. A 6-year-old girl is brought to see her GP by her mother because she started to have vaginal bleeding. Clinical examination is normal. She has previously been prescribed steroid hormonal cream by a local GP in Pakistan, to be applied in the vulval area, because she had itching 6 months ago.

Questions 16–20

Options for Questions 16–20

A   Angelman's syndrome
B   Androgen insensitivity syndrome
C   Congenital adrenal hyperplasia
D   Gonadal dysgenesis
E   Hypothyroidism
F   Hyperprolactinaemia
G   Noonan's syndrome
H   Klinefelter's syndrome
I   Mayer–Rokitansky–Küster–Hauser syndrome

J   Fragile X syndrome
K   Pituitary tumour
L   Pituitary prolactinoma
M   Turner's syndrome (45XO)
N   Mosaic Turner's syndrome (45XO/46XX)
O   von Hippel–Lindau disease

Instructions: For each scenario described below, choose the single most appropriate diagnosis for amenorrhoea from the list of options above. Each option may be used once, more than once, or not at all.

16. A 16-year-old girl presents with primary amenorrhoea. She is tall, and on clinical examination there is normal breast development, sparse axillary and pubic hair, a blind vaginal pouch and an absent uterus.

17. A 16-year-old young girl is referred to the gynaecology clinic by her GP with primary amenorrhoea. She gives a history of excessive weight gain and lethargy. Secondary sexual characteristics are normal on clinical examination. Investigations reveal raised serum thyroid-stimulating hormone and prolactin levels.

18. A 16-year-old tall girl presents with primary amenorrhoea. She has been taking medication for psychosis since the age of 13 years.

19. A 16-year-old tall girl presents with primary amenorrhoea. She gives a history of visual disturbance for the last year. She has changed her glasses twice in the last year and her blood sugars are normal. Clinical examination reveals bitemporal hemianopia.

20. A 16-year-old girl is referred to the gynaecology clinic by her GP with primary amenorrhoea. She has recently been unwell, hospitalised and diagnosed with coarctation of aorta and a renal abnormality. Blood test results are suggestive of autoimmune hypothyroidism.

Questions 21–25

Options for Questions 21–25

A	Adrenal adenoma	I	Hypothyroidism
B	Adrenal carcinoma	J	Hyperthyroidism
C	Anorexia nervosa	K	Hyperprolactinaemia
D	Bulimia nervosa	L	Late-onset congenital adrenal
E	Cushing's disease		hyperplasia
F	Cushing's syndrome	M	Polycystic ovary syndrome
G	Gynandroblastoma	N	Premature menopause
H	Hypothalamic cause	O	Sheehan's syndrome

Instructions: For each clinical scenario described below, choose the single most appropriate cause of amenorrhoea from the list of options above. Each option may be used once, more than once, or not at all.

21. A 22-year-old woman, who is studying at university, presents to her GP with amenorrhoea during the last 6 months. She has a body mass index of 15 but she thinks she is overweight and goes to the gym every day. Her urine pregnancy test is negative. A blood test reveals slightly low follicle-stimulating hormone (FSH) and luteinising hormone (LH) levels.

22. A 30-year-old woman presents to her GP with amenorrhoea lasting a year. She gives a history of an intraductal carcinoma of the breast (T2L2M1) 18 months previously. Subsequently, she received three cycles of chemotherapy followed by a left-sided mastectomy. 4 weeks after that she received radiotherapy to the left breast and axilla. She has one child and wants to conceive.

23. A 20-year-old woman is referred to the gynaecology clinic having had amenorrhoea for the past 6 months and a negative pregnancy test. She has recently noticed an increased growth of hair on the face, chin and chest, with clitoromegaly. Her blood test results show very high levels of 17-hydroxyprogesterone.

24. A 25-year-old woman presents to her GP with a history of amenorrhoea for the last 6 months. She is an athlete and has recently participated in the Olympics. Her serum FSH and LH levels are normal.

25. A 20-year-old woman presents to her GP with facial hirsutism and irregular periods for the past year. She has recently put on weight and her body mass index is 28.

Answers: SBAs

1.   A Explain that you are required to have a chaperone and will wait for the nurse

Intimate examinations can be uncomfortable and embarrassing for the patient and clinician, and you should be sensitive to the patient's needs. Before you carry out the examination, explain the need for it and ask the patient if she has any questions. Explain that the chaperone acts as an impartial observer and should therefore be an allied health professional and not a relative. The chaperone will watch what the doctor is doing and should be present throughout the whole examination. The chaperone's name should then be documented in the notes.

2.   D Situational awareness

Situational awareness is the ability to monitor one's surroundings and detect changes. This is essential on the labour ward where the environment is dynamic, and multitasking and appropriate delegation are necessary. It is also applicable in an operating theatre. Situational awareness is based on experience, expectations and current workload. Team 'huddles' and meetings to plan the work load help to improve situational awareness.

Jackson KS, Hayes K, Hinshaw K. The relevance of non-technical skills in obstetrics and gynaecology. Obstet Gynaecol 2013; 15:269–274.

3.   C Leadership

Effective leadership is essential for a safe environment and to maintain team morale. A good team leader motivates and encourages each team member, while assigning tasks and assessing performance. You will often be the lead, especially on the labour ward, where you have to prioritise and manage your workload. Hence it is essential that you are a good leader.

Jackson KS, Hayes K, Hinshaw K. The relevance of non-technical skills in obstetrics and gynaecology. Obstet Gynaecol 2013; 15:269–274.

4.   B Leave the cyst and arrange follow-up in the gynaecology clinic

A woman must be made aware of any proposed procedure and its possible consequences before surgery. A procedure should only be undertaken without consent if the condition is life threatening; any non-life threatening procedure where consent has not been taken should not go ahead, even if this means that a second procedure is needed at a later date.

In this question, cystectomy has not been discussed with the patient, so the ovarian cyst should not be removed as this is not a life-threatening condition. There is also a risk that an oophorectomy will be needed if there is uncontrollable bleeding during the cystectomy. An injury that occurs during laparoscopy, e.g. a visceral injury, could be potentially life-threatening so should be repaired; it must then be discussed with the woman as soon as she awakens. If, in this case, the cause of the pain was torsion of the ovary, an ovarian cystectomy would be justifiable in the woman's best interest as it would be potentially dangerous to leave a torted ovary without treatment.

5.   C Perform a hysterectomy

This is a life-threatening emergency and the consultant must act in the patient's best interest. The opinion of an experienced colleague should preferably be sought before undertaking the procedure. However, this may not always be possible, as in this situation, and the woman may die if action is not taken immediately. Ideally, the patient should have been consented for a hysterectomy, and this should have been documented.

6.   B Delusions or hallucinations (with violent content)

All hospital staff are likely at some point to face an aggressive patient or partner. Therefore, all staff should be trained in how to manage such situations and learn de-escalation techniques, also known as 'defusing' or 'talking down' strategies. These involve talking to an agitated person in a calm, controlled way and moving them to a less confrontational area. This should be somewhere the staff member feels safe and not trapped. The staff member has to be aware of their own verbal and non-verbal behaviour to avoid becoming agitated with the already aggressive patient. This requires great self-awareness. Recognising developing situations is important so that staff can initiate de-escalation techniques as soon as possible. Conflict management has now become part of induction teaching for all staff working in NHS hospital trusts in England, for example.

Strachan BK, Fuller JB. Dealing with conflict and aggression in obstetrics and gynaecology. Obstet Gynaecol 2009; 11:122–128.

7.   E All of the above

How a person reacts to bad news is very individual, but the reaction will be influenced by the following:

- Obstetric history: as is the case here, having had fertility treatment or recurrent pregnancy loss makes it more difficult to cope
- Perception of the pregnancy: what does the pregnancy and its loss mean to the couple?
- Social situation: does the woman have any support from her family or partner?
- Culture: in some cultures crying is expected, whereas in others a more reserved approach is encountered
- Religion: some people believe that the loss of a pregnancy is 'God's wish' and that they should therefore not mourn the loss

8.   B Clinical effectiveness

The seven pillars of clinical governance are:

1. Risk management
2. Audit
3. Education and training, and continued professional development
4. Clinical effectiveness
5. Strategic leadership, workforce and performance management
6. Patient and public involvement
7. Information management and communication

Clinical effectiveness is ensuring that the right person does the right thing (which is evidence-based) at the right time, in the right place, in the right way and with the right result. It should include holistic care and continuation of care. It should also be carried out in a sensitive manner tailored to the patient's personal needs.

9.   A Audit

Audit is the improvement of patient care by reviewing the current care against a gold standard and then implementing changes to improve care. The changes may be at an individual, team or service level. The audit cycle includes the following steps:

1. Select the topic
2. Identify an appropriate standard (e.g. RCOG guideline) to compare current care with
3. Collect the data to compare the current practice to the standard
4. If necessary, implement changes to improve care
5. Collect data again to see if there have been any improvements

Audits should have a multidisciplinary approach, with involvement of the stakeholders and the local audit department.

10. D To contact the local advocacy and advisory service for hospital patients

Most hospitals have a patient advocacy and advisory service; for example, all hospitals in the UK have a Patient Advice and Liaison Service. It offers patients and their relatives advice, support and information in a confidential manner. Patients' complaints are one way of identifying issues in the system. Complaints should be welcomed with a positive approach and used as feedback to staff. They should not be used to blame individuals.

The complaints process has two stages:

1. The complaint is dealt with at a local level and local resolution is aimed for
2. If local resolution is not possible, the Parliamentary and Health Service Ombudsman undertakes an independent investigation

Answers: EMQs

11. N Turner's syndrome

Turner's syndrome is the most common cause of gonadal failure in young girls. Short stature is the most common clinical presentation in childhood; however, young girls may present with primary amenorrhoea during pubertal age. The most common chromosomal abnormality is 45XO, followed mosaicism and by X isochromosomes.

12. L Noonan's syndrome

Noonan's syndrome is an autosomal dysmorphic syndrome. It is characterised by hypertelorism (an increase in distance between the inner canthi of eyes), downward slanting of the eyes, low set posteriorly rotated ears, short stature and right-sided cardiac anomalies. The incidence is 1 in 2500 live births.

13. D Etoposide

Chemotherapy is one of the most common causes of ovarian failure in peripubertal children. Etoposide, procarbazine and nitrosourea can cause permanent ovarian failure while transient ovarian failure is associated with vincristine.

14. K McCune–Albright syndrome

Breast development corresponding to Tanner stage 2 before the age of 8 years in a girl is considered as precocious puberty. It is also known as central precocious puberty and is caused by the premature activation of the hypothalamic-pituitary–gonadal axis.

McCune–Albright syndrome is caused by a somatic activating mutation of the α subunit of G proteins. Most cases are sporadic but autosomal dominant inheritance has been reported. It is characterised by incomplete sexual precocity, café-au-lait pigmentation and polyostotic fibrous dysplasia. The sexual precocity in this condition is independent of gonadotrophins.

15. F Iatrogenic

Exogenous steroids are a well-known cause of sexual precocity. The most common drugs used are oestrogen-containing creams and pills. Other potential sources of oestrogens include soy formulas and ginseng cream (phyto-oestrogens).

Banerjee K. Puberty delayed. In: Hollingworth T (ed). Differential Diagnosis in Obstetrics and Gynaecology: An A–Z. London: Hodder Arnold, 2008.
Banerjee K. Puberty precocious. In: Hollingworth T (ed). Differential Diagnosis in Obstetrics and Gynaecology: An A–Z. London: Hodder Arnold, 2008.

Balen A. Chapter 14: Disorders of puberty. In: Shaw RW, Luesley D, Monga A (eds). Gynaecology (4th edn). Edinburgh: Churchill Livingstone, 2011.
Critchley HOD, Horne A, Munro K. Chapter 16: Amenorrhoea and oligomenorrhoea, and hypothalamic–pituitary dysfunction. In: Shaw RW, Luesley D, Monga A (eds). Gynaecology (4th edn). Edinburgh: Churchill Livingstone, 2011.

16. B Androgen insensitivity syndrome

Androgen insensitivity syndrome is an X-linked recessive inherited disorder. The karyotype is 46XY (male genotype) and external genitalia usually appear female. Breast development is normal with sparse axillary and pubic hair. Genital examination will reveal a short, blind vaginal pouch with an absent uterus. Cases with partial androgen insensitivity syndrome can present with ambiguous genitalia at birth and this poses real difficulty in gender assignment. The gonads should be removed after puberty in view of the high incidence of developing malignancy (gonadoblastoma) in the future (approximately 5%).

17. E Hypothyroidism

Hypothyroidism can be associated with hyperprolactinaemia in 3–5% of cases.

18. F Hyperprolactinaemia

Drugs used to treat psychosis (e.g. haloperidol, reserpine) can cause hyperprolactinaemia (pharmacological therapy is associated with hyperprolactinaemia in 1–2% of cases). Other drugs that can cause hyperprolactinaemia include metoclopramide, methyldopa, phenothiazines (trifluoperazine, prochlorperazine, chlorpromazine, thioridazine) and cimetidine.

Hyperprolactinaemia is characterised by abnormally high levels of prolactin that is normally down-regulated by dopamine in the hypothalamus. Hence, dopamine agonists are the mainstay of treatment.

Hyperprolactinaemia can be caused by reduced dopamine levels, increased production of prolactin from a prolactinoma or compression of the pituitary stalk by non-prolactin secreting tumours such as craniopharyngiomas, chromophobe adenomas or growth hormone secreting tumours. Prolactinomas can be microadenomas or macroadenomas. 2% of patients with microadenomas develop symptoms or signs of tumour progression during pregnancy, while 15% do so with macroadenomas.

Drugs used in the treatment of hyperprolactinaemia are listed below:

- Bromocriptine
  - dopamine agonist
  - dose: start with the lowest dose of 1.25 mg at bedtime and gradually increase to 7.5 mg in divided doses daily
  - common side effects: nausea, vomiting, headache and postural hypotension
  - may cause adverse psychiatric effects at the beginning of therapy
  - the side effects can be minimised by taking the tablets at bedtime

- Cabergoline:
  - long-acting dopamine agonist
  - dose: start with 0.25–1 mg twice weekly and this can be increased to 1 mg daily
  - fewer side effects compared to bromocriptine
  - can be used in women who cannot tolerate bromocriptine due to its side effects
  - may cause adverse psychiatric effects
  - it is not licensed for use in pregnancy
  - a single dose (1 mg) can be used for breast milk suppression in women with fetal loss
- Quinagolide:
  - long-acting dopamine agonist
  - dose: 25–150 μg daily in divided doses
  - fewer side effects compared to bromocriptine
  - can be used in women who cannot tolerate bromocriptine due to its side effects
  - may cause adverse psychiatric effects
  - it is not licensed for use in pregnancy

19. L Pituitary prolactinoma

The most common causes of hyperprolactinaemia are pituitary prolactinomas (found in 40–50% of cases) and idiopathic hypersecretion. Pituitary prolactinomas can present with visual disturbances especially visual field defects as the prolactinoma presses on the optic chiasma (nasal fibres which represent the temporal field are affected). In view of this, visual field testing will reveal bitemporal hemianopia. Blood tests will reveal hyperprolactinaemia and CT or MRI will show a pituitary tumour.

20. M Turner's syndrome

Turner's syndrome (XO) is associated with congenital heart defects (coarctation of the aorta).

Critchley HOD, Horne A, Munro K. Chapter 16: Amenorrhoea and oligomenorrhoea, and hypothalamic–pituitary dysfunction. In: Shaw RW, Luesley D, Monga A (eds). Gynaecology (4th edn). Edinburgh: Churchill Livingstone, 2011.
Balen A. Chapter 14: Disorders of puberty. In: Shaw RW, Luesley D, Monga A (eds). Gynaecology (4th edn). Edinburgh: Churchill Livingstone, 2011.

21. C Anorexia nervosa

Anorexia nervosa is more commonly seen in adolescent females than males. It is an eating disorder characterised by a low body weight, distortion of the body image and an obsessive fear of gaining weight. It can involve the hypothalamic–pituitary–gonadal axis causing hypothalamic amenorrhoea (usually if the patient's BMI <18).

22. N Premature menopause

Chemotherapy drugs used in the treatment of breast cancer are toxic to the ovary and can cause premature menopause.

23. L Late onset congenital adrenal hyperplasia

An increase in the growth of hair on the face, chin and chest, deepening of the voice clitoromegaly, male pattern hair loss and an increase in muscle bulk are symptoms of virilisation (excessive androgen levels). These can be symptoms of virilising adrenal adenoma, adrenal carcinoma, adrenal hyperplasia and some ovarian tumours. Serum levels for androgens such as testosterone, dehydroepiandrosterone sulphate and urinary 17-ketosteroid excretion, are generally well above the normal range in virilising adrenal tumours. Failure to suppress androgen secretion after the administration of dexamethasone is normally indicative of a virilising adrenal tumour. An MRI scan of the abdomen and pelvis should be arranged to rule out virilising adrenal and ovarian tumours.

Congenital adrenal hyperplasia (CAH) is a form of adrenal insufficiency. About 95% of cases of CAH are caused because of the lack of enzyme 21-hydroxylase, resulting in the inadequate production of two vital hormones; cortisol and aldosterone; but an increase in the production of androgens via alternative pathways in hormone synthesis. CAH can present at birth, early childhood, late childhood and adulthood. The late onset, or non-classical, form is usually milder and may manifest during adolescence or even later in women. It can present with hirsutism, acne, anovulation and infertility. The diagnosis is usually made from very high levels of serum 17-hydroxyprogesterone. The treatment is low dose glucocorticoids.

24. H Hypothalamic cause

Amenorrhoea due to weight loss, excessive exercise and stress are usually due to a hypothalamic cause.

25. M Polycystic ovary syndrome

Polycystic ovaries are seen in 25% of women of reproductive age. They are defined as polycystic ovary syndrome (PCOS) when associated with symptoms such as menstrual irregularity, hirsutism and anovulation.

The definition of PCOS by the Rotterdam European Society for Human Reproduction and Embryology (ESHRE) and the American Society of Reproductive Medicine (ASRM) PCOS Consensus Workshop Group is that two of the three following criteria should be present to diagnose PCOS:

- polycystic ovaries (either 12 or more peripheral follicles or increased ovarian volume (>10 cm^3)
- clinical and/or biochemical signs of hyperandrogenism
- oligo- or anovulation

Women who are overweight or obese should be advised to lose weight (5–10% weight loss can correct menstrual irregularity) as this corrects hormonal imbalance, reduces insulin resistance and initiates ovulation in such women. However, one should treat patients symptomatically (e.g. hirsutism, irregular periods, infertility). All women should be counselled about the short-term (infertility, menstrual irregularity and hirsutism) and the long-term implications (hypertension, type 2 diabetes, ischaemic heart disease and endometrial cancer) of PCOS.

Royal College of Obstetricians and Gynaecologists (RCOG). Green-top Guideline No. 33. Long-term consequences of polycystic ovarian syndrome. London: RCOG Press; 2007.
Critchley HOD, Horne A, Munro K. Chapter 16: Amenorrhoea and oligomenorrhoea, and hypothalamic–pituitary dysfunction. In: Shaw RW, Luesley D, Monga A (eds). Gynaecology (4th edn). Edinburgh: Churchill Livingstone; 2011.

Chapter 2

Teaching, appraisal and assessment

Questions: SBAs

For each question, select the single best answer from the five options listed.

1. Which one of the following is true regarding appraisal as compared with assessment?

    A   Appraisal is primarily for the appraiser, and assessment assesses whether competencies have been met against a set standard

    B   Appraisal is primarily for the appraiser, and assessment is required to practise independently in the form of an Annual Review of Compentence Progression (ARCP) or 'exit interview'

    C   Appraisal is a formal interview where concerns should not be discussed openly; assessment acts to ensure certain standards are met

    D   Appraisal establishes learning goals, and assessment assesses whether competencies have been met in relation to a set standard

    E   Appraisal should be conducted only at the beginning of the year, and assessment in the form of an ARCP or 'exit interview' at the end of the year

2. Which one of the following qualities is required in order to be a good appraiser?

    A   Being a poor listener

    B   Being a hard worker

    C   Being a skilful negotiator

    D   Being an optimist who provides positive feedback only

    E   Keeping everything that is discussed confidential

3. An appraisal interview is required by all doctors in the NHS. Which one of the following is correct regarding the structure of an appraisal interview?

    A   The appraisee should submit their personal development plan and evidence 7–14 days before the meeting

    B   The appraiser and appraisee may meet anywhere that is convenient, even on a busy labour ward where the appraiser is on call

    C   The appraisee should be reassured that, unless it affects patient safety, everything said will remain in confidence, regardless of what the issue is

    D   The appraiser should first review mistakes made by the appraisee and offer constructive criticism as required

    E   Only the appraiser is required to create a list of issues to be discussed

4. Which of the following skills should a good mentor have?

    A   Be a good listener
    B   Be respected among their profession
    C   Be approachable
    D   Be non-judgemental
    E   Be all of the above

5. When should a doctor participate in mentoring?

    A   As a newly appointed consultant
    B   As a specialty trainee year 5–6
    C   As a specialty trainee 1–5
    D   As a foundation-year doctor
    E   All of the above

6. Assessments can be formative or summative.

    Which of the following is an example of a summative assessment?

    A   MRCOG objective structured clinical examination (OSCE)
    B   Mini clinical evaluation exercise
    C   Case-based discussion
    D   Objective structured assessment of technical skills
    E   Multisource feedback

7. The objective structured clinical examination (OSCE) and the clinical skills
    assessment (Part 3 of the MRCOG examination) were created to increase the
    number of different types of testing formats used in the MRCOG examination.

    Which of the following statements is false regarding OSCEs?

    A   An OSCE examines a large number of students
    B   A checklist can be used, which makes it easy to administer and score
    C   The marking is completely subjective
    D   OSCEs and clinical assessments assess the affective and psychomotor domains
    E   Rating scales can be used instead of a checklist

8. Reflection is an essential part of training.

    What grade of reflection ability is level 2?

    A   It identifies and re-evaluates one's own learning needs
    B   It describes evidence of progress from experience
    C   It evaluates experience as evidence of progress
    D   It summarises progress of experience in relation to outcome
    E   None of the above

9. Validity is the determination of whether an assessment is measuring what it is meant to measure.

    Which of the following is a type of validity?

    A   Predictive
    B   Concurrent
    C   Construct
    D   Content
    E   Conduct

10. Six trainees have just joined the obstetrics and gynaecology department. The consultant asks you to teach them various examinations including pelvic examination, speculum examination and taking a cervical smear and swabs.

    Which type of teaching session is most appropriate?

    A   A 10-minute presentation by each trainee for other trainees
    B   Attending the gynaecology clinic
    C   Delivering a lecture to the trainees
    D   Take them to a simulation laboratory with a teaching mannequin
    E   A tutorial format, with the trainees sitting in a circle

11. You have performed a laparoscopic salpingectomy for tubal ectopic pregnancy, with the consultant assisting. You then sit down together and discuss each step of the procedure using a standard proforma, identifying good points and areas for improvement.

    What form of assessment is this?

    A   Case-based discussion
    B   Formative objective structured assessment of technical skills (OSATS)
    C   Mini clinical evaluation exercise
    D   Summative OSATS assessment
    E   360° assessment

12. After taking a history and examining a patient in the gynaecology clinic, you formulate a management plan and then discuss the case with the consultant in the clinic. They assess you and give immediate feedback.

    Which form of assessment is this?

    A   Formative case-based discussion
    B   Formative objective structured assessment of technical skills (OSATS)
    C   Mini clinical evaluation exercise
    D   Summative OSATS assessment
    E   Summative case-based discussion

Questions: EMQs

Questions 13–17

Options for Questions 13–17

A Bedside teaching	J Peer coaching
B Brainstorming	K Problem-based learning
C Complex procedural hierarchy	L Relphi technique
D CTG teaching	M Schema activation
E Delphi technique	N Schema reactivation
F Directly observed procedures	O Schema refinement
G Indirectly observed procedures	P Simplified procedural hierarchy
H Journal club	Q The 1-minute preceptor
I Lectures	

For each of the scenarios described below, choose the single most appropriate teaching method from the list of options above. Each answer maybe used once, more than once or not at all.

13. This is a form of teaching that can be useful for learners when they are at a very early stage in their careers. It is also a form of teaching that most clinicians are happy to deliver and are most comfortable with. In this teaching a lot of information is delivered to a lot of people at once.

14. When a group of medical students is presented with a problem, they create their own learning objectives and answer those objectives through self directed learning.

15. A five-step process that is carried out to structure a teaching opportunity that can arise in a clinical situation.

16. You are the specialist registrar on call for the labour ward and you observe a house officer inserting a Foley catheter. Following this you give a feedback to the house officer if this was correctly performed or not.

17. As a specialist registrar, you are learning how to perform a hysterectomy with your consultant in theatre.

Answers: SBAs

1. **D Appraisal establishes learning goals, and assessment assesses whether competencies have been met in relation to a set standard**

    Appraisal and assessment are often confused, but each has a different role in training. Appraisal between the appraiser and appraisee:

    - Is primarily for the appraisee
    - Aims to establish learning objectives and achievements
    - Is meant to be open and informal
    - Aims to address any concerns in a supportive way
    - Is supposed to occur throughout the year to guide the appraisee

    Assessment, on the other hand, tests that competencies have been met against a certain standard. It is required to ensure safe practice and leads to a licence to practise as a specialist. The evidence for trainees is assessed in the form of an annual review of competence progression or 'exit interview'.

    In simple words, appraisal works to achieve the competencies required, and assessment assess whether they have been achieved. In reality, there is an element of assessment during the appraisal meeting to ensure that safe practice is being maintained, but this should only be a small part of the appraisal process.

2. **C Being a skilful negotiator**

    Trainees sometimes have unrealistic expectations and goals that the trainer needs to mould. This is where negotiation skills are essential. Appraisers do not have to be senior consultants because clinical skills do not equate with the ability to conduct an appraisal. A junior consultant who has been adequately trained and has good personal characteristics can make an excellent appraiser. It is essential that the trainer is a good listener because didactic approaches do not encourage trainees to describe their problems or difficulties. The dialogue that takes place during an appraisal should be confidential. However, the relationship is not legally privileged, so the trainer must inform higher authorities of problems with patient safety, if it is deemed necessary.

    Fox R, Kane S. Appraisal in postgraduate medical education. Obstet Gynaecol 2004; 6:1.

3. **A The appraisee should submit their personal development plan and evidence 7–14 days before the meeting**

    The appraisee's evidence and proposed development plan should be ready 7–14 days before the meeting. The appraiser should prepare for the interview by reading through this portfolio beforehand. This allows them to make a list of the issues they want to discuss; the appraisee should prepare a similar list of issues. The meeting should take place in a mutually convenient, quiet place, at a time when the consultant has no other clinical commitments. At least an hour should be reserved because a rushed meeting may prevent important information being discussed. The appraisee should be reassured that discussions will be treated confidentially unless there is a risk to patient safety, e.g. the trainee has an alcohol problem.

4.   E Be all of the above

The RCOG has noted that doctors feel increasingly isolated because the conventional team structure has disappeared. This may have been a contributing factor for the poor retention and poor recruitment of doctors within the specialty. The RCOG believes that doctors need personal, professional and educational support, and that a mentoring programme is one way to provide this. There are many definitions of mentoring. The UK's Standing Committee on Postgraduate Medical and Dental Education (1998) defines it as 'guiding another individual (the mentee) in the development and re-examination of their own ideas, learning and personal and professional development'. A mentor is a separate role to an advocate, an adviser, a preceptor, a tutor and an educational adviser.

A good mentor should be:

- A good listener
- Respected as a professional
- Approachable and accessible
- Non-judgemental
- Enthusiastic and encouraging
- Wise and experienced
- Able to challenge, but not destructively
- Ethical, honest and trustworthy
- Able to show good interpersonal and communication skills

Standing Committee on Postgraduate Medical and Dental Education (SCOPME). Supporting doctors and dentists at work: an enquiry into mentoring. London: SCOPME; 1998.

5.   E All of the above

The RCOG (2005) recommends that a doctor should have a mentor throughout their career. There will sometimes be less need for this. The need is, however, greater at other times, e.g. after a long period of absence from work (maternity or sick leave) or after being appointed as a new consultant. Ideally, each doctor should identify a mentor within their own hospital at each stage of their career.

Royal College of Obstetricians and Gynaecologists (RCOG). Mentoring for all. London: RCOG Press; 2005.

6.   A MRCOG objective structured clinical examination

A formative assessment is used to keep track of a trainee's progress during a course of learning. The tutor tells the trainee what they are doing well and what needs improvement. It is not used to pass or fail the trainee.

A summative assessment occurs at the end of the course and is used to establish whether the trainee has met the objectives, and to determine what the trainee has learnt.

The MRCOG objective structured clinical examination is therefore a summative assessment.

7. C The marking is completely subjective

The objective structured clinical examination (OSCE) avoids the random questions that occur during an oral assessment. It tests the cognitive, psychomotor and affective domains. A trainee can be assessed against a checklist or rating scale.

A checklist uses clearly defined actions associated with a particular skill. Its advantages include:

- Ease of scoring
- Ability to examine a large number of trainees
- Objective marking

Rating scales can be partially subjective because the examiner has to make a judgement using a continuous scale. Rating scales are useful for assessing attitudes, interpersonal skills and practical skills.

8. C It evaluates experience as evidence of progress

The grading of reflective ability has been developed to assess a trainee's ability to reflect. The three levels of increasing complexity include:

- Level 1: the trainee describes relevant evidence of progress from experience
- Level 2: the trainee evaluates experiences as evidence of progress
- Level 3: the trainee identifies and re-evaluates their learning needs

9. B Concurrent

There are four types of validity:

- Content validity is the degree to which the test measures the content area. It compares what is taught with what is assessed
- Concurrent validity is the extent to which the two scores correlate when a new test and an established test are administered at the same time
- Predictive validity is the degree to which a test can predict future performance. The test is administered and the predictive behaviour awaited. The behaviour is then measured, and the test results and behaviour 'scores' are correlated
- Construct validity is a test that measures a hypothetical construct, e.g. intelligence

10. D Take them to a simulation laboratory with a teaching mannequin

Training students and trainees in a laboratory with a mannequin allows them to learn in a safe environment where any mistakes will not cause harm to patients, and provides the students with hands-on training.

11. B Formative objective structured assessment of technical skills (OSATS)

Objective structured assessment of technical Skills (OSATS) can be either formative or summative:

- Formative OSATS (supervised learning events) give trainees the opportunity to practise and receive feedback for a given procedure
- Summative OSATS (assessments of performance) allow trainees to demonstrate their competence in a procedure and progress in their training

12. C Mini clinical evaluation exercise

The mini clinical evaluation exercise (mini CEX) is a generic tool that is used to test many varied competencies. Trainers can use the mini CEX to directly assess trainees in:

- History-taking
- Clinical examination
- Formulating management plans
- Communicating with patients
- Professional and interpersonal skills

The trainer should provide feedback to the trainee immediately after the assessment. Each mini CEX should take around 20 minutes.

Answers: EMQs

13. I Lectures

Lectures are a form of teaching that clinicians are most comfortable with. It is a useful method if the learners are roughly at the same stage of knowledge, and are at the beginning of their careers in learning. At the same time, the teacher should be an expert in the subject and most likely has limited time to teach the learners. The participation for the learners is minimal in this form of teaching and the teacher can become patronising at times. It has been shown that very little information is retained through this form of teaching, but a strong lecture will provide a framework for further self-directed learning.

Duthie SJ, Garden AS. The teacher, the learner and the method. Obstet Gynaecol 2010; 12:273–280.

14. K Problem-based learning

In problem-based learning, the teacher presents the learner with a problem and the learner explores the problem and creates learning objectives around the scenario. Through self-directed learning, the learner works through the learning objectives and return after 1–2 weeks to share their findings. In this situation, the teacher is the facilitator, and should direct the learners and ensure they stick to the objectives. The facilitator should also ensure that everyone takes part in the sharing of information. The number of objectives depends on the problem being discussed and the experience of the learners.

15. Q The 1-minute preceptor

The 1-minute preceptor is a quick five-step process which creates a structure for teaching in a clinical environment. In order for the teaching to be successful, there must be a strong rapport between the teacher and learner.

The five steps are:

1. Commitment: the learner sees the patient and decides upon a diagnosis and/or treatment
2. Justification: the learner justifies why they came to that decision. The teacher will accept or reject what the learner has said
3. Application: the learning is applied to other situations and other women.
4. Positive reinforcement: the teacher explains to the learner what they did well. This increases the learners' confidence
5. Correction of mistakes: this should be specific

16. F Directly observed procedures

A directly observed procedure is when a teacher observes a learner as they carry out a simple task. It is a three-step process. Firstly, the teacher observes the learner or trainee perform the act. Secondly, the teacher tells the learner or trainee if what was done was correct or incorrect. Thirdly, the learner or the trainee is informed why it was inadequate, if indeed it was, and what could have been done better.

17. C Complex procedural hierarchy

This is used when a learner is being taught a complicated technique which takes time and involves multiple steps. In the example of a hysterectomy, the trainee first assists the consultant in the procedure. Then the learner is asked to verbally recount the steps involved in the procedure. The consultant then assists the trainee with the procedure and the trainee finally carries out the procedure with another trainee, with the consultant immediately available. This takes place against a background of ongoing assessment and regular feedback.

Chapter 3

Information technology, clinical governance and research

Questions: SBAs

For each question, select the single best answer from the five options listed.

1. A 54-year-old patient has had a transvaginal tape inserted the previous day. You are the oncall specialist registrar for the gynaecology team who is seeing her on the gynaecology ward. She is extremely unhappy with the care she received on the ward after the procedure.

   What would you do in this situation?

   A   Advise the patient to contact the Patience Advice and Liaison Service (PALS)
   B   Ask other patients on the ward if they also have been treated poorly
   C   Ask the patient to write a letter of complaint to the ward
   D   Complete an incident form
   E   Talk to the staff involved and find out what exactly happened

2. Which aspect of clinical governance relates to ensuring that patient notes are up to date and accurate, and that patient data are confidential?

   A   Risk management
   B   Research and development
   C   Patient and public involvement
   D   Clinical audit
   E   Information management

3. A baby was stillborn after a delay in performing a category 1 lower segment Caesarean section for acute fetal distress. The subsequent inquiry found that the anaesthetist's arrival had been delayed because the wrong pager had been bleeped, and that this had happened three times in preceding months, although without a serious or fatal outcome.

    Which component of clinical governance might have avoided this tragedy?

    A   Risk management
    B   Research and development
    C   Patient and public involvement
    D   Clinical audit
    E   Information management

4. Clinical audit is part of a quality improvement process that aims to improve patient care.

    Which one of the following describes the audit cycle?

    A   Select a topic, collect data and choose a standard, compare the data with the standard, implement changes if necessary, collect data again
    B   Select a topic, compare data with a standard and implement changes
    C   Select a topic, implement changes, collect data and compare with a standard
    D   Select a topic, identify an appropriate standard, collect data, compare the data with a standard, implement changes if necessary, collect data again
    E   None of the above

5. You are the obstetric specialist registrar on call, and your junior colleagues asks you what the evidence is for using antibiotics in prolonged preterm rupture of membranes.

    Which is the best source to search for the most robust information?

    A   RCOG clinical guidance
    B   Google Scholar
    C   MEDLINE
    D   ClinicalTrials.gov
    E   Cochrane database

6. Which is the most appropriate research design to determine whether oral or intravenous hydration is better in labour?

    A   Randomised control trial
    B   Survey
    C   Cohort
    D   Case–control
    E   Cross-sectional

7. Choosing the correct research design is extremely important. Which is the most appropriate research design to determine the likelihood of an epidural causing lower back pain in the future?

    A   Randomised control trial
    B   Survey
    C   Cohort study
    D   Case–control study
    E   Cross-sectional study

8. Which is the most appropriate research design to determine the incidence of Caesarean section after a previous instrumental delivery?

    A   Randomised control trial
    B   Survey
    C   Cohort study
    D   Case–control study
    E   Cross-sectional study

9. Which is the most appropriate research design to determine the prevalence of cervical cancer?

    A   Randomised control trial
    B   Survey
    C   Cohort study
    D   Case–control study
    E   Cross-sectional study

10. Ethics and conflict of interest are very important in research.

    Which of the following is correct when it comes to a conflict of interest?

    A   It can occur in any part of the team, including the investigators, authors, reviewers or editors
    B   The concept of a financial conflict of interest does not apply to medical research
    C   Only the main authors have to disclose personal or financial relationships with other people or organisations that may affect the reporting of the work submitted
    D   The conflict of interest policy should adopt a closed framework so that only some readers can make objective judgements about the study's conclusions
    E   The researcher is always neutral, therefore there is never any conflict of interest

11. It is essential to put research into practice. What is the correct order of steps in this process?

    A   Knowledge, persuasion, decision, implementation, confirmation
    B   Persuasion, decision, knowledge, implementation, confirmation
    C   Persuasion, knowledge, decision, confirmation, implementation
    D   Persuasion, decision, implementation, confirmation, knowledge
    E   Implementation, confirmation, knowledge, persuasion, decision

12. Evidence-based medicine is the use of the best current evidence to make decisions about the care of individual patients. 'Levels of evidence' refers to a system that classifies evidence into a hierarchy based on scientific rigor and quality.

Which level of evidence includes a case series?

A   Level 1
B   Level 2
C   Level 3
D   Level 4
E   Level 5

13. 'Levels of evidence' refers to a system that classifies evidence into a hierarchy based on scientific rigor and quality.

Which type of study will provide level 2a evidence?

A   Expert opinion without explicit critical appraisal
B   A systematic review of randomised controlled trials
C   A combination of case–control and poor quality cohort studies
D   Individual cohort study
E   A systematic review of cohort studies

14. Clinical guidelines are developed by combining research evidence with the consensus view of experts. There are several methods for developing a guideline.

Which method is described as a questionnaire that is sent out to a panel of people and therefore covers a large geographical area?

A   Delphi survey
B   Nominal group technique
C   Combination of Delphi and nominal techniques
D   'Fish bowl' technique
E   None of the above

15. Which one of the following is a Caldicott principle?

A   Access to patient information should be available to all
B   One must act in the patient's best interest regardless of the law
C   One must justify the reason for every proposed use or transfer of information
D   Only the person ultimately responsible for the patient should have access to the patient's information
E   Use as much information as you want from a patient's records

Questions: EMQs

Questions 16–20

Options for Questions 16–20

A Abortion Act 1967
B The case should be individualised and registered as a stillbirth in case of doubt
C England and Wales: Stillbirth (Definition) Act 1992
D Female Genital Mutilation Act 2003
E Female Genital Mutilation Act 2004
F Stillbirth (Definition) (Northern Ireland) Order 1992
G Registration under the Stillbirth (Definition) Act 1992 not required
H Registration under the Abortion Act 1967 not required
I Scotland: Stillbirth (Definition) Act 1992
J Human Fertilisation and Embryology Act 1990
K Human Fertilisation and Embryology Authority's Code of Practice 1995
L Human Rights Act 1998
M Human Tissue Act 2004
N Human Organ Donation Act 2003

Instructions: For each of the scenarios described below, select the single most appropriate British Act from the list of options above. Each option may be used once, more than once, or not at all.

16. A 39-year-old woman with 3 children presents to the labour ward at 32 weeks' gestation with pre-term labour. She progresses very quickly and proceeds to have a normal vaginal delivery. The baby is admitted to the special care unit for prematurity. Following delivery a fetus papyraceus is found coincidentally.

17. A 25-year-old primiparous woman presents to the labour ward at 23 weeks' gestation with abdominal pain and reduced fetal movements. Clinical examination reveals a soft abdomen and closed cervical os. An ultrasound scan reveals no fetal heart activity. She is in denial and refuses to accept the death of the baby. She goes home and returns 8 days later with abdominal pain and vaginal bleeding. The fetus and the placenta are expelled and the patient is discharged home the following day.

18. A 39-year-old woman with two children presents to the labour ward at 28 weeks' gestation with multiple pregnancies. Clinically, she is contracting four times every 10 minutes with a 4 cm cervical dilatation. An ultrasound scan reveals twin 1 and twin 2 are in breech presentation. Therefore, an emergency Caesarean section is performed. The babies are admitted to the special care baby unit due to extreme prematurity. The woman had triplets and had selective feticide of one baby at 20 weeks' gestation for fetal abnormality.

19. A 28-year-old woman with three children presents to the labour ward. She is unbooked (she has had no prior appintments, scans or blood tests) and is unsure of the first day of her last period. Clinically, the contractions are strong and uterine fundal height measures 25 cm. An ultrasound scan reveals no fetal heart activity. On questioning she gives a history of recent travel to Africa where she was treated for malaria.

20. A 29-year-old woman comes to London for her summer holidays with her 5-year-old child. She is brought to a hospital in an ambulance straight from the airport because she is pregnant and complains of abdominal pain. Clinically, her fundal height measures 39 cm and the midwife calls you because she cannot locate a fetal heartbeat. An ultrasound scan by an obstetric registrar reveals the absence of fetal heart activity. The woman is in denial because she felt fetal movements the previous morning. She is induced the next day followed by delivery of a macerated fetus 16 hours later.

Questions 21–25

Options for Questions 21–25

A	1–2%	I	30–40%
B	2–3%	J	56%
C	5%	K	77%
D	6–10%	L	88%
E	12%	M	85%
F	10–20%	N	99%
G	30%	O	100%
H	32%		

Instructions: For each scenario described below, choose the single most appropriate percentage for the events described from the list of options above. Each option may be used once, more than once, or not at all.

21. A 24-year-old primigravid woman presents to the labour ward at 25 weeks' gestation with contractions. She does not give any history of rupture of membranes. Clinical examination reveals palpable contractions (two to three contractions in 10 minutes) and a cervical dilatation of 2 cm. An ultrasound scan reveals breech presentation. A diagnosis of pre-term labour is made and intravenous atosiban is commenced with steroids in accordance with local protocol because this produces a certain percentage improvement in neonatal survival.

22. A 24-year-old woman presents to the labour ward at 28 weeks' gestation with labour pains. Clinical examination reveals palpable contractions (one to two contractions in 10 minutes) and closed cervical os with minimal effacement. She does not give any history of rupture of membranes. A vaginal fibronectin test is positive. The patient is told the positive predictive value (PPV), expressed as a percentage, this has for pre-term labour (chance of going into labour).

23. A 24-year-old primigravid woman presents to the labour ward at 28 weeks' gestation with labour pains. Clinical examinations reveal palpable contractions (one to two in 10 minutes) and open cervical os. She does not give any history of rupture of membranes. Her C-reactive protein (CRP) is 55 mg/L. It has been explained to her that CRP may predict amniotic fluid infection if a sample is taken for culture (having a particular percentage sensitivity).

24. A 24-year-old multiparous woman presents to the labour ward at 28 weeks' gestation with labour pains. Clinical examination reveals palpable contractions (two to three in 10 minutes) and a 3 cm cervical dilatation. She gives a strong history of rupture of membranes. A discussion is undertaken with the patient as to the chance (expressed as a percentage) of going into premature labour in women with rupture of membranes at this gestation.

25. A 24-year-old primigravid woman presents to the labour ward at 28 weeks' gestation with labour pains. Clinical examination reveals palpable contractions (two to three in 10 minutes) and a 2 cm cervical dilatation. She does not give any history of rupture of membranes. A diagnosis of pre-term labour is made and intravenous atosiban is commenced to buy time for the administration of corticosteroids. Her percentage risk of amniotic infection at this stage is discussed.

Questions 26–30

Options for Questions 26–30

A Abandon surgery and discuss with the patient

B Ask the patient to sign a new consent form

C Ask the hospital solicitor

D Abandon the surgery and arrange a clinic follow-up in 3 months

E Abandon the surgery and contact the partner

F Call consultant for second opinion

G Check the consent form

H Perform a laparotomy to remove the ovary

I Perform a laparotomy to remove the endometriosis

J Perform a laparotomy to do an internal iliac artery ligation

K Do nothing

L Discharge to the GP

M Perform a laparoscopic ovarian cystectomy

N Perform a laparoscopic oophorectomy

O Repeat the scan in 4 months

Instructions: For each scenario described below, choose the single most appropriate course of action from the list of options above. Each option may be used once, more than once, or not at all.

26. A 32-year-old woman with 5 years of infertility is booked for a laparoscopic dye test with or without treatment of endometriosis on a registrar list. While doing the laparoscopy, you are alarmed to see a 4 cm haematoma in the right infundibulopelvic ligament which is expanding and starts bleeding while you are manipulating the uterus.

27. A 40-year-old woman gives consent for laparoscopic sterilisation. You have finished the sterilisation procedure and notice a 3 cm cyst on the left side. Her scan report from 8 months ago showed an incidental finding of a dermoid cyst.

28. A 19-year-old woman presents with pain in the right iliac fossa (RIF). The on-call surgical team performs a diagnostic laparoscopy for suspected appendicitis. On examination the appendix looks normal with few omental adhesions to

the anterior abdominal wall. The surgical team also find a small 3 cm simple left ovarian cyst which is mobile with a smooth surface and looks benign. The surgeons request the removal of the left ovary.

29. A 65-year-old woman presents with postmenopausal bleeding. The ultrasound scan shows endometrial thickness of 2 mm and also a 4 cm simple cyst on the right side. A review of the notes reveals the same findings 1 year ago with a normal CA-125 level and a risk of malignancy index (RMI) of 22.

30. A 50-year-old postmenopausal woman is referred to the fast track gynaecology oncology clinic for an incidental finding of a 4.5 cm right-sided simple ovarian cyst with a CA-125 level of 8 U/mL. She is quite anxious.

Questions 31–35

Options to questions 31–35

A Analysis of variance	J Pearson's correlation test
B Appraisal	K Subanalysis of variance
C Assessment	L Two sample (unpaired) t-test
D χ_2 test	M Three sample (paired) t-test
E Four sample (unpaired) t-test	N Type 1 error
F Fraction regression	O Type 2 error
G Multiple regression	P Type 3 error
H One sample (paired) t-test	Q Type 4 error
I π^2 test	

Instructions: For each question described below, choose the single most appropriate answer from the list of options above. Each option may be used once, more than once, or not at all.

31. What type of error is made when one mistakenly rejects the null hypothesis?

32. What type of error is made when one mistakenly accepts the null hypothesis?

33. Which statistical test would you use to compare the incidence of cervical intra-epithelial neoplasia in a population before and after a smoking cessation programme is introduced?

34. Which statistical test would you use to compare the times taken by a group of senior house officers to conduct a diagnostic laparascopy to the times taken by a group of registrars to do the same procedure?

35. Which statistical test would you use to calculate the strength of the relationship between age and sentinel lymph node count in a sentinel study for cervical cancer?

Answers: SBAs

1 ~~C Clinical effectiveness~~ X A

The NHS has a complaints system which, if used effectively, can result in vast improvements both locally and nationally. Complaints are a good means to identify problematic areas, and should be used as a way of improving the system and not as a means to place blame. Patient advisory service [e.g. the Patient Advice and Liaison Service (PALS), see page 10] are available at all hospitals and offer support and advice in a confidential manner. In this example the patient should be advised to speak to PALS who will advise her appropriately.

2 E Information management

Information management involves ensuring that all patient information is kept up to date and accurate, whilst maintaining confidentiality. The General Medical Council expects doctors to 'keep clear, accurate and legible records' and to 'make records at the same time as the events you are recording or as soon as possible afterwards'.

General Medical Council. Good medical practice. London: General Medical Council; 2013.

3 D Clinical audit

Clinical governance is a systematic approach to maintaining high-quality health care. It is 'a governance system for healthcare organisations that promotes an integrated approach towards management of inputs, structures and processes to improve the outcome of healthcare service delivery where health staff work in an environment of greater accountability for clinical quality' (Som, 2004).

Clinical governance ensures accountability for quality of care, an integrated approach and an enabling environment for implementing change. It is made up of seven pillars:

- Clinical effectiveness and research: the refinement of practice in view of new evidence. It ensures that the right person does the right thing (evidence-based practice), in the right way (using skills and competencies), at the right time (when the patient needs it), in the right place and with the right result for the patient. It encompasses holistic care and continuity of care, and is sensitive to patients' needs
- Risk management: a robust system that aims to understand, monitor and minimise the risks to patients and staff by learning from mistakes. One example is carrying out root cause analysis of a mistake to discover if there were avoidable issues and then rectify them to avoid repeating the mistake
- Information management: ensures that patient data are accurate and up to date, and that patient confidentiality is respected
- Education: also known as continuing professional development. The RCOG defines this as a 'continuing process, outside formal undergraduate and

postgraduate training, that enables individual doctors to maintain and improve standards of medical practice through the development of knowledge, skills, attitudes and behaviour'. Continuing professional development is a mandatory requirement for all obstetricians and gynaecologists.

- Clinical audit: this is defined by the RCOG as 'a quality improvement process that seeks to improve patient care and outcomes through systematic review of care against explicit criteria and the implementation of change'. It is a cyclical process in which local clinical performance is compared with an agreed standard. Changes are implemented to enhance performance, and performance is then reassessed. It usually assesses one or more of: the structure of care, process of care or outcome of care.
- Patient and public involvement: ensures that the services suit the patients' needs. Patient and public feedback is used to improve and develop services. This could be in the form of local questionnaires, involvement of the local hospital patient advisory service (e.g. PALS) or national patient surveys organised by the Care Quality Commission.
- Staffing and staff management: the appropriate recruitment of staff, ensuring that underperformance is identified and that there are good working conditions.

Som C. Clinical governance: a fresh look at its definition. Clinical Governance 2004; 9:87.
Royal College of Obstetricians and Gynaecologists (RCOG). CPD guide: a guide to RCOG continuing professional development. London: RCOG Press; 2010.

4. D Select a topic, identify an appropriate standard, collect data, compare the data with a standard, implement changes if necessary, collect data again.

The RCOG (2003) defines clinical audit is 'a quality improvement process that seeks to improve patient care and outcomes through systematic review of care against explicit criteria and the implementation of change'. It is a cyclical process in which local clinical performance is compared with an agreed standard, changes are implemented to enhance performance, and performance is then reassessed. It usually assesses one or more of the structure of care, process of care or outcome of care.

Royal College of Obstetricians and Gynaecologists (RCOG). Understanding audit. Clinical governance advice 5. London: RCOG Press, 2003.

5. E Cochrane database

Cochrane reviews are systematic reviews of research in health care. They are internationally recognised and are the highest standards of evidence-based health care. They investigate the effect of investigations, prevention, treatment and rehabilitation on patients, as well as the accuracy of a diagnostic test on a specific patient group. Each systematic review answers a clearly formulated question.

6. A Randomised control trial

This is an experimental study whereby participants are randomly assigned to different intervention groups to assess their effectiveness. It may be double-blinded, whereby the subjects and the researcher do not know what each subject is receiving. This is the gold standard of clinical trials.

Sibbald B, Roland M. Understanding controlled trials: why are randomised controlled trials important? BMJ 1998; 316:201.

7. D Case–control study

In this approach, the cases, i.e. people with the disease, are compared with controls, i.e. people without the disease, and examined for exposure to certain attributes. This study can be completed quickly and is relatively cheap to run. However, it is prone to bias as confounding factors cannot be controlled for. It is a good study type for rare diseases and conditions with a long latency between exposure and manifestation.

8. C Cohort study

Cohort studies are longitudinal studies and follow subjects over a period of time, with or without exposure to a certain elements. The two sets of participants are then compared on, for example, the development of a certain disease. Cohort studies are time-consuming, and participants are often lost to follow-up over time. They are, however, good for measuring incidence rates and relative risks.

9. E Cross-sectional study

A cross-sectional study collects data at a single defined timepoint from a whole study population. It can be used to assess the prevalence of a disease and can calculate absolute risks, relative risks and odds ratios.

10. A It can occur in any part of the team, including the investigators, authors, reviewers or editors

A conflict of interest occurs when influences other than science affect the research in any way. It can occur at any point of the research and therefore may involve investigators, authors, editor's reviewers, etc. There are different types of conflict of interest:

- It may be financial, e.g. one drug being given more importance over another because the manufacturer has invested more in the research
- There may be a negative or positive bias of the researcher towards the subject
- The reviewers or the editors may have a negative or positive bias towards the author
- The conflict of interest policy recommended by the International Committee of Medical Journal Editors states that all authors must disclose financial or personal relationships that might affect the conduct or results of the study. The policy aims to create transparency so that readers can make an objective judgement about the study. Reviewers must not, for example, accept work from authors with whom they have either a positive or negative relationship.

11. A Knowledge, persuasion, decision, implementation, confirmation

When research has proven the benefits of a certain diagnostic tool or treatment, this information must be transferred into clinical practice. This is done in a step-by-step process:

1. Knowledge. People must be made aware of new trials, guidelines or systematic reviews and then be convinced of their value and recommendations that they be initiated.
2. Persuasion
3. Decision. The people with authority in a department must then be persuaded and convinced to develop a care pathway or protocol that can lead to a change of practice
4. Implementation. This is when these pathways or protocols are put into practice. Clinicians will need to be reminded of their presence and encouraged to use them
5. Confirmation. The practice will then need to be audited to ensure compliance

12. D Level 4

Level 4 evidence includes a case series. **Table 3.1** describes levels of evidence.

Table 3.1 Levels of evidence relating to therapy or therapeutic studies	
Level of evidence	Type of study
1a	Systematic review of RCTs
1b	Individual RCTs with narrow confidence intervals
2a	Systematic reviews of cohort studies
2b	Individual cohort studies and low-quality RCTs
3a	Systematic review of case-controlled studies
3b	Case-controlled studies
4	Case series
5	Expert opinion

RCT, randomised controlled trial.

13. E A systematic review of cohort studies

A systematic review of cohort studies is Level 2a evidence.

Burns PB, Rohrich RJ, Chung KC. The levels of evidence and their role in evidence-based medicine. Plast Reconstr Surg 2011; 128:305–310.

14. A Delphi survey

There are different ways to develop a guideline. The most common are:

- Nominal group technique. A group of experts and consumers meet, decide what questions need to be answered in the guideline, express their views and then

come to a consensus agreement. The organiser summaries and presents the group's view
- Delphi survey. A questionnaire is sent to a panel of people across a large geographical area asking for opinions and questions. This method is more time-consuming
- A combination of these two techniques. A postal approach is initially used to gain access to a large population, and a meeting is then set up for clarification

15. C One must justify the reason for every proposed use or transfer of information

The Caldicott guardian is the person in an organisation who is responsible for protecting patients' confidential information, and is in charge of ensuring appropriate information-sharing. The principles of the Caldicott guardian are:

- There must be justification of purpose. Every use or transfer of patient information within or from an organisation must be justified
- No patient-identifiable information should be used unless necessary
- The minimal necessary patient identifiable information should be used
- Access to patient identifiable information should be only on a need-to-know basis
- Everyone who has access to patient-identifiable information should be aware of their responsibilities
- Everyone must comply with the law
- The duty to share information can be as valuable as the need to protect patient confidentiality

Crook MA. The Caldicott report and patient confidentiality. J Clin Pathol 2003; 56:426–428.
Department of Health. Information: to share or not to share. Government response to the Caldicott review. Department of Health; 2013.

Answers: EMQs

16. G Registration under the Stillbirth (Definition) Act 1992 not required

In the case of a fetus papyraceus, it is known that the fetus must have died before 24 weeks' gestation and thus it would be incorrect to register it as a stillbirth. Also, when a fetus papyraceus is present at the birth of a live baby born after 24 weeks' gestation, it would be clear from its stage of development that the fetus papyraceus had died in the womb at a stage prior to the 24 weeks' gestation. Thus, the woman can be taken not to have been pregnant with that fetus on giving birth to the surviving child or for the purpose of the legislation after 24 weeks' gestation.

17. G Registration under the Stillbirth (Definition) Act 1992 not required

Fetuses which have died prior to 24 weeks' gestation would not be registered as stillbirths.

18. G Registration under the Stillbirth (Definition) Act 1992 not required

Fetuses known to have died prior to the 24 weeks' gestation (e.g. where there has been a delay between a diagnosed intrauterine death and delivery, vanishing twins or selective or multifetal pregnancy reduction in multiple pregnancies) would not be registered as stillbirths.

19. B The case should be individualised and registered as a stillbirth in case of doubt

In cases where one or more fetuses have been born dead after 24 weeks' gestation but it was not known prior to their birth that they had died, and it is not known precisely when they died, it may be appropriate to use the stage of development of the fetus as an indicator of when death occurred and as a basis for determining when that particular pregnancy ended relative to the 24-week limit. This would need to be agreed on a case-by-case basis by the medical professionals involved; this responsibility should not be left to the attending midwife. The decision and the basis on which it was made would need to be clearly detailed in the mother's notes in case any queries arise at a later date.

Where there is any doubt about the gestational age at which the fetus died, the default position would be for medical professionals to register the birth as a stillbirth.

20. C England and Wales: Stillbirth (Definition) Act 1992

The current English and Welsh law on stillbirth registration set out in the Births and Deaths Registration Act 1953 (as amended by the Still-Birth (Definition) Act 1992), Section 41, is that for:

> ... a child which has issued forth from its mother after the twenty-fourth week of pregnancy and which did not at any time after being completely expelled from its mother breathe or show any other signs of life, the expression "still-birth" shall be construed accordingly.

The law in England and Wales (Section 41 of the Births and Deaths Registration Act 1953 as amended by the Stillbirth Definition Act 1992), Scotland [Section 56(1) of the Registration of Births, Deaths and Marriages (Scotland) Act 1965 as amended by the Stillbirth Definition Act 1992] and Northern Ireland (Births and Deaths Registration Order 1976 as amended by the Stillbirth Definition Northern Ireland Order 1992), requires that any 'child' expelled or issued forth from its mother after the 24th week of pregnancy that did not breathe or show any other signs of life be registered as a stillbirth.

Royal College of Obstetricians and Gynaecologists (RCOG). Good Practice Guideline No. 4. Registration of stillbirth and certification for pregnancy loss before 24 weeks' gestation. Good practice guideline no. 4. London: RCOG Press; 2005.

21. B 2–3%

The incidence of pre-term labour is between 6% and 10% of all pregnancies. About 30% of these are due to medical intervention. A 2–3% improvement in fetal survival is noted by postponing delivery for 24 hours around the period of viability. However, survival of infants is not much different at 32 weeks compared to term babies.

22. K 77%

A fibronectin test is performed in women suspected of being in pre-term labour. It has a PPV of 77% in predicting pre-term labour. On the other hand, less than 3% of women with a negative test will go into labour in the next 3 weeks.

23. J 56%

Inflammatory markers are poor predictors of infection. The sensitivities of the white blood count and CRP for predicting amniotic fluid infection are 32% and 56%, respectively.

24. I 30–40%

The majority of pre-term labour is preceded by premature rupture of membranes (30–40%). The aetiological factors for pre-term labour include infection, multiple pregnancy, low socioeconomic status, smoking, low prepregnancy weight, young maternal age (<18 years), previous pre-term labour, incompetent cervix, Müllerian duct anomalies and early pregnancy bleeding.

25. E 12%

Infection is one of the most common causes of pre-term labour. 12% of cases of preterm labour with intact membranes and 34% of cases with premature rupture of membranes are associated with intraamniotic infection when amniocentesis is performed.

Howe DC, Calder AA. Preterm labour. Pace review. London: Royal College of Obstetricians and Gynaecologists Press 2003; 4:14–15.

26. F Call the consultant for second opinion

The broad ligament is a potential space which can expand with blood. The ureter runs closely at the base of the broad ligament before entering into the bladder laterally in front of the uterus.

As the haematoma is expanding, the bleeding will need to be stopped and you will need the help of a consultant.

27. K Do nothing

She is asymptomatic and has not consented to a cystectomy. A conservative approach with a follow-up appointment in the gynaecology clinic to discuss further management is important.

Small asymptomatic dermoid cysts can be managed conservatively with follow-up ultrasound scans following a discussion of the complications (cyst accidents such as torsion and rupture). If the cyst is significantly growing in size or if the patient develops symptoms, she would need a surgical approach to treat. However, both options (conservative as well as surgical) should be discussed with the patient to make an informed choice.

28. K Do nothing

This woman has RIF pain and the ovarian cyst is on the left side which is totally unrelated to the pain. This woman has not consented to any ovarian procedure, which is unnecessary considering the intraoperative findings. However, if the ovarian cyst was twisted or bleeding due a haemorrhagic cyst, it would have been dealt with at the same time in the patient's best interests.

29. L Discharge to the GP

A RMI of 22 indicates a low risk of ovarian malignancy. In asymptomatic women, ovarian cysts can be managed conservatively with follow-up scans and repeated tests for CA-125 levels every 3–4 months for 1 year before they can be discharged back to their GP.

Since this woman already had a scan 1 year ago with similar findings she can be discharged back to the GP.

Protocol for triaging women:

- Low risk – RMI <25 = <3% risk of cancer
- Moderate risk – RMI 25–250 = 20% risk of cancer
- High risk – RMI >250 = 75% risk of cancer

RMI = menopausal status × results of ultrasound scan findings × absolute CA-125

30. O Repeat the scan in 4 months

A RMI of 24 indicates low risk of malignancy. This patient is asymptomatic and the ultrasound scan features indicate a benign appearance (simple unilocular cyst). She needs follow-up repeat scans and tests for CA-125 levels for 1 year and then if the clinical situation remains the same she can be discharged to her GP.

Royal College of Obstetricians and Gynaecologists (RCOG). Ovarian cysts in postmenopausal women. Green-top guideline no. 34. London: RCOG Press, 2003.
Royal College of Obstetricians and Gynaecologists (RCOG). Management of suspected ovarian masses in premenopausal women. Green-top guideline no. 62. London: RCOG Press, 2011.
National Institute of Health and Care Excellence (NICE). Guidelines on ovarian cancer: the recognition and initial management [CG122]. Manchester: NICE; 2011.

31. N Type 1 error

A type 1 error occurs when the null hypothesis is mistakenly rejected.

Scally AJ. A practical introduction to medical statistics. Obstet Gynaecol 2014; 16:121–128.

32. O Type 2 error

A type 2 error occurs when the null hypothesis is mistakenly accepted. This can occur when the sample size is too small and power of study is not appropriately calculated.

When you have a set of data, the rate of type 1 and type 2 errors correlates inversely: the smaller the risk of one type of error, the greater the risk of the other type of error. It is more important to avoid a type 1 error than a type 2 error.

33. H One sample (paired) t-test

In this situation, the one sample (paired) t-test is most appropriate because it quantifies the difference between two dependent samples taken from the same group. They can be used to compare the performance of a population before and after an intervention is put into place.

34. L Two sample (unpaired) t-test

In this situation, the unpaired t-test is most appropriate because it quantifies the difference between two independent samples (time taken to perform a diagnostic laparoscopy) taken from two groups (the senior house officers and registrars).

35. G Multiple regression

A multiple regression test is used to calculate the relationship between more than one independent variable (obesity and age) and a dependent variable (sentinel lymph node count). Variables can be on a continuous spectrum, e.g. age or time, or represent discreet groups, e.g. smoking status. The variables can then be divided into nominal variables, where the variable has no order, e.g. eye colour, and ordinal variables, e.g. parity.

Chapter 4

Core surgical skills

Questions: SBAs

For each question, select the single best answer from the five options listed.

1. You are seeing a 14-year-old girl in the emergency department because she is complaining of acute lower abdominal pain. Examination reveals signs of peritonism. US reveals a 10 cm dermoid cyst. She is accompanied by her mother's partner because her mother is at work. You have discussed with the girl the need for urgent surgical management, the surgical procedure and the benefits and risks of surgery. She appears to understand all that has been said and is happy to proceed with a laparoscopic ovarian cystectomy as an emergency procedure.

    How should consent be obtained in this case?

    A The biological father has to be called to sign the consent form
    B The mother has to asked to come in to sign the consent form
    C The consent form only requires the consent of the patient
    D The mother's partner should sign the consent form because the patient is only 14 years old
    E Both biological parents should be asked to come in to sign the consent form

2. You are the gynaecology registrar on call. You have been asked by the surgeons to come to theatre because they have incidentally identified a cyst on a patient's ovary during an elective laparoscopic removal of her appendix. When you arrive, you find that the patient has a 5 cm dermoid cyst on her left ovary.

    Which of the following is the correct surgical management?

    A Call your consultant for help
    B Leave the appendix, cyst and left ovary alone
    C Completely remove the left ovary
    D Remove the cyst from the left ovary
    E Remove the appendix and arrange an outpatient gynaecology clinic appointment for the patient

3. You are the registrar on call. A patient with a confirmed ectopic pregnancy has just been admitted. She is stable, and the first-year specialty trainee (ST1) has gained her consent for a laparoscopic salpingectomy. She has had a previous laparoscopic appendectomy. You take her to theatre and complete the procedure with the ST1 as your assistant. You are just about to remove the ports when you notice that there is a 2 cm bowel perforation. The nurse notes that the patient has not consented for repair of any inadvertent organ damage.

    What is the appropriate immediate management?

    A   Ask the patient's next of kin for consent
    B   Remove the ports, close the abdomen and refer to the surgical team
    C   Ask the hospital's lawyers for legal advice
    D   Repair should take place because consent is not required
    E   None of the above

4. A 40-year-old woman has been trying to conceive for the past 3 years without success. She has undergone in vitro fertilisation treatment and is now 8 weeks' pregnant. It is 3 a.m. and she has been brought to hospital by ambulance. She had collapsed at home, was found to be bleeding heavily and was not responding to verbal commands. In the emergency department, you see that she is bleeding heavily and is hypotensive and tachycardic. You perform an abdominal ultrasound scan and find a viable intrauterine pregnancy with a fetal heartbeat. The haemoglobin concentration derived from a venous gas sample is 50 g/L. She requires an urgent evacuation of retained products of conception to stop the bleeding.

    What is best practice for obtaining consent?

    A   No consent is required
    B   Consent is required from the patient
    C   Consent should be obtained from the next of kin
    D   The consultant should be called for advice
    E   The hospital's lawyers should be called for advice

5. An 80-year-old woman who has heart disease, hypertension, chronic obstructive pulmonary disease and dementia is living in a nursing home because she needs 24-hour care. Her daughter occasionally visits her. The nurses in the home noticed that the woman's abdomen was distended. She was brought to hospital, and ascites was identified. CT of the abdomen and pelvis has revealed bilateral ovarian masses, most likely to be ovarian cancer. Due to her dementia, the patient is unaware of her surroundings and is not competent to give consent for any investigation.

    Who is able to make the decision regarding her care?

    A   The daughter, whose mother previously told her that she does not want to suffer
    B   An advance directive explaining what care she wants should be become ill
    C   The next of kin
    D   The nurses at the nursing home
    E   The consultant, using the best interest principle

6. It is 9 p.m. and you have just finished your shift as the registrar on call. You are walking to your car when you notice a piece of paper on the floor headed 'Gynaecology ward handover list'. This contains patients' names, dates of birth and clinical information, including that one patient is HIV positive and another has a complication secondary to a termination. It is unclear which doctor wrote the list.

    What is the most appropriate action to take?

    A   Inform the Caldicott guardian
    B   Inform the college tutor
    C   Send an email to all the doctors telling them what you have found
    D   Dispose of the list in a confidential wastepaper bin
    E   Leave the list on the floor and ignore it

7. You are the gynaecology registrar seeing patients before starting the operating list. You are confirming consent from a patient who is about to undergo a laparoscopic sterilisation. She suffers from obsessive compulsive disorder, anxiety and panic disorder and wants to know what her chances are of dying as a result of the procedure.

    What is the chance of a patient dying as a result of a laparoscopic sterilisation?

    A   1/100,000 to 2/100,000
    B   3/100,000 to 8/100,000
    C   9/100,000 to 12/100,000
    D   1/10,000 to 2/10,000
    E   3/10,000 to 8/10,000

8. You are the gynaecology registrar seeing patients prior to starting the operating list. One patient is going to have an abdominal hysterectomy because of menorrhagia. The second-year specialty trainee asks whether she should cross-match blood because she is wondering what the chances are of haemorrhage at the time of the operation.

    What is the chance of the patient having a haemorrhage that would require a blood transfusion?

    A   1/100
    B   2/100
    C   3/100
    D   4/100
    E   5/100

9. A 60-year-old woman is being investigated for an episode of postmenopausal bleeding. Her ultrasound scan shows an endometrial thickness of 10 mm. An outpatient hysteroscopy was attempted, but the clinician was unable to gain entry to the uterine cavity. The patient has now consented to have a hysteroscopy and endometrial biopsy, but under a general anaesthetic.

    She wants to know what chance there is of failure to enter the uterine cavity.

    A   >1/10
    B   1/10–1/100
    C   1/100–1/1000
    D   1/1000–1/10,000
    E   <1/10,000

10. A 20-year-old woman is undergoing a diagnostic laparoscopy for pelvic pain.

    Which statement is correct regarding consenting this woman about complications arising during surgery?

    A   The risk of damage to major blood vessels is around 1/100,000 cases
    B   The overall risk of serious complications is around 2/1000 cases
    C   The risk of bowel damage is around 1/100,000 cases
    D   The risk of death during diagnostic laparoscopy is 1/100,000 cases
    E   Bowel injury is always identified in all cases during laparoscopic surgery

11. When selecting an ideal suture material, many factors must be taken into consideration.

    Which one of the following is correct regarding the characteristics of polyglecaprone?

    A   Twisted, moderate tissue reaction, poor tensile strength, absorbed over 80 days
    B   Braided, low tissue reaction, good tensile strength, absorbed over 60–90 days
    C   Braided or monofilament, low tissue reaction, good tensile strength, absorbed over 90–120 days
    D   Monofilament, low tissue reaction, good tensile strength, absorbed over 90–120 days
    E   Monofilament, low tissue reaction, good tensile strength, absorbed over 7–14 days

12. When selecting an ideal suture material, many factors must be taken into consideration.

    What are the characteristics of polyglactin?

    A   Twisted, moderate tissue reaction, poor tensile strength, absorbed over 80 days
    B   Braided, low tissue reaction, good tensile strength, absorbed over 60–90 days
    C   Braided or monofilament, low tissue reaction, good tensile strength, absorbed over 90–120 days
    D   Monofilament, low tissue reaction, good tensile strength, absorbed over 90–120 days
    E   Monofilament, low tissue reaction, good tensile strength, absorbed over 7–14 days

13. You are the registrar in theatre and are assisting the consultant with a laparoscopic hysterectomy. You notice that the ureter has been divided at the lower third. The consultant agrees with your finding and asks what should be done next.

What is the appropriate surgical management in this case, with involvement of the urologist?

A Uretero-ureterostomy
B Trans-uretero-ureterostomy
C Boari flap
D Utero-neocystostomy
E Psoas hitch

14. You have inadvertently damaged the bladder dome while performing a total abdominal hysterectomy. The consultant has repaired it with an absorbable suture in two layers.

What is the correct postoperative bladder management protocol?

A Urinary catheter for 1 week, retrograde cystography before removing the catheter
B Urinary catheter for 2 weeks, retrograde cystography before removing the catheter
C Urinary catheter for 2 weeks with simple removal of the catheter
D Urinary catheter for 2 weeks, ultrasound of the kidney, ureter and bladder after removing the catheter
E Urinary catheter for 2 weeks, intravenous urethrography after removal of the catheter forming

15. As the specialist registrar, you are going to supervise a second-year specialty trainee doing an evacuation of retained products of conception. The patient is 8 weeks pregnant, and the ultrasound report indicates a missed miscarriage. The specialist trainee is worried about perforating the uterus. She wants to know what the most common area for perforation is, and which instrument is the usual cause of a perforation.

What would your answer be?

A Anterior wall with a suction catheter
B Posterior wall with a suction catheter
C Posterior wall with a Hegar dilator
D Anterior wall with a curette
E Fundus with a Hegar dilator

16. The enhanced recovery programme is aimed at improving patient outcomes. Which of the following is one of the elements of the enhanced recovery programme?

A Assessment on the day of the surgery
B Early use of blood and blood products
C Early mobilisation
D Using fluids preoperatively and postoperatively to aid recovery
E Use only dissolvable sutures

17. A 55-year-old woman is undergoing a total abdominal hysterectomy and bilateral salpingo-oophorectomy for large (15 cm × 14 cm × 12 cm) fibroids.

What percentage of ureteric injuries occur in the lower third of the ureter?

A   10%
B   20%
C   30%
D   40%
E   50%

18. A 50-year-old woman is undergoing a laparoscopic hysterectomy and bilateral salpingo-oophorectomy for stage 1 uterine cancer. She is hypertensive and her body mass index is 34 kg/m^2.

A pneumoperitoneum of >10 mmHg during laparoscopic surgery in this woman will have which one of the following effects on the cardiorespiratory or renal system?

A   A 50% reduction in glomerular filtration rate and urine output
B   A reduction in pulmonary resistance and ventilation/perfusion mismatch
C   An increase in heart rate
D   A reduction in cardiac output from 10% to 30%
E   A decrease in peak inspiratory pressure

Questions: EMQs

Questions 19–23

Options for Questions 19–23

A   Up to 1 woman in 10
B   Up to 1 woman in 100
C   Up to 5 women in 100
D   Up to 1 woman in 1000
E   Up to 2 women in 1000
F   Up to 5 women in 1000
G   Up to 4–8 women in 1000
H   Up to 7–8 women in 1000

I   Up to 1 woman in 12,000
J   Up to 1 woman in 100,000
K   Up to 3–8 women in 100,000
L   Up to 10 women in 100,000
M   Up to 100 women in 100,000
N   Up to 1000 women in 100,000
O   Up to 10,000 women in 100,000

Instructions: For each condition described below, choose the single most likely quoted risk from the list of options above. Each option may be used once, more than once, or not at all.

19. A 24-year-old woman complains of pelvic pain for the last 8 months. She has been booked for diagnostic laparoscopy. A specialist registrar is obtaining consent for the surgery and informing about the risk of serious complications in this procedure.

20. A 40-year-old woman is booked for an elective Caesarean section for breech presentation. She goes into labour before the planned operation date at 38 weeks of gestation. She is concerned about the possibility of losing her womb during Caesarean section.

21. A 34-year-old primiparous woman presents to the labour ward at 40 weeks of gestation with regular contractions every 3 minutes. Abdominal examination reveals ballotable head and vaginal examination reveals early labour. Thirty minutes later she has a spontaneous rupture of membranes and cord prolapse. She is pushed to theatre for crash Caesarean section. She wants to know her risk of bladder injury.

22. A 20-year-old woman presents to the early assessment unit at 9 weeks of gestation with mild vaginal bleeding. An ultrasound scan reveals a missed miscarriage. The doctors discuss with her these options: (1) conservative, (2) medical and (3) surgical management. The woman prefers to have surgical management for missed miscarriage but is concerned about the risk of uterine perforation.

23. A 28-year-old woman is admitted to the day surgery unit for diagnostic laparoscopy. She has been suffering from dysmenorrhoea which has outlasted her periods for the last 2 years. An ultrasound scan reveals normal ovaries and an endometrial polyp. She is scared that she may die while asleep.

Answers: SBAs

1. C The consent form only requires the consent of the patient

Consent may be verbal, written or non-verbal. It is an agreement with a patient for any intervention or management. For consent to be valid, a patient must have capacity, which means that they must understand what has been explained in order to make a decision. The information given to the patient must be detailed and sufficient for understanding so that it helps in making a decision. Patients must not be forced to make a decision regarding any form of treatment. If they make a decision that the doctor thinks is inappropriate, the consent is still valid if the patient understands and makes the decision with capacity.

In this particular question, the consent form only requires consent from the patient. The doctor can make the decision that she is Fraser- or Gillick-competent during their discussion with her, based on the fact that (a) she is 14, (b) she is of normal intelligence and (c) she has no impairment of consciousness. She can therefore consent to treatment, but she cannot refuse it because she is a minor (<18 years old) and it is in her best interest. The mother's partner has no legal rights over the girl.

2. E Remove the appendix and arrange an outpatient gynaecology clinic appointment for the patient

Because the dermoid cyst is not an immediate threat to the patient's life, there is no justification for removing it without the patient's consent. It should therefore be left, and the appendectomy should proceed as planned. Afterwards, the patient should be seen in the gynaecology clinic to discuss further management of the dermoid cyst.

3. D Repair should take place because consent is not required

Because perforation can lead to sepsis and death, it is in the patient's best interest that the damage be repaired.

4. A No consent is required

Because the patient's condition is critical and there is a threat to her life, the doctor can act in the patient's best interest to save life. In this situation, the doctor should follow the principles of medical ethics:

- Autonomy: the obligation to respect the decision of a person who has the ability to make decisions
- Beneficence: the balancing of benefits against risks
- Non-maleficence: the obligation to avoid harm
- Justice: the obligation to ensure fairness and the distribution of benefits

5. E The consultant, using the best interest principle

The best interest policy from the Mental Capacity Act 2005 states that any decision made on behalf of an adult that does not the mental capacity to make the decision themselves must be in the best interest of that adult.

6. B Inform the college tutor

It is a right of every patient to have their information kept confidential by health-care services. All hospitals are bound by Caldicott principles. The Caldicott guardian, responsible for maintaining the confidentiality of patients' information and its appropriate sharing, is usually the medical director.

In this scenario, the college tutor in the gynaecology department must be informed. She will speak to the trainees and make them aware that this is not acceptable and should not be repeated. She can also arrange departmental teaching regarding the Caldicott principles and the importance of patient confidentiality.

7. B 3/100,000 to 8/100,000

Death during laparoscopy is rare, with an incidence of 1/1000 – 1/10,000. Serious complications such as damage to the bowel, bladder, uterus or major vessels is uncommon, with an incidence of 1/100 – 1/1000. Around 15% of bowel injuries are not diagnosed at the time of laparoscopic surgery.

Royal College of Obstetricians and Gynaecologists (RCOG). Consent advice No. 2 [Diagnostic laparoscopy]. London: RCOG; 2008.

8. B 2/100

A haemorrhage requiring blood transfusion is uncommon. Other risks during hysterectomy are:

- Serious complication (4/100 women)
- Damage to the bladder and/or ureter (7/1000 women)
- Damage to the bowel (4/10,000 women)
- Return to theatre for bleeding or wound dehiscence (7/1000 women)
- Pelvic abscess (uncommon, 2/1000 women)
- Postoperative venous thromboembolism (4/1000 women)
- Death within 6 weeks of surgery (32/100,000 women)

Royal College of Obstetricians and Gynaecologists (RCOG). Consent advice No 4 [Diagnostic laparoscopy]. London: RCOG; 2009.

9. C 1/100 to 1/1000

During diagnostic hysteroscopy:

- The risk of a serious complication is uncommon (2/1000 women)
- Uterine damage is uncommon, as is failure to gain entry into the uterine cavity (1–100 to 1–1000 women)

- Organ damage (bowel, bladder, major blood vessels) is rare (1/1000 to 1/10,000 women)
- Death is very rare (between 3 and 8 per 100,000 women)

Royal College of Obstetricians and Gynaecologists (RCOG). Consent advise No. 1 [Diagnostic laparoscopy]. London: RCOG; 2008.

10. B The overall risk of serious complications is around 2/1000 cases

For laparoscopic surgery:

- More than 50% of injuries occur during entry into the abdomen
- Bowel injury may not be identified in all cases during surgery, and up to 15% of cases present during the postoperative period
- Death is very rare (3–8/100,000) during a laparoscopy
- There is no difference in the incidence of major vascular or visceral injuries between Veress needle entry and open/direct entry
- There is a lower incidence of failed entry into the abdomen, subcutaneous emphysema (extraperitoneal insufflation) and omental injury with the open technique
- Palmer's point entry should be considered in women with previous laparotomy (the risk of adhesions is 23% with a previous Pfannensteil incision and 50% with a previous midline incision)

Powell F, Khaund A. Laparoscopy and laparoscopic surgery. Obstet Gynaecol Reprod Med 2016; 26:297–300.
Royal College of Obstetricians and Gynaecologists (RCOG). Consent advice No. 2 [Diagnostic laparoscopy]. London: RCOG; 2008.

11. D Monofilament, low tissue reaction, good tensile strength, absorbed over 90–120 days

Monofilament, also known as poliglecaprone, has low tissue reaction, good tensile strength and is absorbed over 90–120 days.

Raghavan R, Arya P, Arya P, China S. Abdominal incision and sutures in obstetrics and gynaecology. Obstet Gynaecol 2014; 16:13–18.

12. B Braided, low tissue reaction, good tensile strength, absorbed over 60–90 days

Polyglactin is braided, has a low tissue reaction and good tensile strength, and is absorbed over 60–90 days. Polyglycolic acid is braided or a monofilament, has a low tissue reaction and good tensile strength, and is absorbed over 90–120 days. Polyglecaprone is a monofilament with a low tissue reaction and good tensile strength; it is absorbed over 90–120 days. Polyglactic 910 is a monofilament with low tissue reaction and good tensile strength, and is absorbed over 7–14 days.

Raghavan R, Arya P, Arya P, China S. Abdominal incision and sutures in obstetrics and gynaecology. Obstet Gynaecol 2014; 16:13–18.

13. D Uretero-neocystostomy

Ureteric injury management depends on the site of injury:

- If there is a ureteric injury, further management depends on the site of the injury. If the damage is in the upper third of the ureter, an end-to-end anastomosis (uretero-ureterostomy) is usually recommended
- If the middle third of the ureter is injured, consider an uretero-ureterostomy or trans-uretero-ureterostomy (i.e. implantation of the ureter into the contralateral ureter)
- If the damage is in the lower third of the ureter, the recommendation is to implant the ureter into the bladder (uretero-neocystostomy). Tension should be avoided at the site of anastomosis. If it is impossible to avoid tension caused by a short ureter, a Boari flap or psoas hitch should be used.

Minas V, Gul N, Aust T, et al. Urinary tract injuries in laparoscopic gynaeolcogical surgery; prevention, recognition, management. Obstet Gynaecol 2014; 16:19–28.

14. B Urinary catheter for 2 weeks, retrograde cystography before removing the catheter

Bladder repairs should be watertight; this is usually tested intraoperatively by filling the bladder with an injection of methylene blue diluted in normal saline. Indigo carmine can also be used. If there is no leak, a Foley catheter should be inserted and left in the bladder for 2 weeks to avoid tension during bladder healing. To ensure that there is no leak, a retrograde cystogram should be performed postoperatively before removing the Foley catheter. If a leak is identified on cystography, the catheter should be left in for another week and a repeat cystogram then performed.

Minas V, Gul N, Aust T, et al. Urinary tract injuries in laparoscopic gynaecological surgery; prevention, recognition, management. Obstet Gynaecol 2014; 16:19–28.

15. A Anterior wall with a suction catheter

The most common sites of perforation are shown in **Table 4.1**, and the frequency of perforation by instrument is shown in **Table 4.2**.

Shakir F, Diab Y. The perforated uterus. Obstet Gynaecol 2013; 15:256–261.

Table 4.1 Incidence of perforation according to site	
Site of perforation	Incidence (%)
Anterior wall	40
Cervical canal	36
Right lateral wall	21
Left lateral wall	17
Posterior wall	13
Fundus	13

Table 4.2 Incidence of perforation according to instrument	
Instrument	Incidence of perforation (%)
Suction cannula	51
Hegar dilator	24
Curette	16

16. C Early mobilisation

The enhanced recovery programme focuses on improving patient outcomes and speeding up patients' recovery. It aims to ensure that patients are active participants in their recovery and that they receive evidence-based care at the right times. The four elements of the enhanced recovery programme are:

- Preoperative assessment
- Reducing the physical stress of an operation
- A structured intraoperative and postoperative management plan, including pain relief
- Early mobilisation

This is helped by ensuring that staff are adequately trained, that there are improved processes and room layouts, and that procedure-specific care plans have been formulated.

The anticipated outcomes of the programme are:

- Better outcomes and a reduced length of stay
- An increase in the number of patients being treated, and a reduced level of resources required
- A better staffing environment

17. E 50%

Ureteric injuries can occur with any gynaecological operation.

- The risk of vesicovaginal fistula is around 1/1000 cases of total abdominal hysterectomy
- The risk of bladder injury increases to 4.7% and 2.1%, respectively, with previous Caesarean section and previous laparotomy
- Around 51% ureteric injuries occur in lower third of the ureter, 19% in the middle third and 30% in the upper third
- The ureter lies <2 cm away at the lateral to lateral vaginal fornix
- Opening the retroperitoneum to identify the ureter before uterine artery clamping reduces the risk of ureteric injury from 0.7% to 0.2%
- The detection of ureteric injury increased from 1.6/1000 cases to 6.2/1000 cases with routine cystoscopy
- The detection of bladder injury improved from 2.6/1000 to 10.4/1000 cases with routine cystoscopy

Gopinath D, Jha S. Urological complications following gynaecological surgery. Obstet Gynaecol Reprod Med 2016.

18. A 50% reduction in glomerular filtrate rate and urine output

Effects of pneumoperitoneum include:

- Reduction in lung compliance
- Reduction in lung volume
- Increase in arterial pressure
- Increase in pulmonary and systemic vascular resistance

Heart rate does not usually change.

Royal College of Obstetricians and Gynaecologists (RCOG). Consent advice No. 2 [Diagnostic laparoscopy]. London: RCOG; 2008.
Royal College of Obstetricians and Gynaecologists (RCOG). Green-top Guideline No. 49 [Preventing entry-lreated gynaecological laparascopic injuries]. London: RCOG; 2008.

Answers: EMQs

19. E Up to 2 women in 1000

The risks associated with diagnostic laparoscopy are divided into frequent (wound bruising, shoulder tip pain, wound gaping and wound infection) and serious risks (serious complications in up to 2 women in every 1000 undergoing laparoscopy – damage to the bowel, bladder, uterer or major blood vessels which would require immediate repair by laparoscopy, or laparotomy, failure to gain entry to abdominal cavity and to complete intended procedure, hernia at site of entry, death); 3–8 women in every 100,000 undergoing laparoscopy die as a result of complications.

Additional procedures which may be necessary during the procedure include laparotomy, repair of damage to the bowel, bladder, uterer or blood vessels and blood transfusion.

20. H Up to 7–8 women in 1000

Risks of Caesarean section are as follows:

Serious risks: maternal

- emergency hysterectomy, 7–8 women in every 1000 undergoing Caesarean section
- need for further surgery at a later date, including curettage, 5 in 1000 women
- admission to intensive care unit (highly dependent on the reason for Caesarean section), 9 in 1000 women
- thromboembolic disease, 4–16 in 10,000 women
- bladder injury, 1 in 1000 women
- ureteric injury, 3 in 10,000 women
- death, approximately 1 in 12,000 women

Frequent risks: maternal

- persistent wound and abdominal discomfort in the first few months after surgery, 9 in 100 women
- increased risk of a repeat Caesarean section when vaginal delivery is attempted in subsequent pregnancies, 1 in 4 women
- readmission to hospital, 5 in 100 women
- haemorrhage, 5 in 1000 women
- infection, 6 in 100 women

Frequent risk: fetal

- lacerations, 1–2 in 100 babies

Risks for future pregnancies include:

- increased risk of uterine rupture during subsequent pregnancies/deliveries, 2–7 in 1000 women

- increased risk of ante partum stillbirth, 2–4 in 1000 women
- increased risk in subsequent pregnancies of placenta praevia and placenta accreta, 4–8 in 1000 women

Additional procedures during Caesarean section which may become necessary include hysterectomy, repair of injured organs and blood transfusion.

21. D Up to 1 woman in 1000

Serious risks associated with Caesarean section are:

- bladder injury, 1 in 1000 women
- ureteric injury, 3 in 10,000 women

22. F Up to 5 women in 1000

Serious risks include:

- uterine perforation, up to 5 in 1000 women
- significant trauma to the cervix
- there is no substantiated evidence in the literature of any impact on future fertility

Frequent risks include:

- bleeding that lasts for up to 2 weeks is very common but blood transfusion is uncommon (1–2 in 1000 women)
- need for repeat surgical evacuation, up to 5 in 100 women
- localised pelvic infection, 3 in 100 women

The additional procedures that may be necessary during the procedure include laparoscopy or laparotomy to diagnose or repair organ injury, or uterine perforation.

23. K Up to 3–8 women in 100,000

3–8 women in every 100,000 undergoing laparoscopy die as a result of complications.

Royal College of Obstetricians and Gynaecologists (RCOG). Consent Advice No. 2. Diagnostic laparoscopy. London: RCOG Press, 2008.
Royal College of Obstetricians and Gynaecologists (RCOG). Consent Advice No. 7. Caesarean section. London: RCOG Press, 2009.
Royal College of Obstetricians and Gynaecologists (RCOG). Consent Advice No. 10. Surgical evacuation of uterus for early pregnancy loss. London: RCOG Press, 2010.

Chapter 5

Postoperative care

Questions: SBAs

For each question, select the single best answer from the five options listed.

1. The optimisation of preoperative fluid management is essential to reduce postoperative mortality and morbidity.

    What is the 30-day mortality risk in high-risk patients with an inadequate fluid balance, compared with those who have an adequate fluid balance?

    A   5%
    B   10%
    C   15%
    D   20%
    E   25%

2. Patients who are high risk perioperatively (multiple co-morbidities) are high risk intraoperatively.

    How many times higher is the mortality with inadequate intraoperative monitoring compared with adequate intraoperative monitoring?

    A   2 times higher
    B   3 times higher
    C   4 times higher
    D   5 times higher
    E   6 times higher

3. A 46-year-old woman is to undergo a laparoscopic hysterectomy. She has a body mass index of 22 kg/m^2 and no medical conditions.

    With regard to her peri- and postoperative thromboprophylaxis, which of the following is the most accurate statement?

    A   There is no difference between low molecular weight heparin and unfractionated heparin in the prevention of venous thromboembolism
    B   There is no difference between low molecular weight heparin and unfractionated heparin in reducing the incidence of fatal venous thromboembolism
    C   Both low molecular weight heparin and unfractionated heparin prevent wound haematomas

D   There is no difference between the effect of low molecular weight heparin and the effect of unfractionated heparin on the incidence of bleeding complications intraoperatively and postoperatively

E   In the prevention of asymptomatic venous thromboembolism, intermittent pneumatic compression is not as effective as heparin

4.   A 32-year-old woman underwent a myomectomy, during which she lost approximately 700 mL of blood. 12 hours after the procedure, she developed a spike in temperature of 38°C but remained well. Her temperature following that episode remained normal.

What is the most likely cause of her high temperature?

A   Pelvic collection
B   Pulmonary atelectasis
C   Pulmonary embolism
D   Urinary tract infection
E   Wound infection

5.   A 50-year-old woman underwent an open total abdominal hysterectomy and a bilateral salpingo-oophorectomy for grade 1 endometrioid carcinoma. The procedure was uncomplicated, with an approximate blood loss of 300 mL. The patient developed persistent vomiting 36 hours after the operation. Her clinical observations were stable. Bloods tests showed a sodium concentration of 135 mmol/L and potassium concentration of 3.2 mmol/L.

What is the most likely cause of her vomiting?

A   Bowel injury
B   Paralytic ileus
C   Pneumonia
D   Vesicovaginal fistula
E   Ureteric injury

6.   A 60-year-old woman underwent vaginal hysterectomy for a third-degree uterovaginal prolapse. She was discharged home on day 2 after surgery. She attended gynaecology emergency services on day 11 after surgery with lower abdominal pain, a temperature of 37.7°C and an offensive brownish vaginal discharge.

What is the most likely diagnosis?

A   Bowel obstruction
B   Chest infection
C   Rectovaginal fistula
D   Urinary tract infection
E   Vault haematoma

7. A 60-year-old woman underwent a vaginal hysterectomy for a third-degree uterovaginal prolapse. She complained of a brownish vaginal discharge on day 2 after the operation. Abdominal ultrasound scan of the pelvis has revealed a vault haematoma measuring 5 cm × 5 cm. She is otherwise clinically well and stable.

What is the most appropriate management?

A   Antibiotics (broad spectrum)
B   Incision and drainage under ultrasound scan guidance
C   Observation
D   Laparotomy and drainage
E   Laparoscopic drainage

8. You are a specialist registrar allocated to a gynaecology theatre list. While assisting the consultant, who is performing a laparoscopic hysterectomy, you notice that he has accidentally perforated the terminal ileum, creating a 5 mm tear.

What is the most appropriate step?

A   Laparotomy and repair by the general surgeons
B   Laparoscopic repair by the general surgeons
C   Conservative management
D   Antibiotics
E   Rectosigmoidoscopy

9. A 36-year-old woman is electively booked for a Caesarean section for placenta praevia. She has a history of previous laparoscopic salpingectomy for an ectopic pregnancy, and two emergency previous Caesarean sections for failure to progress. You are the senior registrar, operating the consultant's supervision. At the end of the procedure, you notice a 1 cm tear in the bladder dome.

What is the correct management intraoperatively and what is your advice postoperatively?

A   Interrupted non-absorbable sutures, catheter for 7 days and a cystogram
B   Continuous absorbable sutures, catheter for 7 days and a cystogram
C   Interrupted absorbable sutures, catheter for 7 days and a cystogram
D   Continuous non-absorbable sutures, catheter for 7 days and a cystogram
E   Interrupted absorbable sutures, catheter for 4 days and a cystogram

10. A 63-year-old woman had prophylactic laparascopic bilateral salpingo-oophorectomy in the private sector. She was discharged home 6 hours after surgery. 12 hours after discharge, she is brought to the emergency department with increasing abdominal pain and dizziness. On admission she looks pale. Her pulse rate is 132 bpm, her blood pressure is 80/42 mmHg and her temperature is 37.2°C. Her respiratory rate is 22 per minute, and saturation levels are 95% on air.

What is the most appropriate definitive management?

A   Conservative management
B   Informing the intensive therapy unit
C   Intravenous fluids and antibiotics

    D Laparotomy and explore
    E Laparoscopy and explore

11. The enhanced recovery programme (ERP) for faster postoperative recovery has been implemented for many aspects of obstetrics and gynaecology.

   Which of the following is not included in ERP?

    A Admission on the same day
    B No wound drains used
    C A 24-hour telephone clinic
    D Use of regional block
    E Use of a nasogastric tube

12. You are the a sixth-year specialist trainee, on call for the gynaecology team, and have been called to theatre by a second-year specialist junior trainee because she needs help with evacuation of retained products of conception for missed miscarriage. When you arrive, the specialist junior trainee tells you that she has probably caused a uterine perforation with the dilator but has not yet used suction. After assessment, you feel that uterus has been perforated by the dilator. There is no bleeding, and the anaesthetist informs you that the patient is stable.

   What is the next appropriate management?

    A Admit, observe, antibiotics
    B Laparoscopy and repair
    C Laparotomy and repair
    D Hysteroscopy
    E Call the general surgeons

13. The World Health Organization considers obesity to be a global epidemic, and a body mass index >40 kg/m^2 is a risk factor for postoperative complications.

   Which one of the following does not reduce the risk of wound complications in obese women?

    A Good haemostasis
    B Extensive use of cautery
    C Mass closure of the rectus sheath
    D Use of antibiotics
    E Closure of the superficial fascia

14. A 35-year-old woman underwent a laparoscopic myomectomy to remove a subserosal fibroid measuring 12 cm × 12 cm. The fibroid was removed with a morcellator.

   Which rare complication is specifically associated with the use of a morcellator during this procedure?

    A Pulmonary atelectasis
    B Patient death
    C Visceral injury
    D Conversion to laparotomy
    E Peritoneal myomatosis

Questions: EMQs

Questions 15–19

Options for questions 15–19

A	Bladder injury	J	Kidney injury
B	Common peroneal nerve	K	Large bowel injury
C	Deep vein thrombosis	L	Lateral cutaneous nerve
D	Disseminated intravascular coagulation	M	Obturator nerve
		N	Peritonitis
E	Femoral nerve damage	O	Primary haemorrhage due to intra-abdominal bleeding
F	Genitofemoral nerve		
G	Genital haematoma		
H	Iliohypogastric nerves	P	Pudendal nerve damage
I	Ilioinguinal nerve and	Q	Pulmonary embolism

Instructions: For each of the following postoperative scenarios, chose the correct diagnosis from the list of options above. Each answer may be used once, more than once or not at all.

15. You are the on-call gynaecology registrar and have been asked to review a patient who had a total abdominal hysterectomy 4 hours ago. Her pulse is 120 bpm and her blood pressure is 80/40 mmHg. She has abdominal pain, feels dizzy and is short of breath. The operative notes reveal that it was a routine hysterectomy with an estimated blood loss of 300 mL. She is not bleeding vaginally.

16. You are on-call gynaecology registrar and have been called to review a patient who is 50 years of age and has presented to the emergency department with haemoptysis. She had a total abdominal hysterectomy 1 week ago. She was discharged on day 3 post-operatively. She has no significant past medical history. Her Wells score is 5.

17. You are the on-call gynaecology registrar and have been asked to review a woman who has had a total abdominal hysterectomy the previous day. The procedure has been documented as an 'uncomplicated hysterectomy' with an estimated blood loss of 400 mL. She has not passed much urine after the removal of catheter and complains of diffuse abdominal pain. On examination, the abdomen appears much distended but there are no points of tenderness.

18. You are the on-call gynaecology registrar and have been asked to review a patient who is very anxious and unable to sleep. She had a total abdominal hysterectomy 2 days ago and has noticed that she is able to walk but is not able to climb up the stairs following this surgery. In her operation notes, it is documented that the surgery was complicated and lasted for 4 hours. The estimated blood loss was 300 mL. On examination you notice that she has lack of sensation over the anterior aspect of her thigh and the medial aspect of her calf. She is unable to extend her knees.

19. You are the on-call gynaecology registrar and you have been asked to review a patient because she is complaining of pain in the perineum and vulval region. This is particularly worse when she is sitting. On reviewing the notes you find that she has had an open sacrospinous fixation the previous day.

Answers: SBAs

1. D 20%

Preoperative fluid optimisation minimises mortality and morbidity, but estimation of fluid depletion and fluid replacement is usually inaccurate. In this situation, physiological compensation helps but can mask hypovolaemia. It is reported that the 30-day mortality risk increases to 20% when fluid management is inadequate.

National Confidential Enquiry into Patient Outcome and Death (NCEPOD). Knowing the risk: a review of the peri-operative care of surgical patients. London: NCEPOD; 2011.

2. B 3 times higher

Adequate monitoring helps appropriate management to avoid complications, especially in high-risk patients. Postoperative mortality increases threefold in patients who are not adequately monitored.

3. A There is no difference between low molecular weight heparin and unfractionated heparin in the prevention of venous thromboembolism

The Scottish Intercollegiate Guidelines Network (2010) reports that there is no difference between low molecular weight heparin and unfractionated heparin in preventing deep venous thrombosis and reducing mortality. There is also no difference in the risk of bleeding.

Scottish Intercollegiate Guidelines Network (SIGN). Prevention and Management of venous thromboembolism. SIGN guideline 122. Edinburgh: SIGN, 2010.

4. B Pulmonary atelectasis

Raised temperature within the first 48 hours of surgery may be indicative of pulmonary atelectasis rather than an infective cause. A episode of raised temperature in a clinically well patient is usually not a concern, and there is no need to prescribe antibiotics. The most common cause is atelectasis, resulting from restricted breathing due to pain after a major operation. This patient needs early referral for chest physiotherapy to prevent further complications such as chest infection. She needs to be taught deep breathing exercises.

5. B Paralytic ileus

The most common postoperative complication of laparotomy is paralytic ileus. Handling of the bowel during surgery can reduce peristaltic activity for >12 hours, and it may not return to normal for several days. This is called paralytic ileus. Clinically, the patient can be symptomatic with abdominal pain, vomiting and inability to pass flatus or stool. On auscultation, the bowel sounds may be sluggish or absent. There may be dilated loops of small bowel on an abdominal radiograph. Paralytic ileus can be managed conservatively by what is conventionally called 'drip and suck' (nasogastric tube aspiration and intravenous fluids).

6. E Vault haematoma

This woman has signs and symptoms of an infected vaginal vault haematoma, a known complication of vaginal hysterectomy. After examination, a vaginal swab must be taken for culture and sensitivity. The patient should be treated with appropriate intravenous antibiotics, fluid resuscitation and drainage of the vaginal vault haematoma.

7. A Antibiotics (broad spectrum)

Vaginal vault haematoma is a known complication of hysterectomy, occurring in 20% of women after surgery. In can usually be managed conservatively with antibiotics. Drainage of the haematoma is required only if there is evidence of infection or pain, or if the patient is unwell. Drainage can be performed vaginally.

8. A Laparotomy and repair by the general surgeons

A laparatomy must be performed to fully assess the bowel, specifically the area that was damaged. The general surgeons should be involved to repair the damaged area.

9. C Interrupted absorbable sutures, catheter for 7 days and a cystogram

The sutures should be absorbable and interrupted. The catheter has to remain in situ for 7 days to help with bladder healing and then a cystogram needs to be arranged to check for any urinary leak from the bladder.

10. D Laparotomy and explore

The patient most likely had an intra-abdominal bleed caused by the inferior epigastric vein being punctured at the time of the laparascopy. Although it is possible to start with a laparascopy, the definitive treatment would be a laparotomy so that site of bleeding can be explored.

11. E Use of a nasogastric tube

The enhanced recovery programme aims for faster postoperative recovery, a shorter hospital stay and an early return to normal activities. Optimisation of the patient starts on the day of referral and lasts until patient follow-up.

Torbe E, Crawford R, Nordin A. Enhanced recovery in gynaecology. Obstet Gynaecol 2013; 15:4.

12. A Admit, observe, antibiotics

Uterine perforation is a specific complication that needs to be discussed when obtaining consent for evacuation of retained products of conception. The management of this complication depends on the cause of the perforation.

First, the consultant on call must be involved. If a perforation is caused by a dilator, the procedure should be abandoned and the perforation managed conservatively with observation, antibiotics and completion of the procedure at a later date. If the perforation occurs with the suction catheter, or suction evacuation is attempted, laparoscopy is necessary to exclude uterine bleeding and injury to adjacent organs. Appropriate repair must be carried out.

Shakir F, Diab Y. The perforated uterus. Obstet Gynaecol 2013; 15:256–261.

13. B Extensive use of cautery

Adequate haemostasis is necessary before wound closure. Inadvertent use of diathermy can cause an increase in non-viable tissue and therefore increase the risk of wound infection. Mass closure of the abdomen using delayed absorbable sutures and closure of the superficial fascial layers reduce the risk of fascial breakdown and wound disruption, respectively. Antibiotics are routinely given at induction of anaesthesia and have been shown to reduce the risk of wound infection.

Biswas N, Hogston P. Review surgical risk from obesity in gynaecology. Obstet Gynaecol 2011; 13:87–91.

14. E Peritoneal myomatosis

Peritoneal myomatosis is a very rare complication; it has been reported in only 3 cases after laparoscopic myomectomy and morcellation.

The conversion rate to laparotomy is reported to be 1.3%. Visceral injuries and patient deaths have been reported with laparoscopic myomectomy involving the use of morcellator.

Royal College of Obstetricians and Gynaecologists (RCOG). Laparoscopic myomectomy using a morcellator (query bank). London: RCOG; 2009.

Answers: EMQs

15. O Primary haemorrhage

Primary haemorrhage occurs within 24 hours after an operation. It is usually due to achieving poor haemostasis or a slipped ligature in the post-operative period. If this diagnosis is missed and therefore not treated, the patient may develop disseminated intravascular coagulation. Bleeding after abdominal surgery or after a laparoscopy leads to intra-abdominal collection or collection within the rectus muscle if the bleeding is from the inferior epigastric artery. Symptoms include shortness of breath, feeling light headed and abdominal pain. The signs include hypotension, tachypnoea, tachycardia and cold clammy skin. The patient's Glasgow Coma Scale may also fall.

16. Q Pulmonary embolism

If a pulmonary embolism (PE) is suspected based on the history and examination findings, then the Wells score should be calculated to estimate the clinical probability of a PE. To calculate the Wells score, the following features are reviewed for which a score is allotted from 1–3:

- Signs and symptoms of deep vein thrombosis – a score of 3 is assigned
- Alternative diagnosis less likely – a score of 3 is assigned
- Heart rate more than 100 bpm – a score of 1.5 is assigned
- Immobility for 3 day or surgery in last 4 weeks – a score of 1.5 is assigned
- Previous deep vein thrombosis/PE – a score of 1.5 is assigned
- Hemoptysis – a score of 1 is assigned
- Malignancy – a score of 1 is assigned

The diagnosis is likely to be due to a PE if the total score is more than 4

National Institute for Health and Care Excellence (NICE). Venous thromboembolic diseases: diagnosis, management and thrombophilia testing [CG144]. London: NICE; 2015.

17. A Bladder injury

The likely clinical diagnosis is a bladder injury. If this is suspected, an ureteric injury cannot be excluded until investigations are performed.

The clinical features of a bladder injury include:

- Haematuria
- Suprapubic pain
- Oliguria and leakage of urine from the vagina
- Urine irritates the peritoneum and can cause uroperitoneum
- A form of chemical peritonitis
- It causes generalised abdominal pain, distension and an ileus, but tenderness is absent

- This can be confused with peritonitis caused by contaminated products such as faeces
- The symptoms of uroperitoneum usually appear within the first 48 hours after an operation, unless it was a thermal injury which can present 10–14 days after the operation
- The blood results show a raised creatinine level, which is due to resorption of creatinine through the peritoneal membrane

A CT urogram scan should be perfomed to confirm the presence of a leak and urine in the peritoneal cavity. To diagnose a fistula, the bladder is filled with methylene blue and vaginal leakage is observed.

MRI can be useful to diagnose a vesico-vaginal fistula

Minas V, Gul N, Aust T, et al. Urinary tract injuries in laparoscopic gynaecological surgery; prevention, recognition and management. Obstet Gynaecol 2014; 16:19–28.

18. E Femoral nerve damage

The origin of the femoral nerve is from the L2–L4 nerve roots. It emerges from the lateral border of the psoas muscle and leaves the pelvis lateral to the femoral vessels, underneath the inguinal ligament. Gynaecological surgery, particularly abdominal hysterectomy, is the most common cause of femoral nerve damage. The incidence of this nerve damage is around 11% in abdominal hysterectomies. The nerve is damaged because it is compressed against the pelvic side wall, as a result of deep retractor blades being used.

Kuponiyi O, Alleemudder DI, Latunde-Dada A, Eedarapalli P. Nerve injuries associated with gynaecological surgery. Obstet Gynaecol 2014; 16:29–36.

19. P Pudendal nerve damage

The pudendal nerve originates from the S2–S4 nerve routes. It exits the pelvis through the greater sciatic foramen, then runs besides the internal pudendal artery behind the lateral third of the sacrospinous ligament and the ischial spine. It then re-enters the pelvis through the lesser sciatic foramen to enter the pudendal canal. This nerve can be damaged during sacrospinous ligament fixation surgery.

The symptoms of pudendal nerve damage include:

- Gluteal pain
- Vulval and perineal pain, especially when sitting
- Sexual dysfunction may occur

Kuponiyi O, Alleemudder DI, Latunde-Dada A, Eedarapalli P. Nerve injuries associated with gynaecological surgery. Obstet Gynaecol 2014; 16:29–36.

Chapter 6

Surgical procedures

Questions: SBAs

For each question, select the single best answer from the five options listed.

1. You are the registrar in the gynaecology clinic and are seeing a patient who requires a diagnostic hysteroscopy under general anaesthetic. You are about to obtain her consent.

    Which one of the following statements is correct regarding risk of diagnostic hysteroscopy?

    A   Damage to the bowel, bladder and blood vessels is frequent
    B   It is very common to fail to gain entry into the uterus and complete the procedure
    C   Infertility is a common complication postoperatively
    D   The overall risk of a serious complication is 2/1000
    E   The risk of death is 10/100,000

2. A 36-year-old woman with 5 children comes to see you in the clinic because she would like a long-term, non-reversible form of contraception. She has read about hysteroscopic sterilisation and would like to know the failure rate of this procedure.

    What do you tell her?

    A   0.1%
    B   0.2%
    C   0.3%
    D   0.4%
    E   0.5%

3. You are the gynaecology on-call registrar and are about to carry out an evacuation of retained products of conception with a senior house officer who is in the second year of training in obstetrics and gynaecology. The dilator is about to be positioned, and the junior trainee asks you which area of the uterus is the most common site for a perforation to occur.

    What is the most common area for a perforation to occur during this procedure?

    A   Anterior wall
    B   Cervical canal
    C   Lateral walls
    D   Fundus
    E   Posterior wall

4. You are the gynaecology on-call registrar and are about to do an evacuation of retained products of conception with the senior house officer, who is in the second year of training in obstetrics and gynaecology. The dilator is about to be placed, and the junior trainee asks you which instrument most commonly causes uterine perforation.

    Which instrument is most likely to cause a uterine perforation?

    A   Curette
    B   Hegar dilator
    C   Sponge-holding forceps
    D   Suction cannula
    E   Vulselum

5. As a registrar, you are assisting your consultant with an elective theatre list. The consultant asks you to perform a hysteroscopy for a patient with a postmenopausal bleed. Pelvic ultrasound has shown an endometrial thickness of 7 mm. You insert a 3 mm width hysteroscope but notice that almost the whole scope has been inserted. Clinically and by the scan, the uterus is small. The consultant suspects that you have perforated the uterus, but there is no bleeding. You have not performed any curettage.

    What is your management in this scenario?

    A   Call the surgeons
    B   Laparoscopy
    C   Laparotomy
    D   Observe and give antibiotics
    E   Stay in theatre and watch for bleeding

6. You are the gynaecology on-call registrar and have been asked to review a 38-year-old woman who is under the care of the general surgeons for a bowel problem. Pelvic ultrasound has shown an incidental finding of a 1.5 cm endometrial polyp. The patient says her periods are regular and normal with no intermenstrual or postcoital bleeding.

    How should she be managed?

    A   Hysteroscopic polyp resection
    B   Insertion of a levonorgestrel-releasing intrauterine system (Mirena coil)
    C   Pipelle biopsy
    D   Repeat ultrasound in 4 months
    E   Repeat ultrasound in 6 months

7. You are the on-call registrar for the labour ward and are about to perform a Caesarean section for failure to progress at 4 cm cervical dilatation. This woman is a primigravida and has a body mass index of 35 kg/m². The consultant wants you to make an incision that will require the least amount of analgesia and result in less febrile morbidity, the shortest operating time, less operative blood loss, the lowest risk of wound infection and a shorter hospital stay.

   Which incision will you choose?

   A   Cherney incision
   B   Joel–Cohen incision
   C   Kustner incision
   D   Maylard incision
   E   Pfannenstiel incision

8. You are the on-call registrar for the labour ward. You are about to perform a Caesarean section for failure to progress at 4 cm cervical dilatation. The woman is a primigravida and has a body mass index of 40 kg/m². The consultant wants you to choose a suture material that is associated with the lowest chance of wound infection.

   Which of the following materials has the lowest association with wound infection?

   A   Braided
   B   Monofilament
   C   Plaited
   D   Shafted
   E   Twisted

9. You are the gynaecology on-call registrar and have been asked to review a 40-year-old woman who has just undergone an ultrasound scan. She has had in vitro fertilisation, with a two-embryo transfer. She has a past history of ectopic pregnancy for which she has undergone a left salpingectomy. The woman has presented with abdominal pain and the scan report is as follows:

   'Normal anteverted uterus. No signs of trophoblastic tissue reaction within the uterine cavity. Endometrial thickness is 4 mm. Left ovary appears normal. Right ovary appears normal; however, adjacent to the right ovary is a 40 mm × 40 mm heterogenous echogenic mass. Free fluid is noted in the recto-uterine pouch (pouch of Douglas), with speckles; it measures 20 mm. Patient complaining of right adnexal tenderness during this scan.'

   The patient's β-human chorionic gonadotrophin concentration is 1600 IU/L, and her haemoglobin 95 g/L.

   What is the recommended management?

   A   Administration of methotrexate
   B   Conservative management
   C   Laparoscopic salpingectomy
   D   Laparoscopic salpingotomy and follow-up
   E   Laparoscopic salpingotomy

10. A 32-year-old woman is undergoing a laparoscopic right ovarian cystectomy for a dermoid cyst. She had a midline laparotomy in her home country (Bulgaria) 3 years ago for the same condition. She has a body mass index of 40 kg/m^2.

Which technique will you use to establish a pneumoperitoneum?

A   Closed-entry Palmer's point
B   Closed-entry umbilical point
C   Hasson technique
D   Transfundal needle insertion
E   Suprapubic needle insertion

Questions: EMQs

Questions 11–15

Options for questions 11–15

A	Bowel anastomosis	J	Uretero-ureterostomy
B	Conservative management	K	Uretero-neocystostomy
C	Drainage	L	Trans-uretero-ureterostomy
D	Laparotomy	M	Intravenous urogram
E	Laparotomy and repair	N	Ultrasound of kidneys, ureter and
F	Pelvic CT		bladder
G	Review in 1 week	O	Abdominal X-ray
H	Pelvic ultrasound	P	Rigid cystoscopy
I	Urethral stenting	Q	Flexible cystoscopy

Instructions: For each of the questions below choose the single most appropriate management plan from the list below. Each answer may be used once, more than once or not at all.

11. You are performing a laparoscopic hysterectomy with the consultant and you are trying to identify the ureters. The consultant inadvertently crushes the left ureter with his nontraumatic grasper (Johans' grasper). Visualisation of the ureter following this crushing reveals peristaltic movements and absence of urinary leak.

12. You are performing a laparoscopic hysterectomy with the consultant and you note that the upper third of the left ureter has accidentally been transected.

13. You are performing a laparoscopic hysterectomy with the consultant and you note that the lower third of the left ureter has accidentally been transected.

14. You are the gynaecology registrar in theatre and you are about to perform a laparoscopy procedure on a patient who has been diagnosed with endometriosis. She has had two laparoscopies for the same reason previously. You use a veress needle, with great difficulty and then insert the primary trocar in the umbilicus. Following insertion of the camera you notice two holes in the bowel. How would you manage her?

15. You are the gynaecology registrar in theatre and you have just performed an endometrial ablation on a 44-year-old woman who was diagnosed to have menorrhagia. She also wants a laparoscopic sterilisation to be performed at the same time. You perform the sterilisation but following this you notice there is an area on the sigmoid bowel which looks white and devascularised. There is no bleeding or faecal soiling. How should she be managed?

Answers: SBAs

1.   D The overall risk of a serious complication is 2/1000

Women should be informed that the cause of their complaint cannot always be diagnosed at hysteroscopy. They must also be informed of serious and frequently occurring risks, such as damage to the uterus, bowel, bladder and major blood vessels. It must be explained that these risks are increased in women who are obese or have a medical condition. The risk of serious complications also increases if it is a therapeutic procedure. The chance of a serious risk is 2/1000 women. Failure to gain entry is uncommon (1/100 to 1/1000), infertility is rare (1/1000 to 1/10,000), and death is very rare, at 3–8/100,000. The frequent but less serious risks are infection and bleeding.

Royal College of Obstetricians and Gynaecologists (RCOG). Diagnostic hysteroscopy under general anaesthesia. Consent advice no 1. London: RCOG, 2008.

2.   C 0.3%

Hysterocopic sterilisation (using Essure, Bayer, Whippany, NJ, USA) is a long-term, non-hormonal, irreversible and effective method of sterilisation. It involves inserting a stainless steel coil with polyester fibres into the intramyometrial part of the fallopian tube. The coil is inserted through a catheter that is passed through the 5 Fr operating channel of a 5.5 mm rigid hysteroscope. Normal saline is used to distend the uterus.

Hysteroscopic sterilisation is an outpatient procedure so avoids general anaesthesia and surgical procedures via an abdominal approach. It only 5–10 minutes to perform, and the patient is discharged within 1 hour. A follow-up ultrasound or radiogram is arranged at or after 3 months to check the placement of the coil.

The Essure birth control system has a success rate of 99.7%; it has been employed more than 500,000 times across Europe, North America and Australasia.

Cooper NAM, Clark TJ. Ambulatory hysteroscopy. Obstet Gynaecol 2013; 15:159–166.

3.   A Anterior wall

The majority of perforations occur in the uterine body. They are usually small and do not bleed very much. If, however, the uterine vessels are involved, e.g. in the lower part of the uterus or at the level of internal cervical os, bleeding can be significant. This can lead to intraperitoneal bleeding or the formation of a haematoma in the broad ligament.

Shakir F, Diab Y. The perforated uterus. Obstet Gynaecol 2013; 15:256–261.

4.   D Suction cannula

The incidence of perforation according to instrument is shown in **Table 4.2**.

Uterine perforation is a known complication of suction evacuation. It can occur during diagnostic hysteroscopy and hysteroscopic operative procedures.

The signs of perforation during the procedure include:

- The instrument entering beyond the limitations of the uterus
- Loss of resistance when the instrument is inserted
- Sudden inability to see the uterus during hysteroscopy because the uterus has collapsed
- Excessive bleeding
- A large deficiency in the distension medium used for hysteroscopic procedures
- Visualisation of the site of perforation at hysteroscopy
- Visualisation of omentum or bowel at hysteroscopy
- Visualisation of fatty tissue omentum while performing suction evacuation

If the perforation is recognised early and managed immediately, morbidity and mortality are significantly reduced.

Shakir F, Diab. Y. The perforated uterus. Obstet Gynaecol 2013; 15:256–261.

5.   D Observe and give antibiotics

The management of a perforation depends on what instrument made the perforation. If this was a small dilator or a hysteroscope of <5 mm width, the patient can be observed and given a 5-day course of antibiotics. If a larger instrument has been used, avulsion of tissue has been attempted, tissue has been grasped or there is bleeding, laparoscopy should be considered. This aims to rule out damage to the surrounding organs and check if the site of perforation is bleeding. In all cases, the patient should be informed the principles of duty of candour must be followed. An incident form must also be completed.

Shakir. F, Diab. Y. The perforated uterus. Obstet Gynaecol 2013; 15:256–261.

6.   A Hysteroscopic polyp resection

Regarding the management of endometrial polyps:

- If the woman is asymptomatic and premenopausal, the endometrial polyp should be removed if it is >1 cm in diameter
- If the polyp is <1 cm in diameter, it is likely to regress. The pros and cons of removal should be discussed with the patient
- If a premenopausal woman is symptomatic, the polyp should be removed regardless of size
- In postmenopusal women, the polyp should always be removed, regardless of size or symptoms; this will allow a histological diagnosis so malignancy can be ruled out.

Annan JJ, Aquilina J, Ball E. The management of endometrial polyps in 21st century. Obstet Gynaecol 2012; 14:33–38.

7.   B Joel–Cohen incision

Caesarean section is the most common operation performed worldwide.

The commonly used Joel–Cohen incision was introduced in 1954 and was initially used for gynaecological procedures. It is a straight transverse incision 3 cm below the anterior superior iliac spines. Blunt dissection is used to extend the subcutaneous tissue and fascia, and to separate the rectus sheath.

The Pfannenstiel incision, introduced in 1900, is generally used to perform gynaecological procedures. It is a curved incision situated 2 cm above the pubic symphysis. The skin is cut with a knife and the rectus sheath is opened using a knife or scissors.

Many studies have been conducted to compare the Pfannenstiel and Joel–Cohen incisions. The latter has been found to be associated with the lowest analgesic requirements, less febrile morbidity, the shortest operating times, less operative blood loss, reduced risk of wound infection and shorter hospital stays.

Raghavan. R, Arya P, Arya P, China S. Abdominal incisions and sutures in obstetrics and gynaecology. Obstet Gynaecol 2014; 16:13–18.

8.   B Monofilament

Various factors have to be considered when deciding which suture material to use. These include the patient's age, the absence or presence of an infection, the surgeon's experience with the sutures and the location of the wound. There are three types of suture: rapidly absorbable, slowly absorbable and non-absorbable. These are further subdivided into monofilament and braided sutures. There are fewer wound infections with monofilament sutures than braided ones. The chances of wound dehiscence are the same for non-absorbable and slowly absorbable sutures, but continuous wound pain is more common with non-absorbable sutures.

Raghavan. R, Arya P, Arya P, China. S. Abdominal incisions and sutures in obstetrics and gynaecology. Obstet Gynaecol 2014; 16:13–18.

9.   D Laparoscopic salpingotomy and follow-up

With the advances in ultrasound and increased operator experience, most ectopic pregnancies are now diagnosed by pelvic ultrasound. An ectopic pregnancy should be seen as a mass that moves separately from the ovary. A serum β-human chorionic gonadotropin (β-hCG) level is helpful when planning the management of an ectopic pregnancy. If this is 1500 IU/L and above, an intrauterine pregnancy should be seen. If an intrauterine pregnancy is not seen, a diagnosis of ectopic pregnancy should be strongly suspected. A serum progesterone level is not routinely recommended, as per National Institute of Health and Care Excellence guidelines concerning ectopic pregancy and miscarriage.

A laparoscopic approach to surgery rather than a laparotomy is recommended if a surgeon is experienced. A symptomatic woman with a large ectopic pregnancy should be managed surgically.

If there is a healthy contralateral tube, a salpingectomy should be performed to remove the ectopic pregnancy. If the contralateral tube is damaged or absent, a salpingotomy should be performed. The patient must be warned of persistent trophoblastic tissue, which occurs in 4–8% of women undergoing a salpingotomy. Postoperative follow-up should involve serial monitoring of β-hCG, which increases in women with persistent trophoblastic disease. This is one of the indications for the use of methotrexate in gynaecology.

The indications for the use of methotrexate in the management of an ectopic pregnancy include a small (<3.5 cm) unruptured ectopic pregnancy in an asymptomatic, haemodynamically stable woman, as well as persistent trophoblastic disease. The success rate after a single dose of methotrexate is up to 94%. When a single dose does not lead to resolution, a second dose can be administered; this increases the success rate to almost 98%.

Methotrexate is hepatotoxic and nephrotoxic. It can cause myelosuppression leading to neutropenia and thrombocytopenia. Therefore baseline blood tests in the form of full blood count, liver function tests and renal function tests should be carried out before starting treatment. The patient should be reliable in terms of following treatment and complying with monitoring during therapy. Monitoring will include repeat blood tests and a symptom review in an early pregnancy assessment unit.

There is no increase in the rate of either miscarriages or congenital anomalies after treatment with methotrexate for an ectopic pregnancy. However, as methotrexate is an antifolate, women should be advised to avoid becoming pregnant for 3 months and to use a reliable form of contraception.

Other side effects of methotrexate include nausea, vomiting, gastritis, diarrhoea, stomatitis, conjunctivitis, photosensitivity and abdominal pain (the latter is seen in 7% of women following methotrexate therapy for ectopic pregnancy).

Lipscomb GH, Stovall TG, Ling FW. Nonsurgical treatment of ectopic pregnancy. N Eng J Med 2000; 343:1325–1329.
Royal College of Obstetricians and Gynaecologists. Diagnosis and Management of Ectopic Pregnancy. Green-top guildine no. 21. London: RCOG, 2016.
National Institute for Health and Care Excellence (NICE). Ectopic pregnancy and miscarriage diagnosis and initial management in early pregnancy and miscarriage [Clinical guideline No. 154]. Manchester: NICE; 2012.

10. A Closed-entry Palmer's point

The rate of adhesion formation after a previous abdominal transverse incision is 23%, and after a midline laparotomy it is is >50%; therefore Palmer's entry point is should be used. This form of entry is also preferred in obese women. Palmer's point is 2–3 cm below the costal margin in the left mid-clavicular line. This is the area where adhesion formation is least likely to occur after surgery, unless surgery has previously taken place in that area.

Frappell J. Laparoscopic entry after previous surgery. Obstet Gynaecol 2012;14:207–209.

Answers: EMQs

11. B Conservative management

A minor crush injury can be managed conservatively as long as there remains ureteric peristalsis, adequate perfusion and no urine leak. A more significant crush injury requires ureteral stenting.

Minas V, Gul N, Aust T, Doyle M, Rowlands D. Urinary tract injuries in laparoscopic gynaecological surgery; prevention, recognition and management. Obstet Gynaecol 2013; 16:19–28.

12. J Uretero-ureterostomy

The patient should be admitted on the day of the surgery because this reduces the pre-operative bed usage. The patient should fast for 2 hours prior to the surgery to avoid dehydration. This is considered safe and unlikely to increase the chances of aspiration. If a major ureteric injury occurs, such as a transection, the repair technique is dependent on the site of injury. If the injury occurs at the upper end of the ureter then an end-to-end anastomosis (uretero-ureterostomy) should be performed. If the middle third is injured then either an uretero-ureterostomy or a trans-uretero-ureterostomy (the injured ureter is anastomosied with the contralateral ureter) can be performed. The latter involves intentionally damaging the contralateral ureter and therefore should not be a first line choice.

Torbe E, Crawford R, Norbin A, Acheson N. Enhanced recovery in gynaecology. Obstet Gynaecol 2013; 15:263–268.

13. K Uretero-neocystostomy

If the damage to the ureter occurs at the lower third then a reimplantation of the ureter into the bladder (uretero-neocystostomy) should be performed.

Aslam N, Moran PA. Catheter use in gynaecological practice. Obstet Gynaecol 2014; 16:161–168.

14. E Laparotomy and repair

The patient requires a laparotomy and repair of the damaged bowel.

15. E Laparotomy and repair

There is a thermal injury on the bowel. This needs to be resected because it is devascularised.

Chapter 7

Antenatal care

Questions: SBAs

For each question, select the single best answer from the five options listed.

1. A 34-year-old woman in her first pregnancy has been referred to the antenatal clinic with an anomaly scan report at 20 weeks' gestation. The scan has reported an echogenic bowel. It has been explained that cytomegalovirus infection in pregnancy is a possible cause for this, and she is worried about fetal infection.

    Which one of the following results will indicate that there is no risk of cytomegalovirus infection to the fetus?

    A   Amniocentesis and polymerase chain reaction negative for cytomegalovirus
    B   A maternal serum test positive for cytomegalovirus IgG and IgM with low avidity
    C   A maternal serum test negative for cytomegalovirus IgG and positive for IgM
    D   A maternal serum test positive for cytomegalovirus IgG and negative for IgM
    E   A repeat ultrasound scan showing resolution of the echogenic bowel in the fetus

2. A 42-year-old woman who conceived after in vitro fertilisation is currently 13 weeks pregnant. The dating scan reports a nuchal translucency of 4 mm and a Down's syndrome risk of 1 in 20. She is referred to the antenatal clinic by the screening midwife to discuss this result.

    What option would you offer her at this stage?

    A   Non-invasive prenatal testing to test for free fetal DNA in a maternal serum sample
    B   Offer chorionic villus sampling as a diagnostic test and explain that there is a 1% procedure-related risk of miscarriage
    C   Reassure the woman that the 'high risk' result of her screening test is due to her age and that no further testing is required
    D   Urgently refer her to the fetal medicine specialist for amniocentesis
    E   Reassure her that there is no further fetal concern if the fetal karyotype result is normal

3. A midwife contacts the antenatal clinic regarding a pregnant woman she is seeing at the community centre who is 22 weeks pregnant. The woman is worried because her 5-year-old son developed a rash the previous day, and this is suggestive of chickenpox. The woman cannot remember having had chickenpox herself.

    What is your advice regarding her further management?

    A   Call the patient in for a blood test for varicella zoster virus (VZV)
    B   If the patient is not immune to VZV, she should be given varicella-zoster immunoglobulin
    C   The patient should attend her local community centre for a blood test for VZV IgM
    D   Prescribe oral acyclovir
    E   Tell the midwife to reassure the patient that potentially susceptible individuals are not at risk of VZV infection once the rash develops, therefore no further management is required

4. A 28-year-old woman is referred at 10 weeks' gestation to the obstetric medicine antenatal clinic because she suffers from epilepsy. She has been seizure-free for the previous year and is taking antiepileptic drugs (AEDs).

    Which of the following is correct regarding her pregnancy care?

    A   In-utero exposure to carbamazepine and lamotrigine can adversely affect the neurodevelopment of the offspring
    B   Monitoring of serum AED levels in pregnancy is recommended
    C   In two thirds of women, seizure control deteriorates during pregnancy
    D   She should be advised to take 400 mcg/day of folic acid in the first trimester to reduce the incidence of major congenital malformations
    E   Serial growth scans are required because she is exposed to AEDs

5. A 32-year-old woman presents to the delivery suite at 39 weeks' gestation in her second pregnancy with a history of ruptured membranes. She had a vaginal delivery 3 years previously, and the baby was treated for neonatal early-onset group B *Streptococcus* (GBS) infection. Vaginal swabs taken in the antenatal period of the current pregnancy were negative for GBS colonisation.

    Which one of the following is appropriate regarding her intrapartum care?

    A   Await a spontaneous onset of labour for 24 hours
    B   Intrapartum antibiotic prophylaxis for GBS infection is not required
    C   If chorioamnionitis is suspected, GBS-specific antibiotics should be commenced
    D   The risk of intrapartum pyrexia (>38°C) is 1.5 per 1000 women with early-onset GBS infection
    E   The risk of neonatal early-onset GBS infection is approximately 0.9 per 1000 births versus 2.3 per 1000 births in women with GBS detected in the current pregnancy

6. A 37-year-old woman in her first pregnancy has attended maternity triage at
    38 weeks' gestation with reduced fetal movements. An utrasound scan by two
    practitioners has confirmed intrauterine fetal death. She has had routine antenatal
    care and the pregnancy has been uneventful up to this point.

    Which one of the following is correct with regards to further management?

    A   A Kleihauer test should be done if she is rhesus negative
    B   Expectant management is advised
    C   The patient's clotting profile should be monitored as there is a risk of maternal
        disseminated intravascular coagulation (20% within 2 weeks)
    D   Systems that use customised weight charts have proved to be useful for
        categorising late intrauterine fetal deaths
    E   Tissue karyotyping is important as approximately 25% of stillborn babies have
        a chromosomal abnormality

7. A 29-year-old woman is reviewed in the antenatal clinic in her second pregnancy
    at 24 weeks' gestation. In the current pregnancy, irregular antibodies were
    detected in the booked blood test. An ultrasound scan at 20 weeks reported a low-
    lying placenta and she has multiple episodes of vaginal bleeding.

    Which of the following statement is true regarding these antibodies?

    A   A blood sample for cross-matching should be taken at least every 2 weeks
    B   If both anti-E and anti-c antibodies are detected, the presence of anti-E
        increases the severity of fetal anaemia
    C   Serial monitoring of anti-Kell antibody titres is recommended, with referral to
        a fetal medicine specialist for levels are >4 IU/mL
    D   If non-invasive fetal genotyping using maternal blood shows the fetus to be
        Kell antigen-negative, weekly ultrasound monitoring for haemolytic disease of
        the fetus and newborn is needed
    E   Referral to a fetal medicine unit should be made once anti-D levels reach
        >15 IU/mL

8. A 29-year-old primigravida at 30 weeks' gestation is referred to the day assessment
    unit for a review of her ultrasound report. This shows a fetal abdominal
    circumference less than the 5th centile and a raised pulsatility index on umbilical
    artery Doppler flow.

    Which one of the following is evidence-based practice regarding the patient's
    further management?

    A   Doppler ultrasound assessment of flow in the ductus stenosus should be used
        for surveillance of a preterm small-for-gestational-age (SGA) fetus with an
        abnormal umbilical artery Doppler ultrasound scan, and to time delivery
    B   In the preterm SGA fetus, a Doppler ultrasound scan of the middle cerebral
        artery has proven accuracy in predicting acidaemia and adverse outcomes,
        and should be used to time delivery
    C   In the SGA fetus with umbilical artery reversed end–diastolic frequency,
        induction of labour is recommended

    D If end diastolic flow is absent, or reversed end-diastolic frequencies are present, repeat surveillance with a fetal Doppler ultrasound scan twice weekly until delivery

    E When delivery is not imminent, a single course of antenatal corticosteroids should be administered to accelerate fetal lung maturation and reduce the risk of neonatal death and morbidity

9. A 19-year-old woman in her first pregnancy attends the emergency department with nausea and vomiting. She is 10 weeks' pregnant according to her last menstrual period. Her urine dipstick is positive (4+) for ketones.

Which of the following is recommended for the treatment of nausea and vomiting in pregnancy?

    A Corticosteroids should be reserved for severe or refractory cases where standard therapies have failed

    B Dextrose infusions with additional potassium chloride in each bag, guided by daily monitoring of electrolytes, is the most appropriate intravenous hydration

    C First-line anti-emetics such as anti-histamines (H_1 receptor antagonists) and phenothiazines are not proven to be safe in pregnancy

    D Metoclopramide is safe and effective, and can be used as a first line therapy

    E Pyridoxine is not recommended for nausea and vomiting in pregnancy

10. A 36-year-old woman in her first pregnancy is referred to the high-risk antenatal clinic at 10 weeks' gestation because she has β-thalassaemia major and established diabetes.

Which of the following is correct regarding the antenatal care plan and counselling?

    A Abdominal ultrasound is required to detect cholelithiasis and evidence of liver cirrhosis caused by iron overload or transfusion-related viral hepatitis

    B Maternal cardiac status should be assessed by echocardiography post-natally

    C Chelation therapy is safe in pregnancy

    D HbA1c is preferred for monitoring glycaemic control over serum fructosamine

    E She should be offered serial fetal biometry scans every 2 weeks from 24 weeks' gestation

11. A 34-year-old woman presents to the maternity day assessment unit with reduced fetal movements. This is her third such presentation in the past 2 weeks and she is currently 35 weeks' pregnant. She had a booking body mass index of 37 kg/m² and has a previous history of depression. An ultrasound scan at 32 weeks confirmed normal fetal growth, liquor volume and umbilical artery Doppler indices.

What is your management plan for her?

    A The test of choice is biophysical profile monitoring

    B Take a cardiotocograph, and if the results are normal, she should be reassured that fetal movements tend to plateau at 32 weeks' gestation

    C Fetal surveillance involving cardiotocograph monitoring, as well as checking maternal blood pressure and testing urine for proteinuria

    D Offer immediate delivery of the baby

E   Ultrasound assessment of fetal growth, liquor volume and umbilical artery
     Doppler indices should be requested within the next 1 week

12. A 27-year-old woman in her second pregnancy has been referred to the maternity
    day assessment unit because she has complained of itching palms and soles at
    32 weeks' gestation.

    Which one of the following is true regarding intrahepatic cholestasis of pregnancy
    (ICP)?

    A   A family history of cholestasis in pregnancy is present in up to 30% of affected
         women
    B   Constitutional symptoms, including dark urine and pale stools, and right
         upper quadrant pain excludes the diagnosis of ICP
    C   Jaundice affects 20% of women with ICP
    D   Serum bile acid concentrations are the most sensitive and specific marker for
         the diagnosis and monitoring of ICP
    E   There is usually a good correlation between transaminase levels and bile acid
         concentration in ICP

13. A 31-year-old woman is hypertensive and is planning for a pregnancy. She had a
    renal transplant 2 years ago and her current medication includes azathioprine,
    mycophenolate mofetil, an angiotensin receptor antagonist and statin. You are
    seeing her in the pre-conception counselling clinic.

    How would you counsel her regarding pregnancy?

    A   Azathioprine is potentially teratogenic and should therefore be avoided in the
         first trimester, and should ideally be stopped 3 months before conception
    B   After switching from mycophenolate mofetil to a replacement drug, a 3-month
         'washout' period prior to becoming pregnant is recommended
    C   As she has significant proteinuric hypertension, an angiotensin receptor
         antagonist should be continued for renal protection
    D   Hypertension predates the pregnancy and persists in more than 20% of
         pregnant women with renal transplants
    E   Statins do not need not be stopped prior to conception

14. A 27-year-old primigravid woman is referred to her antenatal clinic in Edinburgh
    to discuss the results of an anomaly scan, which reported anhydramnios. The fetus
    is in a flexed breech presentation. Neither fetal kidney could be identified on the
    scan, and there is no evidence of renal arteries on colour flow Doppler ultrasound
    bilaterally. Within the limited views, the rest of the fetal anatomy appears normal
    and biometry supports a gestation of 20 weeks. The woman denies a history of
    leaking per vaginam.

    What is the next course of action to take antenatally?

    A   Counsel the woman that the scan findings are incompatible with life and
         discuss termination of the pregnancy as one possible option
    B   Discharge the woman back to midwife-led care
    C   Offer a repeat scan at 28 weeks' gestation to confirm the diagnosis because the
         anhydramnios may be transient

    D   Offer amniocentesis to exclude an underlying chromosomal abnormality

    E   Refer the woman to antenatal triage for a sterile speculum examination to exclude preterm rupture of membranes

15. A 27-year-old primigravid woman is booked under consultant-led care because she suffers from inflammatory bowel disease.

Which one of the following drugs should be avoided in pregnancy?

    A   Aminosalicylates

    B   Azathioprine

    C   Ciclosporin

    D   Fluoroquinolones

    E   Tacrolimus

16. A 36-year-old woman is seen in the antenatal clinic at 17 weeks' gestation. She has an 8-year-old child, who was delivered by a lower segment Caesarean section at 41 weeks, weighing 3.56 kg. Her body mass index is 28 kg/m^2.

What is the management plan for her pregnancy?

    A   Serial growth scans from 26 to 28 weeks' gestation

    B   Serial symphsio–fundal height (SFH) measurements from 26 weeks' gestation

    C   Serial SFH measurements from 28 weeks' gestation

    D   A uterine artery Doppler ultrasound at 20 weeks' gestation, with a single third-trimester growth scan and an umbilical artery Doppler ultrasound

    E   A uterine artery Doppler ultrasound at 22 weeks' gestation and serial growth scans

17. A 26-year-old woman has attended the combined obstetric cardiology clinic for pre-pregnancy counselling. She had a tetralogy of Fallot that was repaired in childhood and is keen to plan a pregnancy. She is currently asymptomatic, and recent echocardiography showed mild pulmonary regurgitation.

What is your advice regarding the likely outcome of pregnancy?

    A   She is at a risk of developing arrhythmias and left heart failure

    B   She is likely to tolerate pregnancy well

    C   Hospital admission will be needed for bed rest and diuretics

    D   A fetal cardiac scan will be needed because the overall risk of the fetus having congenital heart disease is 15%

    E   An elective Caesarean section should take place at term

18. 'Three-person in vitro fertilisation', a technique recently approved by the UK House of Lords, is used in the management of which type of genetic disorder?

    A   Cancer predisposition syndrome

    B   Monogenic disease

    C   Mitochondrial disorders

D   Numerical chromosomal abnormalities (aneuploidy)
E   X-linked disorders

19. Which of the following is not a strict criterion for transabdominal cervical cerclage, either open or laparoscopic?

A   Previous history of mid-trimester pregnancy loss
B   Previous failed elective vaginal cerclage
C   Previous failed rescue/emergency vaginal cerclage
D   2 previous cone biopsies for cervical adenocarcinoma
E   Seriously deficient cervix

20. Thrombotic thrombocytopaenic purpura (TTP) and haemolytic uraemic syndrome (HUS) are very serious conditions which are difficult to diagnose on clinical and laboratory findings.

   Which of the following is seen commonly in HUS but rarely in TTP?

A   Blood pressure variability
B   Defects in complement regulation
C   Drug-related renal toxicity
D   Haemolysis
E   Thrombotic microangiopathy

21. Regarding renal function in pregnancy, which one of the following options is correct?

A   A creatinine concentration >90 µmol/L should be considered diagnostic of kidney injury in pregnancy
B   If the urine output falls to <20 mL/h, a 20% reduction in the dose of magnesium sulphate infusion should be considered
C   Postpartum urinary retention occurs in up to 5% of women
D   Serum creatinine falls by 15 µmol/L
E   The presence or absence of acute kidney injury in pre-eclampsia affects the obstetric management of the condition

22. Biologics (biological molecules) are commonly used to treat young women with rheumatic diseases and other immune-mediated conditions, including Crohn's disease, idiopathic thrombocytopaenic purpura, psoriasis and asthma.

   Which of the following anti-tumour necrosis factor agents does not cross placenta and therefore does not have the potential to affect the fetus?

A   Adalimumab
B   Certolizumab
C   Etanercept
D   Infliximab
E   Rituximab

23. A 36-year-old woman presented with upper abdominal pain at 28 weeks' gestation. An abdominal ultrasound scan reported a 10 cm, well-circumscribed lesion in the liver.

    What is the most common hepatic lesion that can show accelerated growth in pregnancy?

    A   Focal nodular hyperplasia
    B   Hamartoma
    C   Hepatic cell carcinoma
    D   Haemangioma
    E   Liver cell adenoma

24. The latest UK and Ireland *Confidential Enquiry into Maternal Deaths* (2016) includes surveillance of maternal deaths from 2012–14.

    Which of the following key facts and figures is incorrect?

    A   The rate of indirect deaths remains high with an increase in deaths due to influenza
    B   Maternal deaths from hypertensive disorders have slightly increased compared to previous years
    C   Maternal deaths from direct causes have reduced between 2009–11 and 2012–14
    D   Thrombosis and thromboembolism remain the leading causes of direct maternal death
    E   In 2017, suicide has been reclassified as an indirect cause of maternal death

25. Which of the following vaccines can be administered in pregnancy?

    A   BCG vaccine
    B   Measles vaccine
    C   Mumps vaccine
    D   Rubella vaccine
    E   Diphtheria toxoid

26. A 42-year-old woman conceived after in vitro fertilisation and day 5 blastocyst transfer. She attended the antenatal clinic after her dating scan confirmed a viable monochorionic twin pregnancy.

    Which one of the following is correct regarding pregnancy counselling?

    A   Selective growth restriction occurs in up to 5% of monochorionic twins in the absence of twin-to-twin transfusion syndrome (TTTS)
    B   Selective growth restriction occurs in up to 10% of monochorionic twins when TTTS is present
    C   TTTS complicates up to 15% of monochorionic pregnancies
    D   Twin anaemia–polycythaemia sequence occurs in 10% of uncomplicated monochorionic diamniotic pregnancies
    E   Twin reversed arterial perfusion sequence complicates approximately 10% of monochorionic twin pregnancies

27. Ultrasound is routinely used for the assessment of fetal well-being in women with multiple pregnancies.

    Which one of the following statements is correct regarding the use of ultrasound scan in fetal assessment?

    A A detailed anomaly scan of twin pregnancies should take place between weeks 20 and 22
    B Fetal ultrasound assessment should take place every 3–4 weeks in uncomplicated monochorionic pregnancies from 16 weeks + 0 days of gestation onwards until delivery
    C In twin pregnancies showing selective growth restriction, surveillance of fetal growth should be undertaken at least every 3–4 weeks with fetal Doppler ultrasound
    D First trimester nuchal translucency measurements should not be used to screen for twin-to-twin transfusion syndrome in monochorionic pregnancies
    E Women carrying twins should be offered nuchal translucency measurements between 11 weeks + 0 days and 14 weeks + 1 day of gestation

28. Which one of the following statements regarding stillbirth and the current available evidence for its prevention is correct?

    A The use of umbilical artery Doppler ultrasound reduces the risk of perinatal death in high risk women
    B The Thrombophilia in Pregnancy Prophylaxis Study (TIPPS) showed that low molecular weight heparin reduces the risk of placenta-related complications and pregnancy loss in women suffering from thrombophilia
    C The Trial of Umbilical and Foetal Flow in Europe (TRUFFLE), revealed that the use of Doppler ultrasound to monitor flow in the ductus venosus improves the perinatal outcome as compared to computerised assessment of cardiotocography
    D The overall risk of perinatal death is lowest at 39 weeks' gestation
    E The overall risk of stillbirth in the UK is approximately 1 in 500

Questions: EMQs

Questions 29–33

Options for Questions 29–33

A	Bursitis of the knee joint	J	Osteoma of the hip
B	Dislocation of the hip	K	Pregnancy-induced osteomalacia
C	Fracture of sacral promontory	L	Symphysis pubis dysfunction
D	Fracture of the pubic bone	M	Sciatica
E	Lumbosacral disc prolapse	N	Subluxation of the sacral promontory
F	Mechanical back pain	O	Transient osteoporosis of pregnancy affecting the hip joint
G	Osteitis pubis		
H	Osteomyelitis of pubis	P	Tuberculosis of the spine or Pott's disease
I	Osteomyelitis of the hip		

Instructions: For each clinical scenario described below, choose the single most appropriate diagnosis from the list of options above. Each option may be used once, more than once, or not at all.

29. A 42-year-old woman attends her antenatal appointment at 28 weeks' gestation. A waddling gait is seen on entering the examination room. She complains of a burning pain in the pubic region during walking, standing on one leg and parting her legs. Clinical examination reveals tenderness on the sacroiliac joint and restriction of the abduction and lateral rotation of hip.

30. A 42-year-old woman attends the obstetric day assessment unit at 28 weeks' gestation with low grade pyrexia and reduced hip movements due to severe pain. Clinical examination reveals tenderness over the pubic symphysis and pubic rami, painful abduction of the hip and pain on lateral compression of the pelvis. She gives a history of recurrent urinary tract infection in the past and recently had stenting of the ureters for ureteric stricture. An X-ray of the pelvis shows widening as well as bony erosions of the symphysis pubis.

31. A 42-year-old woman attends the obstetric day assessment unit at 28 weeks' gestation. A waddling gait is seen on entering the examination room. She complains of pain in the pubic region which is radiating to the groin and thigh. She also explains that the pain is aggravated on climbing stairs and lying on one side in bed. The other aggravating factors for pain include coughing and sneezing. Examination of her hips reveals tenderness on compression of the right as well as left trochanters.

32. A 42-year-old Asian with five children attends her antenatal appointment at 28 weeks' gestation. She complains of non-specific pain in the lumbosacral and pubic regions. Blood tests reveal low serum calcium but raised alkaline phosphatase. Pseudofractures (Looser zones) are reported on the X-ray of the pubic bone.

33. A 42-year-old Asian woman with three children attends the obstetric day assessment unit at 28 weeks' gestation. She complains of pain in her left hip and the anterior aspect of her left knee (especially during walking). Clinical examination reveals no tenderness on pubic symphysis and an ultrasound scan of the left hip joint shows effusion.

Questions 34–38

Options for Questions 34–38

A	Amniocentesis and viral culture	J	Administer intravenous ganciclovir to the neonate
B	Fetal blood sampling		
C	Intravenous acyclovir	K	Administer intravenous zidovudine to the neonate
D	Offer termination following thorough counselling		
		L	Vaccinate the mother against rubella
E	Offer rubella immunoglobulin	M	Vaccinate the newborn against rubella
F	Refer to fetal medicine unit for special scan	N	Vaccinate the mother against chickenpox
G	Refer to virology department	O	Vaccinate the fetus against chickenpox
H	Reassure		
I	Administer prophylactic intravenous acyclovir to the neonate		

Instructions: For each clinical scenario described below, choose the single most appropriate management option from the list of options above. Each option may be used once, more than once, or not at all.

34. A 40-year-old multiparous woman had a forceps delivery and is very excited about her baby. She was about to be discharged on postnatal day 2 but finds out from her husband that her first child has developed rubella. She is really worried about taking her newborn baby home. Her virology results at booking (her first midwife appointment) revealed that she is immune to rubella.

35. A 30-year-old multiparous woman presents to the early pregnancy assessment unit (EPAU) for advice because she recently had a rash (2 weeks ago) and was found to have rubella. She gives a history of a positive urine pregnancy test and has mild spotting. Clinically, the diagnosis is a threatened miscarriage and an ultrasound scan reveals an 8 week, single, viable, intrauterine pregnancy.

36. A 35-year-old nulliparous woman calls a health service helpline at 35 weeks' gestation. She is very anxious because she had contact with her nephew who developed a rubella rash 1 week ago. She wants to know if her baby will be affected. Her booking virology tests results show an immunity to rubella.

37. A 40-year-old multiparous woman has suffered from epilepsy for the last 20 years. She comes to her GP for preconception counselling. Currently she is on carbamazepine 400 mg per day and has read about the risks to the baby if she gets pregnant. She has recently started taking folic acid (5 g) daily as she is planning to conceive. She gives a history of vaccination against rubella in the past. However, her booking blood tests reveal that she is not immune to rubella.

38. A 30-year-old multiparous woman had a normal vaginal delivery 6 hours ago. She possibly does not want to have more children in the future but is currently considering using reliable contraception. She is about to be discharged home and the midwife finds out that her booking blood tests revealed IgG antibodies to rubella.

Questions 39–43

Options for Questions 39–43

A   Commence intravenous prophylactic unfractionated heparin

B   Change to prophylactic intravenous unfractionated heparin

C   Change to heparinoid danaparoid sodium

D   Change to low-molecular weight heparin (LMWH)

E   Commence prophylactic low molecular heparin

F   Commence dalteparin

G   Monitor anti-Xa levels

H   Remove catheter 3 hours after giving heparin

I   Remove catheter 8 hours after giving the last dose of heparin

J   Remove catheter 12 hours after giving the last dose of heparin

K   Remover catheter 24 hours after giving the last dose of heparin

L   Withhold heparin for 12 hours before giving spinal anaesthesia

M   Withhold heparin 24 hours before giving spinal anaesthesia

N   Withhold heparin for 24 hours before giving epidural anaesthesia

O   Withhold heparin for 48 hours before giving epidural anaesthesia

Instructions: For each scenario described below, choose the single most appropriate management option from the list of options above. Each option may be used once, more than once, or not at all.

39. A 43-year-old multiparous woman presents to the EPAU at 12 weeks' gestation with mild vaginal bleeding. She gives a history of unprovoked deep venous thrombosis (DVT) 1 year prior to this pregnancy and was treated with warfarin for 6 months. Currently, the GP has started her on aspirin in view of a previous history of pre-eclampsia.

40. A 40-year-old multiparous woman presents to the obstetric day assessment unit at 28 weeks' gestation with reduced fetal movements [normal cardiotocograph (CTG)]. Her notes indicate that she had DVT at 20 weeks' gestation during her current pregnancy and is on 80 mg LMWH twice daily. Her booking blood results were normal. However, her recent blood test reveals a platelet count of 60×10^9/L.

41. A 30-year-old woman who delivered 8 hours ago gives a history of previous thrombophilia. Her mode of delivery was Caesarean section for a prolonged second stage of labour. She had a massive postpartum haemorrhage and her current haemoglobin level is 80 g/L. The midwife comes to you to inform you about the minimal soakage of the Caesarean section wound dressing.

42. A 33-year-old multiparous woman is reviewed by the senior house officer in the postnatal ward. She had a Caesarean section for failure to progress and has been using an epidural for pain relief for the last 4 hours following Caesarean section. The midwife has just given her the first dose of prophylactic LMWH postnatally.

43. A 38-year-old multiparous woman is admitted to the antenatal ward for an elective Caesarean section for breech presentation. She had a pulmonary embolism during this pregnancy and has been on a therapeutic dose of LMWH (90 mg twice daily) for the last 3 months. She took her last dose just before coming into the ward.

Questions 44–48

Options for Questions 44–48

A Low-molecular-weight heparin (LMWH) plus low dose heparin
B LMWH not recommended
C LMWH during antenatal period
D Low dose aspirin only
E Prophylactic LMWH during labour
F Prophylactic LMWH postnatally for 10 days
G Prophylactic LMWH postnatally for 6 weeks
H Prophylactic LMWH antenatally plus postnatally for 6 weeks
I Prophylactic LMWH antenatally plus postnatally for 5 days

J Therapeutic dose of LMWH antenatally
K Therapeutic dose of LMWH antenatally and postnatally
L Therapeutic dose of LMWH antenatally and prophylactic dose postnatally
M Unfractionated heparin all through the antenatal period
N Unfractionated heparin during the postnatal period
O Unfractionated heparin during labour

Instructions: For each scenario described below, choose the single most appropriate management from the list of options above. Each option may be used once, more than once, or not at all.

44. A 36-year-old obese nulliparous woman (body mass index >30 kg/m²) attends the maternal medicine obstetric clinic for a review at 38 weeks' gestation to discuss mode of delivery, because her ultrasound scan shows a breech presentation. Subsequently, she undergoes an elective Caesarean section at 39 weeks' gestation and is discharged home on the second postoperative day.

45. A 36-year-old nulliparous woman attends the early pregnancy assessment unit at 10 weeks' gestation with minimal vaginal bleeding. A transvaginal scan reveals triplets. Medical history unveils that she had single episode of axillary venous thrombosis 3 years ago. She was investigated adequately but no cause was found.

46. A 36-year-old obese nulliparous woman attended the antenatal clinic for her first consultation with the doctor at 20 weeks' gestation (her ultrasound scan shows a low-lying placenta). A further review was carried out at 34 weeks' gestation because her repeat scan also showed a low lying placenta. Subsequently, she underwent an elective Caesarean section at 38 weeks' gestation because of the increased vaginal bleeding (She loses 2000 mL of blood). She recovered well following 3 units of blood transfusion. The senior house officer discharged her on postnatal day 3. However, 5 days later she presents to the emergency department with a spiking temperature due to a Caesarean section wound infection and is admitted to the gynaecology ward for intravenous antibiotic therapy.

47. A 36-year-old multiparous woman attends the antenatal clinic for a review at 20 weeks' gestation. A general examination reveals a body mass index of 41 and varicose veins. Her anomaly scan and booking bloods are normal.

48. A 31-year-old woman attends the antenatal clinic for review at 20 weeks' gestation. She suddenly remembers to tell you that she had superficial thrombophlebitis 6 months prior to pregnancy which resolved with no residual signs.

Questions 49–53

Options for Questions 49–53

A   Anti-D immunoglobulin 50 IU
B   Anti-D immunoglobulin 100 IU
C   Anti-D immunoglobulin 200 IU
D   Anti-D immunoglobulin 250 IU
E   Anti-D immunoglobulin 500 IU
F   Anti-D immunoglobulin 1000 IU
G   Anti-D immunoglobulin 1500 IU
H   Anti-D immunoglobulin 2000 IU
I   Anti-D immunoglobulin is not recommended or indicated
J   Anti-D immunoglobulin is indicated in next pregnancy
K   Anti-D immunoglobulin is not indicated in next pregnancy
L   Anti-D immunoglobulin is indicated in all future miscarriages
M   Anti-D immunoglobulin is indicated in all future pregnancies
N   Anti-D immunoglobulin to all her family members
O   Anti-D immunoglobulin to all her siblings

Instructions: For each scenario described below, choose the single most appropriate action from the list of options above. Each option may be used once, more than once, or not at all.

49. A 20-year-old woman presents to her GP in Cambridge requesting a termination of an unwanted pregnancy. She had some vaginal bleeding 1 week ago and attended the EPAU at her local hospital. A scan showed a single viable intrauterine pregnancy of 11 week's gestation. The GP refers her to a clinic for a termination of pregnancy. She undergoes a termination 2 weeks later. However, her blood tests reveal that she is Rhesus (RhD)-negative and positive for antibodies to Rhesus D antigen.

50. A 20-year-old woman attends the EPAU with mild vaginal bleeding. She has just missed her period and the urine pregnancy test is positive. An ultrasound scan shows a single viable intrauterine pregnancy of 5 weeks' gestation. Her blood group is 'AB' negative and has anti-Kell antibodies.

51. A 20-year-old woman attends the obstetric day assessment unit at 21 weeks' gestation with minimal vaginal bleeding. Clinically, her abdomen is soft with no contractions. Her cervix, vagina and vulva are normal. An obstetric ultrasound scan reveals a fetus of 22 weeks with an anterior, low lying placenta. Her booking blood tests reveal 'O' negative blood group with no antibodies.

52. A 20-year-old woman attends the EPAU at 8 weeks' gestation. She complains of very minimal lower abdominal pain and mild vaginal bleeding. An ultrasound scan shows a left-sided ectopic pregnancy (2×2 cm in size) with no free fluid in the pelvis. Clinically, she is stable and comfortable. Following appropriate counselling, she decides to have medical management by methotrexate and is willing to be followed up closely by the EPAU to review her symptoms and test for β-hCG. Her blood tests reveal haemoglobin 14 g/L and 'B' negative blood group. There are antibodies to Duffy antigen.

53. A 20-year-woman attends the obstetric day assessment unit at 36 weeks of pregnancy with an antepartum haemorrhage. She had received anti-D immunoglobulin at 32 weeks' gestation because her blood group is 'O' negative

with no antibodies. Clinically, she is stable and speculum examination reveals minimal vaginal bleeding but closed cervical os. An ultrasound scan reveals a viable baby with normal growth, liquor and placental location.

Questions 54–58

Options for Questions 54–58

A   Anti-D immunoglobulin injection
B   Allow vaginal breech delivery
C   Abandon external cephalic version
D   Conduct vaginal breech delivery
E   Elective Caesarean section
F   Emergency Caesarean section
G   Emergency Caesarean section not indicated
H   External cephalic version (ECV) contraindicated

I   ECV not indicated
J   Offer ECV at 36 weeks' gestation
K   Offer ECV at 37 weeks' gestation
L   Follow up in 1 week in the antenatal clinic
M   Repeat ECV in 1 week
N   Repeat ECV after tocolysis
O   Vaginal breech delivery contraindicated

Instructions: For each clinical scenario described below, choose the single most appropriate intervention with regards to breech presentation from the list of options above. Each option may be used once, more than once, or not at all.

54. A 39-year-old multiparous woman presents to the antenatal clinic at 36 weeks of gestation for a routine review. Abdominal examination reveals breech presentation and an ultrasound scan reveals footling breech presentation with normal amniotic fluid.

55. A 39-year-old nulliparous woman presents to the antenatal clinic at 36 weeks' gestation for a routine review. Clinical examination reveals breech presentation. An ultrasound reveals extended breech with normal amniotic fluid.

56. A 39-year-old multiparous woman comes into the labour ward at 39 weeks' gestation for an ECV. After 15 minutes of abdominal manipulation, the ECV is successful. However, post-ECV, the CTG reveals bradycardia which recovers to baseline after 3 minutes followed by a normal trace. Clinically, her abdomen is soft with no tenderness.

57. A 39-year-old nulliparous woman presents to the obstetric day assessment unit at 36 weeks' gestation with mild to moderate vaginal bleeding. Clinical examination reveals a soft abdomen with a normal cervix and vagina, with no active vaginal bleeding. A formal departmental ultrasound scan shows breech presentation with normal growth and liquor with a posterior low lying placenta. She is admitted for 24 hours for observation and is then discharged home. 3 days later she attends the labour ward because she is booked for an ECV. You are the registrar on call for the labour ward on that day.

58. A 39-year-old multiparous woman presents to the labour ward at 40 weeks' gestation with contractions. You are called to review the woman because the midwife is not sure about the presentation. A clinical examination reveals 4 cm cervical dilatation and footling breech presentation. She has a history of precipitous delivery with her last two deliveries.

Questions 59–63

Options for Questions 59–63

A	*Actinomyces*	I	*Plasmodium vivax*
B	*Bacillus anthracis*	J	*Plasmodium ovale*
C	*Chlamydia trachomatis*	K	*Plasmodium falciparum*
D	*Escherichia coli*	L	*Staphylococcus aureus*
E	*Gardnerella vaginalis*	M	*Treponema pallidum*
F	Group B *Streptococcus*	N	*Mycobacterium tuberculosis*
G	Molluscum contagiosum	O	*Treponema pallidum pertenue* (yaws)
H	*Mycoplasma hominis*		

Instructions: For each fact described below, choose the single most likely organism from the list of options above. Each option may be used once, more than once, or not at all.

59. Afro-Caribbeans with a Duffy negative blood group antigen are less susceptible to this particular bacterial infection.

60. Women with sickle cell trait are less susceptible to this particular bacterial infection.

61. Fetal ingestion of infected fluid, aspiration of infected amniotic fluid and haematogenous infection via umbilical vein are proposed mechanisms of infection.

62. Antibiotic prophylaxis is recommended for pregnant women during the intrapartum period with this particular infection.

63. This particular organism can cause neonatal conjunctivitis and pneumonia.

Questions 64–68

Options for Questions 64–68

A Aortic dissection	I Mitral valve prolapse
B Aortic stenosis	J Peripartum cardiomyopathy
C Aortic regurgitation	K Patent ductus arteriosus
D Coarctation of the aorta	L Rheumatic heart disease
E Epstein anomaly	M Transposition of aorta
F Eisenmenger's syndrome	N Tricuspid regurgitation
G Hypertrophic cardiomyopathy	O Ventricular septal defect
H Mitral regurgitation	

Instructions: For each scenario described below, choose the single most appropriate diagnosis from the list of options above. Each option may be used once, more than once, or not at all.

64. A 42-year-old Bangladeshi woman presents to the emergency department at 32 weeks' gestation with distension of the abdomen. An abdominal scan reveals a congested liver and minimal ascites. An echocardiogram shows left ventricular dilatation with an ejection fraction of 15%. Clinical examination reveals a respiratory rate of 26 breaths/minute and an oxygen saturation of 95%. She is para 10 with all normal vaginal deliveries. She speaks no English.

65. A 28-year-old woman is brought to the emergency department at 25 weeks' gestation with acute severe chest pain radiating to the back. She has a lifelong history of Marfan's syndrome but has remained well for the last 18 years. She is hypertensive and currently on methyldopa 250 mg 3 times a day. General examination reveals a blood pressure of 180/80 mmHg, pulse 120 bpm and respiratory rate 22 breaths/minute.

66. A 20-year-old Asian woman presents to the obstetric day assessment unit at 24 weeks' gestation with palpitations. A cardiovascular system examination reveals a mid systolic click and late systolic murmur.

67. A 42-year-old Asian woman presents to the emergency department 4 weeks post delivery with increasing shortness of breath while lying flat. On cardiovascular examination the apical impulse is diffuse and displaced downwards. A chest radiograph shows cardiomegaly and respiratory system examination reveals vesicular breath sounds with fine basal crepitations.

68. A 35-year-old primiparous woman presents with syncope at 20 weeks' gestation. A cardiovascular examination reveals an ejection systolic murmur, double apical pulsation and arrhythmia. She is started on β-blockers following which her symptoms improve gradually. She gives a history of the sudden death of her cousin who was 18 years old.

Questions 69–73

Options for Questions 69–73

A Intravenous artesunate
B Antiemetic plus repeat oral quinine
C Antiemetic plus repeat oral quinine and clindamycin
D Intravenous quinine
E Intravenous clindamycin
F Intravenous quinine plus oral clindamycin
G Intravenous quinine plus intravenous clindamycin

H Oral quinine
I Oral clindamycin
J Oral quinine plus oral clindamycin
K Oral chloroquine for 3 days
L Oral chloroquine 300 mg weekly until delivery
M Pyrimethamine
N Primaquine
O Sulphadiazine

Instructions: For each scenario described below, choose the single most appropriate treatment from the list of options above. Each option may be used once, more than once, or not at all.

69. A 28-year-old Afro-Caribbean woman with four children presents to the obstetric day assessment unit with these vague symptoms: malaise, fever and headache. She had travelled to Ghana 4 weeks ago and was perfectly fine. She is currently 30 weeks pregnant and has good fetal movements. Her blood tests and peripheral smear reveal anaemia, thrombocytopaenia, and hyperparasitaemia with *Plasmodium falciparum*.

70. A 28-year-old Afro-Caribbean woman with two children presents to the day assessment unit at 29 weeks' gestation with fever, malaise and musculoskeletal pain. She gives a history of malaria 4 years ago during her visit to Nigeria. A peripheral blood smear shows *P. falciparum*. Clinically, haematologically and biochemically there are no symptoms or signs of severe complications.

71. A 28-year-old primiparous African woman presents to the day assessment unit at 37 weeks' gestation with fever, malaise and muscle pain. She gives a history of malaria during childhood and has been physically fit so far. A peripheral blood smear shows *P. falciparum*. Clinically, haematologically and biochemically there are no symptoms or signs of severe complications. She vomits after receiving the first dose of oral quinine and clindamycin.

72. A 28-year-old nulliparous Asian woman presents to the day assessment unit at 20 weeks' gestation with fever, malaise and muscle pain. She returned to the UK 2 weeks ago from India. A peripheral blood smear shows *Plasmodium vivax*. She receives anti-malarial treatment for 7 days and is cured. 4 weeks later, she comes to see her GP for advice because she is about to go on holiday to Africa.

73. A 28-year-old Afro-Caribbean woman with three children presents to the day assessment unit at 37 weeks' gestation with fever, malaise and muscle pain. Her peripheral smear shows *Plasmodium ovale*. Clinically, haematologically and biochemically there are no symptoms or signs of severe complications.

Answers: SBAs

1. D A maternal serum test positive for cytomegalovirus IgG and negative for IgM

Diagnosis of primary maternal CMV infection in pregnancy should be based on a positive test for immunoglobulin G (IgG) specific to CMV in the serum of pregnant women who did not exhibit these antibodies previously, or upon detection of virus-specific immunoglobulin M (IgM) and IgG antibodies in association with low IgG avidity. Diagnosis of prenatal fetal CMV infection is more difficult and is based on amniocentesis performed >7 weeks after maternal infection and >21 weeks' gestation.

Navti O, Hughes BL, Tang JW, Konje J. Comprehensive review and update of cytomegalovirus infection in pregnancy. Obstet Gynaecol 2016; 18:301–307.

2. B Offer chorionic villus sampling as a diagnostic test, explaining that there is a 1% procedure-related risk of miscarriage

Chorionic villus sampling is performed between 11 (11+0) and 13 (13+6) weeks whereas amniocentesis is usually performed from 15 weeks. A fetal nuchal translucency of 4 mm or more is associated with a poor pregnancy outcome even when the fetal karyotype is normal.

Royal College of Obstetricians and Gynaecologists (RCOG). Amniocentesis and chorionic villus sampling. Green-top guideline no. 8. London: RCOG; 2010.

3. B If the patient is not immune to VZV, she should be given varicella-zoster immunoglobulin

Pregnant women need to avoid contact with women who have chicken pox until the lesions have crusted because at this point infectivity becomes almost nil (lesions crust about five days after the onset of rash). If women present for medical advice within 24 hours of onset of rash, and if they are 20 weeks or more, then oral acyclovir should be prescribed.

If the pregnant women present later after contact then varicella zoster immunoglobulin (VZIG) can be administered up to 10 days after contact (especially in cases of continuous exposures).

Pregnant women who are non-immune and have encountered women with chicken pox should be treated as infectious until the incubation period which is 8–28 days after exposure if they receive VZIG and for 8–21 days if they do not receive VZIG.

Royal College of Obstetricians and Gynaecologists (RCOG). Chickenpox in pregnancy. Green-top guideline no. 13. London: RCOG; 2015.

4.   E Serial growth scans are required because she is exposed to AEDs

To detect a small-for-gestational-age fetus, serial growth scans are required, and because the patient is exposed to anti-epileptic drugs (AEDs), these scans will also aid in the planning of further management.

Evidence suggests that in-utero exposure to carbamazepine and lamotrigine does not impact the neurodevelopment of children negatively, therefore regular monitoring of serum AED levels in pregnancy is not recommended.

To reduce the likelihood of major congenital malformation, women on AEDs are recommended to take 5 mg/day of folic acid until at least the end of the first trimester.

Royal College of Obstetricians and Gynaecologists (RCOG). Epilepsy in pregnancy. Green-top guideline no. 68. London: RCOG; 2016.

5.   E The risk of neonatal early-onset GBS infection is approximately 0.9 per 1000 births versus 2.3 per 1000 births in women with GBS detected in the current pregnancy

Intrapartum antibiotic prophylaxis (IAP) to protect against group B *Streptococcus* (GBS) infection is recommended because an increase in the risk of neonatal infection may be caused by the persistence of low levels of maternal anti-GBS antibodies. If a vaginal swab is positive for GBS, the risk of neonatal disease becomes 2.3 per 1000 births (the overall UK rate of infection is 0.5 per 1000).

If GBS was present in a previous pregnancy, the likelihood that a subsequent pregnancy will also be associated with GBS is approximately 38%. Therefore, the risk of early-onset GBS infection in neonates is approximately 0.9 per 1000 births.

Intrapartum pyrexia (>38°C) is associated with a risk of early onset GBS infection of 5.3 per 1000 births.

Royal College of Obstetricians and Gynaecologists (RCOG) The prevention of early-onset neonatal group B streptococcal disease. Green-top guideline no. 36. London: RCOG; 2012.

6.   D Systems that use customised weight charts have proved to be useful for categorising late intrauterine fetal deaths

In all cases, a Kleihauer test should be undertaken immediately in case a large fetomaternal haemorrhage has occurred. Pre-eclampsia, chorioamnionitis and placental abruption should be excluded before following expectant management. Clotting profile, platelet count and fibrinogen levels should be monitored because there is a risk of maternal disseminated intravascular coagulation (10% within 4 weeks after the date of late intra-uterine fetal demise (IUFD), increasing to 30% thereafter).

Systems that use customised weight charts have proved to be useful to categorise late IUFDs.

Tissue karyotyping is important as approximately 6% of stillborn babies have a chromosomal abnormality.

Royal College of Obstetricians and Gynaecologists (RCOG). Late intrauterine fetal death and stillbirth. Green-top guideline no. 55. London: RCOG; 2010.

7. B If both anti-E and anti-c antibodies are detected, the presence of anti-E increases the severity of fetal anaemia

The indications for referral to fetal medicine specialist include:

- a history of previous significant haemolytic disease of the fetus and newborn (HDFN)
- intrauterine transfusion
- a titre of 1:32 or above
- rising titres as it indicates the risk of severe fetal anaemia.
- anti-D, anti-c and anti-K antibodies

Anti-K, anti-D and anti-c antibodies

In case of detection of anti-K antibodies on investigation, the referral should be immediate because severe fetal anaemia occurs even at low titres.

Anti-D antibody levels of <4 IU/mL usually indicated anti-D immunoglobulin administration. This should be ascertained by history and documentation.

When antibody levels are >4 IU/mL, a fetal medicine referral is indicated.

When anti-d antibody levels are <15 IU/mL and >4 IU/mL, there is moderate risk of developing HDFN and if this level increases to >15 IU/mL then it is likely that severe HDFN can develop. These levels should prompt sincere urgent referral to fetal medicine specialist. It is recommended the such women have weekly ultrasound with assessment of fetal middle cerebral artery peak systolic velocities (MCA PSV).

In situations where women have red cell antibodies and at risk of needing blood transfusion during pregnancy and labour, (e.g. women with sickle cell disease or diagnosed with placenta praevia) a cross match sample should be taken every week.

Royal College of Obstetricians and Gynaecologists (RCOG). The management of women with red cell antibodies during pregnancy. Green-top guideline no. 65. London: RCOG; 2014.

8. A Doppler ultrasound assessment of flow in the ductus stenosus should be used for surveillance of a preterm small-for-gestational-age (SGA) fetus with an abnormal umbilical artery Doppler ultrasound, and to time delivery

In the preterm SGA fetus, middle cerebral artery (MCA) Doppler has limited accuracy to predict acidaemia and adverse outcome and should therefore not be used to time delivery. Conduct surveillance with fetal Dopplers twice weekly if end–diastolic flow is positive, or daily until delivery if there is absent or reversed end–diastolic velocity (AREDV). In the SGA fetus with umbilical artery AREDV, delivery by Caesarean section is recommended, and when delivery is being considered, a single course of antenatal corticosteroids should be administered to accelerate fetal lung maturation and reduce neonatal death and morbidity.

9. A Corticosteroids should be reserved for severe or refractory cases where standard therapies have failed

The appropriate intravenous hydration is intravenous fluid normal saline with potassium chloride in the bag is administered with daily electrolyte monitoring. Dextrose infusions are not appropriate.

First-line anti-emetics H1 receptor antagonists (anti-histamines) and phenothiazines are recommended to be used because they are safe in pregnancy. Metochlopramide is safe but is used as a second line in view of extrapyramidal effects. Pyridoxine should be used for nausea and vomiting in pregnancy and hyperemesis gravidarum.

Royal College of Obstetricians and Gynaecologists (RCOG). The management of nausea and vomiting of pregnancy and hyperemesis gravidarum. Green-top guideline no. 69. London: RCOG; 2016.

10. A Abdominal ultrasound is required to detect cholelithiasis and evidence of liver cirrhosis caused by iron overload or transfusion-related viral hepatitis

In women with thalassaemia and established diabetes, serum fructosamine measurement is more reliable than HbA1c. HbA1c is suggested not to be reliable as marker for glycaemic control because it is diluted in the serum by transfused blood and thus measurement may find low levels.

It is recommended that the patient's serum fructosamine concentrations should be <300 nmol/L and HbA1c <43 mmol/L for at least 3 months prior to conception.

Prior to conception, if the iron levels exceed 15 mg/gm then there is risk on the myocardium of the heart (iron loading). Therefore, chelation of iron with low dose desferrioxamine should be used in these women between 20 and 28 weeks' gestation with haematologist input (use of iron in the first trimester is thought to be teratogenic and therefore is not recommended).

Royal College of Obstetricians and Gynaecologists (RCOG). Management of beta thalassaemia in pregnancy. Green-top guideline no. 66. London: RCOG; 2014.

11. C Fetal surveillance involving cardiotocograph monitoring, as well as checking maternal blood pressure and testing urine for proteinuria

The number of spontaneous movements increases until the 32nd week of gestation and after this the frequency of fetal movements tends to plateau until the beginning of labour, but not in the later part of third trimester. In women with reduced fetal movements and pre-eclampsia where there is potential placental dysfunction, it is recommended that blood pressure is measured and a urine dipstick for proteins is undertaken to assess severity and need for delivery.

Biophysical profile is a test of fetal wellbeing which was used conventionally in high-risk pregnancies. However, the evidence currently available is limited and does not support its use.

If there is a single episode of reduced fetal movement, the mother should be reassured and informed that most pregnancies are uncomplicated (70%).

If the reduced fetal movement happens on two or more occasions then there is an increased risk of poor outcome in comparison to reduced fetal movement on one occasion (e.g stillbirth, fetal growth restriction and preterm birth). Ultrasound should be performed in these cases.

Royal College of Obstetricians and Gynaecologists (RCOG). Reduced fetal movements. Green-top guideline no. 57. London: RCOG; 2011.

12. D Serum bile acid concentrations are the most sensitive and specific marker for the diagnosis and monitoring of ICP

Jaundice is rare, affecting <10% of women with intrahepatic cholestasis of pregnancy. A family history of cholestasis in pregnancy supports the diagnosis and is present in up to 14% of affected women. The increase in liver transaminase levels may occur before or after the increase in serum bile acids. There is poor correlation between the transaminases levels and bile acid concentration.

Geenes V, Williamson C, Chappell LC. Intrahepatic cholestasis of pregnancy. Obstet Gynaecol 2016; 18:273–281.

13. B After switching from mycophenolate mofetil to a replacement drug, a 3-month 'washout' period prior to becoming pregnant is recommended

Teratogenic drugs include (**Table 7.1**):

- Mycophenolate mofetil
- Angiotensin-converting enzyme inhibitors
- Angiotensin receptor antagonists

These drugs should be stopped prior to pregnancy. Mycophenolate mofetil is substituted with azathioprine and is considered safe during pregnancy.

In women with a renal transplant, hypertension generally starts prior to pregnancy and persists in more than 50%.

Wiles K, Tillett A, Harding K. Solid organ transplantation in pregnancy. Obstet Gynaecol 2016; 18:189–197.

Table 7.1 Medications commonly prescribed in solid organ transplant recipients			
Pregnancy			Breastfeeding
Considered safe	More data needed	Teratogenic	Considered safe
Aspirin	Amlodipine	Angiotensin receptor antagonists	Amlodipine
Azathioprine	Doxazosin	Angiotensin-converting enzyme	Aspirin
Ciclosporin	Everolimus	inhibitors	Azathioprine
Clopidogrel	Rituximab	Mycophenolate	Captopril
Erythropoietin	Sirolimus	Warfarin	Ciclosporin
Hydralazine	Statins		Enalapril
Hydrocortisone			Erythropoietin
Hydroxychloroquine			Hydrocortisone
Labetalol			Hydroxychloroquine
Low molecular weight heparin			Labetalol
Nifedipine			Low molecular weight heparin
Prednisolone			Nifedipine
Tacrolimus			Prednisolone
β-agonist and steroid inhalers			Tacrolimus
			Warfarin
			β-agonist and steroid inhalers

14. A Counsel the woman that the scan findings are incompatible with life and discuss termination of the pregnancy as one possible option

The findings are diagnostic of bilateral renal agenesis, which is incompatible with life. As the fetus does not produce urine, there is complete anhydramnios and associated lung hypoplasia. Termination of pregnancy can be offered in this situation. Most individuals who have unilateral renal agenesis lead normal lives but are at increased risk of renal failure, hypertension and recurrent infections.

15. D Fluoroquinolones

Mild to moderate ulcerative colitis is usually treated with aminosalicylates, and for maintenance therapy of remission, sulfasalazine is considered safe both during pregnancy and breastfeeding. The recommended upper limit is 3 g/L.

Azathioprine can also be used during pregnancy and breastfeeding. The active metabolite is mercaptopurine, and since the fetus lacks the enzyme which converts azathioprine to mercaptopurine, the fetus is not exposed to the active metabolites and therefore the harm to the fetus is reduced.

Tacrolimus and cyclosporin are used mainly for fulminant colitis during pregnancy when women with UC fails to respond to steroid therapy. There is a possibility of the following risks with these drug usage: preterm birth, low birth weight and small-for-gestational-age neonates.

One should avoid fluroquinolones during pregnancy as there is association with bone and cartilage damage in animal studies.

Kapoor D, Teahon K, Wallace SVF. Inflammatory bowel disease in pregnancy. Obstet Gynaecol 2016; 18:205–212.

16. D A uterine artery Doppler ultrasound at 20 weeks' gestation, with a single third-trimester growth scan and an umbilical artery Doppler ultrasound

This woman has three three minor risk factors for a small-for-gestational-age fetus: pregnancy interval, age and body mass index.

Royal College of Obstetricians and Gynaecologists (RCOG). The investigation and management of the small-for-gestational-age fetus. Green-top guideline no. 31. London: RCOG; 2014.

17. B She is likely to tolerate pregnancy well

A Caesarean section is indicated for obstetric reasons in women with surgically corrected tetralogy of Fallot with the view that they tolerate pregnancy well. Having said that, cardiac complications during pregnancy may occur and the reported incidence is 12%. These include arrhythmias and right heart failure. Moderate to severe pulmonary regurgitation can lead to an increase in right ventricular size and right ventricular dysfunction and failure. The use of diuretics and bed rest is recommended if right ventricular failure occurs during pregnancy. Early delivery or transcatheter valve implantation are the next steps to be considered in these women if conservative therapy as above fails and if they do not respond to medical therapy. Congenital heart disease is a risk in 6% of fetuses.

Vause S, Thorne S, Clarke B. Preconceptual counselling for women with cardiac disease. In: Steer PJ, Gatzoulis MA, Baker P (eds), Heart diseases and pregnancy. London: RCOG Press, 2006: 3–8.

18. C Mitochondrial disorder

Mitochondrial disorders are the most commonly reported inborn errors of metabolism. These arise because of mitochondrial genome mutations and are purely from maternal inheritance. The UK House of Lords has approved 'three-person IVF' to allow fertility clinics to undertake mitochondrial donation. The advances in technology in IVF therapy aids to eradicate mitochondrial diseases by substituting maternal DNA with DNA from an anonymous female donor.

Ben-Nagi J, Serhal P, SenGupta S, et al. Preimplantation genetic diagnosis: an overview and recent advances. Obstet Gynaecol 2016; 18:99–106.

19. C Previous failed rescue/emergency vaginal cerclage

Transabdominal cerclage is indicated when either a transvaginal cerclage is cannot be performed because of extreme shortening, scarring or laceration of the cervix with cervical insufficiency, or when a patient has had multiple failed previous elective transvaginal cerclages.

Gibb D, Saridogan E. The role of transabdominal cervical cerclage techniques in maternity care. Obstet Gynaecol 2016; 18:117–125.

20. B Defects in complement regulation

Complement-mediated haemolytic uremic syndrome (HUS) is caused by dysregulation of the alternative pathway of the complement system.

Fakhouri F, Roumenina L, Provot F, et al. Pregnancy-associated hemolytic uremic syndrome revisited in the era of complement gene mutations. J Am Soc Nephrol 2010; 21:859–867.
Wiles KS, Banerjee A. Acute kidney injury in pregnancy and the use of non-steroidal anti-inflammatory drugs. Obstet Gynaecol 2016; 18:127–135.

21. A A creatinine concentration >90 µmol/L should be considered diagnostic of kidney injury in pregnancy

Kidney injury is diagnosed when the creatinine concerntration is >90 µmol/L in pregnancy. When the urine output falls to <20 mL/hr, the dose of magnesium sulphate should be reduced by 50%. The obstetric management in pre-eclampsia as such is not affected in the presence of acute kidney injury, however one may need to consider delivery if there is anuria. Retention of urine occurs following delivery in up to 15% of women and the causes can be neurological, mechanical or physiological. The serum creatinine following delivery falls.

Wiles KS, Banerjee A. Acute kidney injury in pregnancy and the use of non-steroidal anti-inflammatory drugs. Obstet Gynaecol 2016; 18:127–135.

22. B Certolizumab

The terminology biologics comprises a variety of biologic molecules. This includes both murine and human monoclonal antibodies and soluble cytokine receptors. These cross the placenta to varying degrees and consequently affect the fetus.

The agent peglylated anti-TNF certolizumad crosses the placenta relatively and may become the main biologic treatment in women of reproductive age in future.

Ching Soh M, MacKillop L. Biologics in pregnancy – for the obstetrician. Obstet Gynaecol 2016; 18:25–32.

23. D Haemangioma

Haemangiomas in the liver are the most common benign tumours occurring in the liver. These are seen in 2–20% of individuals who are healthy. They predominately occurr in middle-aged women. Generally, their growth is slow but occasionally may speed up in the presence of oestrogen receptors and excessive hormonal presence in pregnancy.

Milburn J, Black M, Ahmed I, et al. Diagnosis and management of liver masses in pregnancy. Obstet Gynaecol 2016; 18:43–51.

24. D Thrombosis and thromboembolism remain the leading causes of direct maternal death

There was no significant change in the rate of maternal deaths from direct causes between 2009–11 and 2012–14. The rate of maternal deaths from hypertensive disorders is at its lowest ever, with fewer than one death for every million women giving birth. The World Health Organization has reclassified maternal suicides as a direct cause of maternal death.

Knight M, Nair M, Tuffnell D, Kenyon S, Shakespeare J, Brocklehurst P, Kurinczuk JJ (Eds.) on behalf of MBRRACE-UK. Saving lives, improving mothers' care - surveillance of maternal deaths in the UK 2012–14 and lessons learned to inform maternity care from the UK and Ireland Confidential Enquiries into

Maternal Deaths and Morbidity 2009–14. Oxford: National Perinatal Epidemiology Unit, University of Oxford; 2016.

25. E Diphtheria toxoid

The use of attenuated live viral and bacterial vaccines use is contraindicated in pregnancy because of the increased risks to the fetus.

Inactivated viral and bacterial vaccines use poses no fetal risks and therefore can be used during pregnancy.

Arunakumari PS, Kalburgi S. Vaccination in pregnancy. Obstet Gynaecol 2015; 17:257–263.

26. C Twin-to-twin transfusion syndrome (TTTS) complicates up to 15% of monochorionic pregnancies

Twin-to-twin transfusion syndrome (TTTS) complicates up to 15% of monochorionic pregnancies. Twin anaemia–polycythaemia sequence is an important association in complicated monochorionic pregnancies, especially those with TTTS, occurring in up to 13% of cases after laser ablation. It is relatively rarely associated with apparently uncomplicated monochorionic diamniotic twin pregnancies.

Kilby MD, Bricker L on behalf of the Royal College of Obstetricians and Gynaecologists. Management of monochorionic twin pregnancy. BJOG 2016; 124:e1–e45.

27. E Women carrying twins should be offered nuchal translucency measurements between 11 weeks + 0 days and 14 weeks + 1 day of gestation

A detailed anomaly ultrasound scan of twin pregnancies should take place between 18 weeks and 20 weeks + 6 days of gestation, and in uncomplicated monochorionic pregnancies, fetal ultrasound should take place fortnightly from 16 weeks + 0 days onwards. In twin pregnancies showing selective growth restriction, surveillance of growth should be undertaken at least every 2 weeks with fetal Doppler ultrasound. Screening for twin-to-twin transfusion syndrome in monochorionic pregnancies should not be carried out by first trimester nuchal translucency measurements. Women carrying twins should be offered nuchal translucency measurements between 11 weeks + 0 days and 14 weeks + 1 day of gestation.

Royal College of Obstetricians and Gynaecologists (RCOG). Management of monochorionic twin pregnancy. Green-top guideline no. 51. London: RCOG; 2016.

28. A Cochrane review has indicated that the use of umbilical artery Doppler ultrasound is associated with a reduced risk of perinatal death in high risk women

The lowest risk of perinatal death is at 39 weeks' gestation and the risk of stillbirth in the UK is 1 in 200 pregnant women.

In high risk pregnant women, the use of umbilical artery Doppler is suggested to reduce the risk of perinatal death. The study thrombophilia in pregnancy prophylaxis did not show benefit of low molecular weight heparin (LMWH) usage on either risk of placenta realated complications or pregnancy loss in women with thrombophilia.

The trial of umbilical and fetal flow in Europe (TRUFFLE) found little difference on the fetal outcome when ductus venosus Doppler measurement on ultrasound was comparted to computerised assessment of cardiotocography. The risk of perinatal death is lowest at 39 weeks' gestation, and the overall risk of stillbirth in the UK is around 1 in 200, not 1 in 500.

Smith G. Prevention of stillbirth. Obstet Gynaecol 2015; 17:183–187.

Answers: EMQs

29. L Symphysis pubic dysfunction

Symphysis pubis dysfunction is common during pregnancy and results from instability of the pelvic girdle owing to laxity or diastasis of the pubic symphysis joint. The incidence varies from 1 in 36 to 1 in 300 pregnancies in the UK (the variation is related to a deficiency in objective criteria for diagnosing this condition). Symptoms include pubic bone pain (burning, stabbing or shooting) during walking, turning over in bed, standing on one leg and lifting and parting of legs. The pain can also radiate to the lower abdomen, perineum, groin, thigh, leg and lower back.

Clinical examination usually reveals tenderness over the pubic symphysis or sacroiliac joint, positive Trendelenburg sign (sagging of the opposite buttock when the patient is asked to stand on one leg) and positive Patrick's Fabere sign. (With one iliac spine held in a fixed position by the doctor who is examining, the woman lies in a supine position, placing her opposite heel on the ipsilateral knee with the leg falling passively outwards. The test is positive if pain occurs in either sacroiliac joint.) A waddling gait is seen in extreme cases.

30. H Osteomyelitis of the pubis

Osteomyelitis of the pubis is a rare condition and is caused by low grade infection of the pubic bone. It may occur following gynaecological surgery (2–12 weeks later), urogenital procedures or operative delivery. Common symptoms include tenderness over the pubic rami or symphysis pubis, reduced painful hip movements (especially abduction) and pain on the lateral compression of the pelvis. Low grade pyrexia is a systemic feature. Haematological investigations reveal normocytic normochromic anaemia, increased white blood cell count and C-reactive protein. Blood and urine cultures are positive in 50% of cases.

Radioisotope bone scans show an increase in uptake but are not recommended for use during pregnancy.

31. G Osteitis pubis

Osteitis pubis is a painful inflammatory condition involving the pubic region in a symmetrical fashion. The cause is mostly idiopathic although it can be associated with pregnancy, seronegative spondyloarthritis, urogenital procedures and trauma. The symptoms are pain in the pubic region, which is aggravated by climbing stairs, kicking and pivoting (rotating or spin) on one leg. X-rays of the pubic bone reveal erosions, cystic changes and rarefaction of the medial margins of the pubic rami. Also, when the patient is asked to stand on one leg, diastasis of the pubic symphysis with displacement is seen on a pelvic X-ray. Blood tests usually reveal normal inflammatory markers.

32. K Pregnancy-induced osteomalacia

Pregnancy-induced osteomalacia is a metabolic disorder caused by vitamin D deficiency. The increased requirements of vitamin D during pregnancy are normally met by an increased dietary intake. If this is not the case, it can result in osteomalacia. The woman presents with vague symptoms (aches and pains) and these may lead to misdiagnoses. The pain described is usually in the spinal area and localised pain in the pubic area can occur due to pseudo fractures (Looser zones seen in pubic bone and ischial rami). A waddling gait may be seen due to proximal myopathy. Low serum calcium and a raised alkaline phosphatase are invariably seen in almost all patients. A reduced serum vitamin D level confirms the diagnosis. Biochemistry is normalised following replacement of vitamin D orally. If there is no improvement with this treatment, malabsorption needs to be ruled out.

33. O Transient osteoporosis of pregnancy affecting the hip joint

Transient osteoporosis of pregnancy affecting the hip joint is a rare condition of the hip. It typically affects the left hip in pregnant women although the right hip and other joints may be involved. Symptoms include pain in the hip, localised either to the groin or referred to the anterior aspect of knee. Pain is elicited especially during walking or on weight bearing. Lack of tenderness on pressure on the pubic symphysis distinguishes this condition from other painful conditions affecting the pubic bone.

Haematological tests reveal marginally raised inflammatory markers.

X-rays of the hip reveal osteopenia that is localised and involves the femoral head and acetabulum.

Williams S. Pubic pain during pregnancy. In: Hollingworth T (ed). Differential Diagnosis in Obstetrics and Gynaecology: An A–Z. London: Hodder Arnold, 2008:297–301.
Jain S, Eedarapalli P, Jamjute P, Sawdy R. Symphysis pubis dysfunction: a practical approach to management. Obstet Gynaecol 2006; 8:153–158.

34. H Reassure

The mother is immune and passive transfer of immunity (antibodies) is expected from mother to baby. Therefore reassure the mother.

35. D Offer termination following thorough counselling

The incubation period for rubella is 14–21 days. Most women (50–70%) with rubella will present with maculopapular rash, lymphadenopathy and arthritis. The period of infectivity is 7 days before and 7 days after the appearance of the rash.

Maternal infection affects most fetuses during the first trimester of pregnancy. The risk is small at 13–16 weeks' gestation and very small after 16 weeks' gestation. The major fetal effects include congenital heart defects (patent ductus arteriosus), ocular defects (cataract, glaucoma and microphthalmia), hearing problems (sensorineural deafness) and mental retardation. It also causes haemolytic anaemia, thrombocytopaenia, viraemia, jaundice, transient hepato-splenomegaly, purpura and diabetes.

36. H Reassure

The mother has been in contact with a person who had rubella but she is immune to rubella so reassurance is all that is required.

37. L Vaccinate the mother against rubella

Women should be advised routinely about rubella vaccination during preconception counselling. In this scenario, she can be offered and vaccinated against rubella because she would be at risk of developing rubella and also wants to get pregnant. However, women should be advised to avoid pregnancy until 1 month post vaccination because the fetus is at risk in view of the live virus in the vaccine (US Center for Disease Control recommendations).

38. H Reassure

This woman is immune to rubella and therefore no further action is necessary. Reassure the woman.

Nelson-Piercy C. Handbook of Obstetric Medicine (4th edn). London: Informa Healthcare, 2010.

39. E Commence prophylactic low-molecular heparin

She had a previous history of DVT and therefore warrants commencement of prophylactic low-molecular-weight during pregnancy. Any woman with a previous venous thromboembolism (VTE), except those who had a VTE after major surgery and have no other risk factors, should be offered low molecular weight heparin in the antenatal period. It should be started in early pregnancy or as soon as the risk is identified and continued for 6 weeks during puerperium.

40. C Change to heparinoid danaparoid sodium

Pregnant women who develop heparin-induced thrombocytopaenia and require further anticoagulant therapy, can be managed by changing LMWH to heparinoid danaparoid sodium during the antenatal period. During the postnatal period LMWH can be changed to warfarin therapy.

41. A Commence intravenous prophylactic unfractionated heparin

If there is need for heparin treatment in a woman considered to be at increased risk of bleeding, intravenous unfractionated heparin can be given while awaiting the resolution of risk factors for bleeding (because unfractionated heparin is short acting).

42. J Remove catheter 12 hours after giving the last dose of heparin

At least 12 hours should pass after the last prophylactic dose of LMWH and the introduction or removal of epidural or spinal catheter.

43. M Withhold heparin 24 hours before giving spinal anaesthesia

A therapeutic dose of heparin should be withheld 24 hours before spinal or epidural anaesthesia is given. The woman in this scenario has just received a therapeutic dose and will be at risk of bleeding and epidural haematoma if a spinal or epidural anaesthesia is given to her now. Thus, it is recommended to withhold the heparin for 24 hours before spinal anaesthesia is given. In case of emergency before 24 hours, general anaesthesia is preferred.

Letsky E, Murphy MF, Ramsay JE, Walker I. Haemorrhagic disease and hereditary bleeding disorders. London: RCOG Press; 2005.
Royal College of Obstetricians and Gynaecologists (RCOG). Reducing the risk of venous thromboembolism during pregnancy and the puerperium. Green-top guideline no. 37a. London: RCOG Press; 2015.

44. F Prophylactic LMWH postnatally for 10 days

All women who have had an elective Caesarean section (category 4) and have one or more additional risk factors (such as age over 35 years, body mass index >30) should be considered for thromboprophylaxis with LMWH for 10 days after delivery.

All women who have had an emergency Caesarean section (category 1, 2 or 3) should be considered for thromboprophylaxis with LMWH for 10 days after delivery.

A daily dose of 40 mg clexane is recommended for women who have had a Caesarean section. However, a higher thromboprophylactic dose needs to be considered with a body mass index >35. In the *Confidential Enquiry into Maternal Deaths* report (2016), the majority of morbidly obese women who died of thromboembolism did not receive thromboprophylaxis and those who did either had an inadequate dose or received it for an insufficient amount of time post-Caesarean section.

45. H Prophylactic LMWH antenatally plus postnatally for 6 weeks

Women with previous recurrent venous thromboembolism (VTE), a previous unprovoked, oestrogen or pregnancy-related VTE, a previous VTE and a history of VTE in a first-degree relative (or a documented thrombophilia) or other risk factors should be offered antenatal thromboprophylaxis with LMWH. Also recommended is the use of graduated elastic compression stockings in all women with a previous VTE or thrombophilia during pregnancy and for 6–12 weeks postpartum.

Women with a previous single provoked VTE, for instance a VTE related to surgery, and no other risk factors require close surveillance; antenatal LMWH is not routinely recommended.

46. G Prophylactic LMWH postnatally for 6 weeks

Any woman with 2 or more current persisting risk factors shown (other than a previous venous thromboembolism or thrombophilia) should be considered for prophylactic LMWH for at least 7 days postpartum. Women with 3 or more current or persisting risk factors (other than venous thromboembolism or thrombophilia) should be considered for prophylactic LMWH before giving birth and this is usually continued for 6 weeks postpartum.

In women who have additional persistent risk factors (lasting more than 7 days postpartum), such as prolonged admission or wound infection, thromboprophylaxis should be extended for up to 6 weeks or until the additional risk factors are no longer present.

47. H Prophylactic LMWH antenatally plus postnatally for 6 weeks

The incidence of pulmonary embolism reported during the antenatal period is 1.3 in 10,000 maternities with a case fatality rate of 3.5%. It remains the leading direct cause of maternal death in the UK (1.56 in 100,000 maternities). However, according to the recent *Confidential Enquiry into Maternal Deaths* report (2016), it is the second most common cause of overall maternal deaths (11% of maternal deaths). In 2003–2005, 79% of women who died from pulmonary embolism in the UK had identifiable risk factors. Therefore, it is possible to prevent venous thromboembolism (VTE) in obstetric patients with appropriate thromboprophylaxis.

RCOG recommendations are in **Table 7.2**.

Women should be reassessed before or during labour for risk factors for VTE. Age over 35 years and body mass index >30 or body weight >90 kg are important independent risk factors for postpartum VTE even after vaginal delivery.

Any woman with 4 or more current or persisting risk factors (other than previous VTE or thrombophilia) should be considered for prophylactic LMWH antenatally and will usually require prophylactic LMWH for 6 weeks postnatally.

Any woman with 2 or more current or persisting risk factors shown (other than previous VTE or thrombophilia) should be considered for prophylactic LMWH for at least 10 days postpartum.

Table 7.2 RCOG recommendations for women with a previous venous thromboembolism with or without thrombophilia

Scenario	Recommendations
Women with previous recurrent VTE Women with previous VTE + family history of VTE Women with previous VTE + thrombophilia Women with thrombophilia: anti-thrombin deficiency or more than 1 thrombophilia defect (homozygous factor V Leiden deficiency, prothrombin gene defect, compound heterozygotes) or presence of other risk factors	Antenatal and 6 weeks postnatal prophylactic LMWH
Women with low risk thrombophilia (other than above): asymptomatic and with family history of thrombophilia	Postnatal thromboprophylaxis with LMWH should be extended to 6 weeks
Single previous provoked VTE without thrombophilia, family history and other factors	Close surveillance antenatally and thromboprophylaxis with LMWH for 6 weeks postpartum
Women with previous VTE and on long-term warfarin	Antenatal high dose prophylactic or therapeutic LMWH and postnatal warfarin
VTE, venous thromboembolism	

48. B LMWH not recommended

A past history of superficial thrombophlebitis is not an indication for the administration of LMWH during pregnancy.

Royal College of Obstetricians and Gynaecologists (RCOG). Reducing the risk of thromboembolism during pregnancy and the puerperium. Green-top guideline no. 37a. London: RCOG Press; 2015. Calderwood CJ and Thanoon OI. Thromboembolism and thrombophilia in pregnancy. Obstet Gynecol Reprod Med 2009; 19:339–343.

49. I Anti-D immunoglobulin is not recommended or indicated

Anti-D immunoglobulin should be given to all non-sensitised RhD-negative women having a therapeutic abortion or termination of pregnancy, whether surgical or medical regardless of gestational age. It is not recommended for women who are already sensitised.

50. I Anti-D immunoglobulin is not recommended or indicated

The diagnosis in this case is threatened miscarriage and she is less than 12 weeks pregnant. She has antibodies to Kell antigen which are entirely unrelated to antibodies to D antigen. Hence, if she continues with this pregnancy uneventfully, she would need either a single dose of prophylactic anti-D immunoglobulin at 28 weeks or 2 doses at 28 weeks' and 34 weeks' gestation.

The RCOG does not recommend the routine administration of anti-D immunoglobulin before 12 weeks of pregnancy, unless there is heavy, recurrent bleeding or bleeding associated with abdominal pain. Anti-D immunoglobulin should be given to all non-sensitised RhD-negative women diagnosed with threatened miscarriage after 12 weeks of pregnancy. Where bleeding continues intermittently after 12 weeks' gestation, anti-D immunoglobulin should be given at 6-weekly intervals.

Anti-D immunoglobulin should be given to all non-sensitised RhD-negative women who have a spontaneous complete or incomplete miscarriage after 12 weeks of pregnancy.

It is not indicated for women who have a spontaneous miscarriage before 12 weeks of pregnancy or for women with minimal vaginal bleeding before 12 weeks of pregnancy.

Anti-D immunoglobulin administration should be considered in non-sensitised Rhesus-negative women if there is heavy or repeated bleeding or associated with abdominal pain as gestation approaches 12 weeks. Gestational age should be confirmed by ultrasound.

51. E Anti-D immunoglobulin 500 IU

A dose of 250 IU is recommended for prophylaxis following sensitising events up to 20 weeks of pregnancy. For all events after 20 weeks, at least 500 IU anti-D immunoglobulin should be given followed by a test to identify fetomaternal haemorrhage greater than 4 mL red cells; additional anti-D immunoglobulin should be given as required.

A test for fetomaternal haemorrhage is not required before 20 weeks' gestation.

52. D Anti-D immunoglobulin 250 IU

Anti-D immunoglobulin should be given to all non-sensitised rhesus-D negative women who have an ectopic pregnancy, regardless of mode of treatment, because there is a significant chance of sensitisation.

Women with indeterminate rhesus D typing results should be treated as rhesus D negative until final results are obtained and completed.

53. E Anti-D immunoglobulin 500 IU

Anti-D immunoglobulin should be given to all non-sensitised rhesus-D negative women after the following potentially sensitising events during pregnancy:

- Amniocentesis, chorionic villus sampling, cordocentesis
- Other intrauterine procedures (e.g. insertion of shunts, embryo reduction)
- Antepartum haemorrhage
- External cephalic version for breech presentation
- Abdominal injury (sharp/blunt, closed/open)
- Intrauterine death
  - An appropriate dose of prophylactic anti-D Ig should be administered to rhesus D negative, previously non-sensitised women within 72 hours of the

diagnosis of IUD, irrespective of the time of subsequent delivery in the event of intrauterine death if no sample can be obtained to test the baby's rhesus status
- Ectopic pregnancy
- Evacuation of molar pregnancy
- Termination of pregnancy
- Delivery of baby – instrumental, normal or by Caesarean section
- Cell salvage use
  - Where intraoperative cell salvage (ICS) is used during a Caesarean section in rhesus D negative, previously non-sensitised women, and where cord blood group is confirmed as rhesus-D positive or is unknown, a minimum dose of 1500 IU anti-D Ig should be administered following the re-infusion of salvaged red cells. A maternal sample should also be taken for estimation of feto-maternal haemorrhage 30–45 min after reinfusion in case more anti-D Ig is indicated.

Following the above sensitising events, women should receive a minimum of 500 IU anti-D within 72 hours of the event whether the woman has received anti-D during pregnancy or not.

In addition, further doses of anti-D will be necessary if the volume of feto-maternal haemorrhage exceeds 4 mL of fetal cells. If more than 4 mL is detected, a follow-up sample should be obtained at 48 hours following an IV dose of anti-D and again at 72 hours following an intramuscular dose of anti-D to check if the fetal cells have cleared from the maternal blood.

Qureshi H, Massey E, Kirwan D, et al. BSCH guideline for the use of anti-D immunoglobulin for the prevention of haemolytic disease of the fetus and newborn. British Committee for Standards in Haematology (BCSH) guideline on anti-D administration in pregnancy. London: BCSH; 2014.
National Institute for Health and Clinical Excellence (NICE). Ectopic pregnancy and miscarriage: diagnosis and initial management [CG154]. London: NICE; 2012.
Royal College of Obstetrics and Gynaecologists (RCOG). The management of gestational trophoblastic disease. Green-top guideline no. 38. London: RCOG; 2010.

54. K ECV offer for 37 weeks' gestation

External cephalic version (ECV) before 36 weeks' gestation is not associated with a significant reduction in non-cephalic births or caesarean section. ECV should be offered from 36 weeks in nulliparous women and from 37 weeks in multiparous women. The overall success rate of ECV has been described to be 50% (30–80%), 40% in nulliparous women and 60% in multiparous women. The spontaneous reversion rate to breech presentation is 5%.

55. J ECV offer for 36 weeks' gestation

Spontaneous version rates for nulliparous women are approximately 8% after 36 weeks but less than 5% after unsuccessful external cephalic version (ECV). Success rates of ECV are 30–80%. Spontaneous reversion to breech presentation after successful ECV occurs in less than 5% of cases. Therefore, ECV from 36 weeks' gestation in nulliparous women seems reasonable; however, there is no upper time limit on the appropriate gestation for ECV. Successes have been reported at 42 weeks' gestation and can be performed in early labour provided that the membranes are intact.

56. G Emergency Caesarean section not indicated

External cephalic version (ECV) is associated with alterations in fetal parameters. Fetal bradycardia and a non-reactive cardiotocograph can occur but are usually transient findings. One should not rush to theatre if the bradycardia recovers within a few minutes. Alterations in the umbilical and middle cerebral artery waveforms have been reported and also an increase in amniotic fluid volume. However, the significance of these changes is unknown.

While taking consent, women should be warned about a 0.5% risk of emergency Caesarean section associated with complications (e.g. fetal distress, abruption placenta and uterine rupture) during ECV.

57. H ECV contraindicated

RCOG guidelines describe antepartum haemorrhage within 7 days as an absolute contraindication to external cephalic version (ECV).

The absolute contraindications to ECV include:

- where Caesarean delivery is necessary
- abnormal CTG
- major uterine anomaly
- ruptured membranes
- multiple pregnancies (except delivery of second twin)
- placenta praevia

Relative contraindications to ECV include:

- fetal growth restriction
- proteinuric pre-eclampsia
- oligohydramnios
- major fetal anomalies
- scarred uterus
- unstable lie

58. F Emergency Caesarean section

Footling breech presentation in labour is an indication for Caesarean section. The feet normally enter the vagina with less than full dilatation of the cervix and it is more likely to be associated with cord prolapse (7%) than otherwise. Also, it is almost impossible to deliver the aftercoming fetal head with less than full dilatation of the cervix.

Royal College of Obstetricians and Gynaecologists (RCOG). External cephalic version (ECV) and reducing the incidence of breech presentation. Green-top guideline no 20a. London: RCOG Press, 2006.

59. I *Plasmodium vivax*

A Duffy blood group antigen acts as an erythrocyte receptor for *Plasmodium vivax* merozoites. This is absent in certain Afro-Caribbean populations and therefore they are less susceptible to *P. vivax* infection.

60. K *Plasmodium falciparum*

Women with haemoglobinopathies (e.g. sickle cell trait) and erythrocyte enzyme defects (glucose-6-phosphate dehydrogenase deficiency) are less susceptible and resistant to severe and complicated malaria. If they acquire *Plasmodium falciparum* infection, the disease is less severe because the parasite is less able to divide in the abnormal erythrocyte. This may be due to the physical characteristics of the HbAS erythrocytes or due to the acquisition of natural immunity.

61. N *Mycobacterium tuberculosis*

Congenital tuberculosis is rare but carries a high mortality rate (around 50%). It is frequently under-diagnosed and is more common in the offspring of a mother if she has miliary tuberculosis with involvement of the endometrium.

The following women should be screened for tuberculosis prior to pregnancy:

- women with human immunodeficiency virus (HIV)
- women in close contact with a person having or suspected to have tuberculosis
- women born in countries with a high prevalence of tuberculosis, e.g. Asia and Africa
- women of low socioeconomic status including certain racial and ethnic minority populations
- women with certain medical disorders which are known to increase the risk of infection
- alcoholics and intravenous drug users (IVDU)
- residents of long-term and residential care facilities

62. F Group B *Streptococcus*

Streptococci are facultative anaerobic gram-positive cocci (usually arranged in chains) and may be cultured from the genital tract in up to 30% (6–30%) of pregnant women at some point during pregnancy. It causes no problems most of the time. In view of this, screening all women involves treating 30% of them, and treating 30% of them will cause two maternal death a year due to a penicillin allergy.

Overall 3–12% of all neonates are colonised with group B *Streptococcus* (GBS) in the first week of life. It can cause severe neonatal sepsis in 1 in 1000 deliveries and is also a recognised cause of neonatal infection (meningitis) and postpartum endometritis. The pregnancies at risk include: (a) vaginal swab culture positive for GBS infection in the current pregnancy; and (b) a previous baby affected by neonatal GBS infection. Therefore, prophylactic benzylpenicillin (if given more than

4 hours before delivery it decreases the risk of neonatal infection by 70%) has been recommended to be given during the intrapartum period for pregnant women identified as GBS carriers, GBS bacteriuria in the current pregnancy and previous neonate with GBS infection or delivering before 37 weeks' gestation irrespective of maternal GBS colonisation. If no treatment is given or if there is less than 4 hours of treatment before delivery, then the baby should have swabs taken and the paediatricians should be informed.

In women without GBS colonisation or unknown status, prophylactic antibiotics should be offered if the following risk factors are present (risk factors for developing early onset neonatal GBS infection):

- prolonged rupture of membranes >18 hours
- premature delivery (<37 weeks' gestation)
- intrapartum fever (>38°C)

63. C *Chlamydia trachomatis*

The baby can acquire *Chlamydia* infection during the passage through the birth canal. This can cause neonatal conjunctivitis (5–14 days postnatally) and neonatal pneumonia.

James D, Steer PJ, Weiner CP, Gonik B, Crowther C, Robson S (eds). High Risk Pregnancy: Management Options (4th edn). St Louis: Saunders, 2011.
Magowan B. Churchill's Pocketbook of Obstetrics and Gynaecology (3rd edn). Edinburgh: Churchill Livingstone, 2005.
Royal College of Obstetricians and Gynaecologists. Green-top Guideline No. 36. Group B streptococcal disease: Early onset. London: RCOG Press, 2003.

64. J Peripartum cardiomyopathy

The aetiology of peripartum cardiomyopathy is unclear. Women usually present late in pregnancy or early in the postpartum period (it can occur up to 6 months postpartum). It is more common in older multiparous Afro-Caribbean women but is also associated with multiple pregnancies, hypertension and pre-eclampsia. Women may present with symptoms and signs of biventricular failure (tachycardia, pulmonary oedema and peripheral oedema).

The above diagnosis should be considered in pregnant or puerperal women presenting with worsening breathlessness especially while lying flat or at night. It can be confused with pre-eclampsia because 25% of affected women will be hypertensive. RCOG recommends all such women should have an electrocardiogram and a chest X-ray. The treatment aims at reducing the preload and afterload (β-blockers, diuretics and angiotensin-converting enzyme inhibitors).

50% of women will have a spontaneous recovery. The prognosis is related to left ventricular size and function within 6 months after delivery. The maternal mortality rate is reported to be 25–50%, although a 95% survival rate after 5 years has been reported. Also, 25% of the maternal deaths due to cardiac causes are associated with cardiomyopathy.

65. A Aortic dissection

Marfan's syndrome is inherited as an autosomal dominant disease. The majority of patients (80%) with Marfan's syndrome will have cardiac involvement, the most common being mitral valve prolapse, mitral regurgitation and aortic root dilatation.

During pregnancy, Marfan's syndrome carries a risk of aortic dissection and aortic rupture. The predictors for dissection and rupture include systolic hypertension, pre-existing aortic root dilatation (10% if the size of the root is more than 4 cm) or if there is a strong family history of rupture or dissection. Pregnancy is contraindicated in women with an aortic root that is more than 4–4.5 cm.

Because systolic hypertension has been a key factor in the majority of deaths from aortic dissection, there has been an emphasis on monitoring and adequate control of hypertension with antihypertensive therapy during pregnancy.

In women who are at high risk, aortic root replacement should be offered prior to pregnancy. β-blockers used in these women (with aortic dilatation or hypertension) have been shown to reduce the rate of aortic dilatation and the risk of adverse effects in patients with Marfan's syndrome. Repeated echocardiograms are advocated in order to assess aortic root dilatation.

Planned Caesarean section is usually recommended for women with progressive aortic root dilatation of more than 4.5 cm.

Aortic dissection is a serious complication and one should have a high index of suspicion in women with a history of Marfan's syndrome. The presentation is usually acute with central chest pain radiating to the back. It is diagnosed by a CT scan of the chest.

The other risk factors for aortic dissection include coarctation of aorta and Ehlers–Danlos syndrome type IV.

66. I Mitral valve prolapse

If a woman with mitral valve prolapse is asymptomatic she should be left alone. However, if she is symptomatic one should consider mitral valve repair (balloon valvuloplasty).

67. J Peripartum cardiomyopathy

Peripartum cardiomyopathy can present late in the pregnancy or in the first 6 months of the postpartum period. If the woman presents with increasing shortness of breath on lying down flat or at night the above diagnosis should seriously be considered.

68. G Hypertrophic cardiomyopathy

Hypertrophic cardiomyopathy is a rare disease with an incidence of 0.1–0.5% in women. The spectrum of presentation is broad and is associated with sudden death. 70% are familial with autosomal dominant inheritance. There is usually a family history of sudden death in a first-degree relative following which other family members are screened or the woman is investigated for a murmur or symptoms during pregnancy.

The symptoms and signs are mainly due to a left ventricular outflow obstruction. These include:

- syncope
- chest pain
- ejection systolic murmur
- pan-systolic murmur
- heart failure
- arrhythmias
- effect of pregnancy on hypertrophic cardiomyopathy

Women usually tolerate this condition well in pregnancy (due to an increase in left ventricular size and stroke volume). If the woman is symptomatic, β-blockers should be commenced. One should avoid hypotension and hypovolaemia because this would increase left ventricular outflow obstruction. Therefore, be overcautious if considering regional anaesthesia and treat hypovolaemia immediately and adequately.

Royal College of Obstetricians and Gynaecologists. Good Practice Series No. 13. Cardiac disease and pregnancy. London: RCOG Press, 2011.
Nelson-Piercy C. Handbook of Obstetric Medicine (4th edn). London: Informa Healthcare, 2010.
Knight M, Kurinczuk JJ, Spark P, Brocklehurst P. United Kingdom Obstetric Surveillance System (UKOSS) Annual Report 2007. National Perinatal Epidemiology Unit, 2007.
Lewis G (ed). The Confidential Enquiry into Maternal and Child Health (CEMACH). Saving Mothers' Lives: reviewing material deaths to make motherhood safer: 2003–2005. The seventh report on confidential enquiries into maternal deaths in the United Kingdom. CEMACH, 2007.
Roth A and Elkayam U. Acute myocardial infarction associated with pregnancy. Ann Int Med 1996; 125:751–762.
Webber MD, Halligan RE, Schumacher JA. Acute infarction, intracoronary thrombolysis, and primary PTCA in pregnancy. Cathet Cardiovasc Diag 1997; 42:28–43.

69. A Intravenous artesunate

Malaria can present with non-specific flu-like illness. The symptoms include headache, fever with chills, nausea, vomiting, diarrhoea, coughing and general malaise. The signs include raised temperature, splenomegaly, jaundice, pallor, sweating and respiratory distress.

The features of complicated or severe malaria include prostration, impaired consciousness, respiratory distress (acute respiratory distress syndrome), pulmonary oedema, convulsions, collapse, abnormal bleeding, disseminated intravascular coagulation, jaundice and haemoglobinuria.

Laboratory findings include severe anaemia, thrombocytopaenia, hypoglycaemia, acidosis, renal impairment, hyperlactataemia, hyperparasitaemia, algid malaria (gram-negative septicaemia) and meningitis.

Microscopic diagnosis allows for species identification and estimation of parasitaemia. Pregnant women with 2% or more parasitised red blood cells are at higher risk of developing severe malaria and should be treated by following the severe malaria protocol.

The RCOG recommends:

- Admission of women with uncomplicated malaria to hospital
- Admission of women with complicated malaria to the intensive care unit
- Intravenous artesunate as the first line for the treatment of severe falciparum malaria
- Intravenous quinine if artesunate is not available
- To use quinine and clindamycin to treat uncomplicated *Plasmodium falciparum* (or mixed, such as *P. falciparum* and *Plasmodium vivax*)
- Use chloroquine to treat *P. vivax*, *Plasmodium ovale* or *Plasmodium malariae*
- Primaquine use should be avoided in pregnancy
- Involve infectious diseases specialists, especially for severe and recurrent cases
- If vomiting persists, oral therapy should be stopped and intravenous therapy should be instituted
- Treat the fever with antipyretics
- Screen for anaemia and treat appropriately
- Follow-up to ensure detection of relapse

70. J Oral quinine plus oral clindamycin

Uncomplicated malaria in the UK is defined as fewer than 2% parasitised red blood cells in a woman with no signs of severity and no complicating features.

The treatment is one of the following:

- Oral quinine 600 mg every 8 hours and oral clindamycin 450 mg every 8 hours for 7 days (they can be given together) or
- Combination artemether–lumefantrine 4 tablets/dose for weight >35 kg, twice daily for 3 days (with fat) or
- Combination atovaquone–proguanil 4 standard tablets daily for 3 days

71. C Antiemetic plus repeat oral quinine and clindamycin

Vomiting is a known adverse effect of quinine and is associated with malarial treatment failure. Use an antiemetic if the patient vomits and repeat the antimalarial medication. Repeat vomiting after an antiemetic is an indication for parenteral therapy.

Treatment for uncomplicated falciparum malaria with vomiting:

- Quinine 10 mg/kg dose intravenous in 5% dextrose over 4 hours every 8 hours plus intravenous clindamycin 450 mg every 8 hours
- Once the patient stops vomiting she can be switched to oral quinine 600 mg 3 times a day to complete 5–7 days and if needed oral clindamycin can be switched to 450 mg 3 times a day for 7 days

72. L Oral chloroquine 300 mg weekly until delivery

Relapse during pregnancy can be prevented by administering chloroquine oral 300 mg weekly until delivery.

73. K Oral chloroquine for 3 days

The treatment for non-falciparum malaria, *Plasmodium vivax*, *Plasmodium ovale* and *Plasmodium malariae* is oral chloroquine (base) 600 mg followed by 300 mg 6 hours later. Then 300 mg on day 2 and again on day 3.

Royal College of Obstetricians and Gynaecologists (RCOG). The diagnosis and treatment of malaria in pregnancy. Green-top guideline No. 54B. London: RCOG Press; 2010.

Chapter 8

Maternal medicine

Questions: SBAs

For each question, select the single best answer from the five options listed.

1. Which one of the following is not a risk factor for myocardial infarction in pregnancy?

    A   Antepartum infections
    B   Blood transfusion
    C   Eclampsia
    D   Migraine headaches
    E   Thrombophilia

2. A 25-year-old parous Asian woman who had a vaginal delivery 5 months previously is brought by ambulance to the emergency department with complaints of breathlessness, palpitations and gross peripheral oedema. Pulse rate is 120 bpm, blood pressure 100/60 mmHg and temperature 37°C. An ECG reveals supraventricular tachycardia. The recent pregnancy was low risk and had no antenatal or postnatal complications. The patient reports similar breathlessness after her first delivery, but because she was in Pakistan, she did not attend for medical advice. The symptoms improved with bed rest.

    What is the most likely diagnosis?

    A   Dilated cardiomyopathy
    B   Hypertrophic cardiomyopathy
    C   Peripartum cardiomyopathy
    D   Pre-eclamspia
    E   Pulmonary embolism

3. A 32-year-old nulliparous woman attends the emergency department at 34 weeks' gestation with complaints of severe dyspnoea. She is known to suffer from asthma and currently uses salbutamol and beclomethasone inhalers. She also gives a history of cough with green sputum for the previous 4 days. Examination reveals bilateral wheeze and crackles at the left lung base. Pulse rate is 120 bpm, temperature 38.1°C and oxygen saturation on air 91%.

   What should be the initial management?

   A   Intravenous antibiotics
   B   Nebulised salbutamol
   C   Nebulised ipratropium bromide
   D   Oxygen
   E   Prednisolone

4. A 32-year-old woman moved to the UK 2 months ago from Pakistan. She is nulliparous and is currently 22 weeks pregnant. On arrival from Pakistan, she saw a GP because she had symptoms of cough, fever and conjunctivitis. She told the GP that she was diagnosed with tuberculosis in Pakistan 5 months ago. You are the specialist registrar in the antenatal clinic and see her during an antenatal visit. She is taking anti-tubercular medication and is anxious because her cousin was treated with anti-tubercular medication in Pakistan and delivered a child who was diagnosed with permanent deafness.

   The use of which anti-tubercular medication during pregnancy can cause deafness in the child?

   A   Ethambutol
   B   Isoniazid
   C   Pyrazinamide
   D   Rifampicin
   E   Streptomycin

5. A 32-year-old nulliparous woman presents to the maternity day assessment unit at 33 weeks' gestation with itching, particularly on the palms and feet. This is affecting her quality of life because she is unable to sleep at night. She is still working in an office but has not been able to focus at work due to lack of sleep. Clinical examination has not revealed a rash, and her baby is moving well. Blood tests reveal a raised alanine aminotransferase of 90 IU/L and bile acids of 38 mg/L.

   What is the initial management?

   A   Alternate-day cardiotocography
   B   Booking induction of labour for 37–38 weeks' gestation
   C   Weekly liver function tests (LFTs) and 2-weekly growth scans
   D   Weekly LFTs and start ursodeoxycholic acid
   E   Weekly LFTs, and start ursodeoxycholic acid and antihistamine tablets

6. A 28-year-old nulliparous woman attends the maternity day assessment unit at 36 weeks' gestation with because she thought she appeared yellow when she looked in the mirror. She has been vomiting for a week and feels very thirsty. On general

examination, the bulbar conjunctiva appears yellowish bilaterally. Abdominal examination shows tenderness in the right upper quadrant. Her pulse rate is 95 bpm, temperature 37.8°C, blood pressure 143/92 mmHg and oxygen saturation 100% on air. A urine dipstick test shows +1 of protein and +1 of leucocytes. Blood test results reveal conjugated bilirubin of 200 mg/L, alanine aminotransferase of 150 IU/L, alkaline phosphatase of 150 IU/L, raised white cell count of 14×10^9/L and prothrombin time of 20 seconds. Her blood glucose level ascertained by a fingerprick blood sugar is 2.1 mmol/L.

What is the most likely diagnosis?

A   Acute fatty liver disease
B   Cholecystitis
C   Haemolysis, elevated liver enzymes, low platelet count (HELLP) syndrome
D   Hepatitis
E   Pre-eclampsia

7. A 28-year-old woman had a vaginal delivery at 39 weeks' gestation. She suffers from Crohn's disease and is taking sulfasalazine, prednisolone and azathioprine. She is keen to start breastfeeding and asks your advice, as the specialist registrar, on taking these medications during breastfeeding.

What is your advice?

A   Continue with prednisolone and azathioprine but stop sulfasalazine or avoid breastfeeding
B   Continue with sulfasalazine and azathioprine but stop prednisolone or avoid breastfeeding
C   Continue with sulfasalazine and prednisolone but stop azathioprine or avoid breastfeeding
D   Halve the dose of all medications and continue breastfeeding
E   Stop all medications or avoid breastfeeding

8. A 29-year-old primigravid patient presents to the maternity day assessment unit at 20 weeks' gestation with localised right iliac fossa pain, vomiting and diarrhoea. On examination, there is guarding and rebound tenderness in the right iliac fossa. Her temperature is 38.1°C, pulse 110 bpm, respiratory rate 17 per minute and blood pressure 126/76 mmHg. Her white cell count is 23×10^9/L and a C-reactive protein concentration of 176 mg/L. Ultrasound identifies a non-compressible, enlarged (8 mm), blind-ending tubular structure in the right iliac fossa and a fluid collection. Cardiotocography is normal. The mother is extremely anxious.

What is the chance that the fetus will survive?

A   1.5%
B   6%
C   10%
D   36%
E   40%

9. A 21-year-old primigravid woman attends the maternity day assessment unit at 28 weeks' gestation with a raised temperature, a cough and chest and hip pain. She is known to have sickle cell disease but has so far had no problems during pregnancy. A growth scan shows fetal growth is normal. A general examination reveals crackles and reduced air entry over the left lung. Her pulse rate is 120 bpm, temperature 38.1°C, respiratory rate 30 per minute and oxygen saturation 92% on air.

    What is the initial management?

    A   Oxygen, antibiotics, analgesia, prophylactic low molecular weight heparin
    B   Oxygen, antibiotics, analgesia, prophylactic low molecular weight heparin, exchange transfusion
    C   Oxygen, antibiotics, analgesia
    D   Oxygen, antibiotics, analgesia, exchange transfusion
    E   Oxygen, antibiotics, analgesia, unfractionated heparin

10. A 21-year-old nulliparous woman attends the emergency gynaecology department with lower abdominal pain. A urinary pregnancy test is positive but she is not aware that she could be pregnant. An emergency transvaginal scan shows a viable fetal pole of 6 weeks' gestation. Because there is a history of β-thalassaemia major, the sonographer requests you, as the on-call specialist registrar, to see the woman before she is discharged. You note that she is taking iron chelation therapy, vitamin C and prophylactic penicillin in view of a history of splenectomy in the past. She is also up to date with her vaccinations. She would like to continue with this pregnancy. However, she is anxious that she has been taking medication and asks your advice on the current and any potential new medications.

    What is your advice?

    A   Continue chelation therapy, stop vitamin C, start folic acid 5 mg, continue penicillin
    B   Stop chelation therapy, stop vitamin C, start folic acid 5 mg, continue penicillin
    C   Stop chelation therapy, continue vitamin C, start folic acid 5 mg, continue penicillin
    D   Stop chelation therapy, stop vitamin C, start folic acid 5 mg, stop penicillin
    E   Stop chelation therapy, stop vitamin C, start folic acid 5 mg, continue penicillin, start thromboprophylaxis

11. A 30-year-old Romanian parous woman attends the emergency gynaecology unit at 26 weeks' gestation with left iliac fossa pain but no vaginal bleeding. As the on-call specialist registrar, you suspect that she may have an ectopic pregnancy and therefore arrange urgent pelvic ultrasound. The report is as follows:

    'Anteverted uterus. Well-defined gestational sac, yolk sac and fetal pole with cardiac activity seen at the uterine fundus corresponding to pregnancy of 6 weeks + 3 days. Right ovary contains the corpus luteum. On the left ovary, there is a 9 cm × 8 cm × 7 cm multiloculated cyst with solid components, and papillary projections. No adnexal tenderness or cervical excitation is elicited, and there are no signs of torsion or free fluid in the recto-uterine pouch (pouch of Douglas)'.

What tumour markers do you request on the blood test request form?

A α-Fetoprotein (α-FP), lactate dehydrogenase (LDH), β-human chorionic gonadotropin (β-hCG)

B LDH, α-FP, C-reactive protein

C LDH, α-FP, CA-125

D LDH, α-FP, CA-19.9

E LDH, β-hCG

12. A 36-year-old woman who had 2 previous normal deliveries attends her appointment with the breast surgeon. She is 33 weeks pregnant and noticed a palpable lump in her right breast the previous night. She is extremely worried that this might be cancer. She says that her mother died of breast cancer at 60 years of age. On examination, the lump is found to be round, firm, immobile and tender on palpation.

What is the appropriate initial management?

A Genetic testing for the *BRCA1* and *BRCA2* gene

B Reassure the patient and discharge her

C Request urgent CA-125, carcino-embryonic antigen and CA-15.3 values

D Urgent ultrasound-guided biopsy for cytology, and an antenatal clinic appointment

E Urgent ultrasound of the breast, and an antenatal clinic appointment with the consultant

13. A 34-year-old primigravid woman is seen by the community midwife at 30 weeks' gestation. For the first time during this pregnancy, the blood pressure reading is high (154/103 mmHg), and it remains high (151/104 mmHg) She woman is otherwise asymptomatic. The midwife refers her to the maternity day assessment unit for review and discussion of a management plan. You are the registrar on call for the maternity assessment unit and review her. The general examination is normal other than pedal oedema. A repeat blood pressure reading is 155/100 mmHg. Urinary assessment reveals an absence of protein. All blood test results, including renal function, liver function and platelets, are normal. There is no history of allergy to any medication.

How will you manage her in line with NICE guidelines?

A Admit her and give labetolol, and upon discharge measure blood pressure twice a week, test for proteinuria at each visit and take weekly blood tests

B Admit her and give labetolol, and upon discharge measure blood pressure twice a week and test for proteinuria at each visit with no further blood tests if there is no proteinuria

C Do not admit her, give labetolol, measure blood pressure twice a week, test for proteinuria at each visit with no further blood tests if there is no proteinuria

D Do not admit her, give nifedipine, measure blood pressure twice a week, test for proteinuria at each visit with no further blood tests if there is no proteinuria

E Do not admit her, give labetolol, measure blood pressure 3 times a week, test for proteinuria at each visit with no further blood tests if there is no proteinuria

14 A 30-year-old primigravid woman is seen by the community midwife at 30 weeks' gestation. The pregnancy has so far been low risk. Blood pressure measures 140/90 mmHg with a value of 142/93 mmHg when repeated after 30 minutes. The midwife therefore refers her to maternity day assessment unit. Blood pressure on arrival at hospital is 149/99 mmHg. She is asymptomatic and the general and fetal examination are normal. A urine dipstick test reveals 2+ of protein. All blood tests results, including renal function, liver function and platelets, are normal. She is not allergic to any medication.

How will you manage her in line with NICE guidelines?

A   Admit to hospital, do not treat the hypertension, measure blood pressure 4 times a day, do not repeat quantification for proteinuria, take blood tests twice weekly

B   Admit to hospital, treat the hypertension with labetolol, measure blood pressure 4 times a day, do not repeat quantification for proteinuria, take blood tests twice weekly

C   Admit to hospital, treat the hypertension with nifedipine, measure blood pressure 4 times a day, do not repeat quantification for proteinuria, take blood tests twice weekly

D   Do not admit to hospital, do not treat the hypertension, measure blood pressure 4 times a day, do not repeat quantification for proteinuria, take blood tests twice weekly

E   Do not admit to hospital, treat hypertension with nifedipine, measure blood pressure 4 times a day, do not repeat quantification for proteinuria, take blood tests twice weekly

15. A 34-year-old nulliparous woman attends the preconception antenatal clinic, which you, as a specialist registrar, are taking. She gives a history of systemic lupus erythematosis diagnosed 3 years previously and is now complaining of fatigue, aching joints, a rash and cold fingers. She attributes her joint symptoms to sitting typing for long hours in her job as a medical secretary. Blood tests reveal high titres of antinuclear factor and double-stranded DNA antibodies. She is taking prednisolone, candesartan and hydroxycholoroquine. She has been in good health with no clinical relapse for the past year and is keen to start a family soon. She would like to know what factors could affect or not affect her pregnancy outcome.

Which one of the following factors does not affect pregnancy outcome?

A   Active disease within 12 months but not within in 6 months before conception
B   Chronic hypertension
C   Hypocomplementaemia
D   Serum creatinine level >280 mg/L at conception
E   Thrombocytopenia

16. A 32-year-old woman has been diagnosed with antiphospholipid syndrome after investigation for three unexplained recurrent miscarriages at <10 weeks' gestation. Lupus anticoagulant has tested positive on two occasions 12 weeks apart. She has no risk of a thrombotic event. You, as the specialist registrar, review her in the high-

risk pregnancy antenatal clinic at 7 weeks' gestation. She expresses anxiety that she will have another miscarriage.

How will you manage her at this gestation?

A   Aspirin 75 mg once a day
B   Aspirin 75 mg once a day with low molecular weight heparin at a low prophylactic dosage
C   Aspirin 75 mg once a day plus low molecular weight heparin at a therapeutic dosage
D   Aspirin 75 mg once a day plus low molecular weight heparin at a treatment dosage, and consider warfarin
E   No treatment

Questions: EMQs

Questions 17–21

Options for Questions 17–21

A	Hepatitis B	H	Cytomegalovirus
B	Hepatitis C	I	Epstein–Barr virus
C	Hepatitis E	J	Influenza A
D	Herpes simplex type 1	K	Measles
E	Herpes simplex type 2	L	Parvovirus B19
F	Human immunodeficiency virus (HIV)	M	Rubella
		N	Rhinovirus
G	Human papilloma virus	O	Varicella

Instructions: For each fetal or neonatal condition described below, choose the single most appropriate maternal viral infection from the list of options above. Each option may be used once, more than once, or not at all.

17. Laryngeal papilloma in infants.

18. Patent ductus arteriosus.

19. Cutaneous scarring in the fetus.

20. Ventriculomegaly in the fetus.

21. Limb hypoplasia in the fetus.

Questions 22–26

Options for Questions 22–26

A	Amitriptyline	I	Lithium
B	Benzodiazepines	J	Olanzapine
C	Citalopram	K	Paroxetine
D	Clozapine	L	Risperidone
E	Domperidone	M	Sertraline
F	Fluoxetine	N	Sulpiride
G	Haloperidol	O	Venlafaxine
H	Imipramine		

Instructions: For each abnormality described below, choose the single drug most likely to be the cause from the list of options above. Each option may be used once, more than once, or not at all.

22. Risk of raised blood pressure on higher dose.

23. Right ventricular outflow tract obstruction.

24. Risk of gestational diabetes and weight gain.

25. Agranulocytosis in the fetus and breastfed infant.

26. Cleft palate.

Questions 27–31

Options for Questions 27–31

A	Avoid amniocentesis in the third trimester
B	Amniocentesis of a single twin sac
C	Biophysical profile
D	Chorionic villus sampling before 10 weeks
E	Chorionic villus sampling after 10 weeks
F	Cordocentesis
G	Detailed fetal anomaly scan and fetal cardiac scan
H	First trimester amniocentesis
I	Fetal growth scan
J	Fetal scalp blood sampling
K	In utero fetal blood transfusion
L	Middle cerebral artery doppler
M	Peritoneal shunt
N	Second trimester amniocentesis
O	Third trimester amniocentesis

Instructions: For each clinical scenario described below, choose the single most appropriate initial intervention from the list of options above. Each option may be used once, more than once, or not at all.

27. A 29-year-old Asian woman presents to the day assessment unit at 35 weeks' gestation with reduced fetal movements. An anomaly scan performed in another country at 20 weeks' gestation was normal. A fetal cardiotocograph (CTG) reveals reduced variability for 60 minutes followed by a normal CTG. A detailed ultrasound scan performed by the fetal medicine department reveals polyhydramnios and double bubble sign with no other abnormality. Booking blood results (her first midwife appointment) show that she is positive for the HIV antigen.

28. A 29-year-old white woman attends the antenatal clinic at 15 weeks for a review of her booking antenatal investigations. Her haematological, biochemical and virology results are normal and she is Rhesus positive with no antibodies. However, her screening (quadruple) tests for trisomies showed an increased risk of trisomy 21 (more than 1 in 100) and an ultrasound at 13 weeks and 5 days revealed an increased nuchal translucency.

29. A 29-year-old European woman, para 1, attends for her dating scan (at 12 weeks) which reveals normal morphological features of the baby but 5 mm nuchal translucency. Her serum screening tests reveal decreased pregnancy-associated plasma protein A (PAPP-A) levels.

30. A 29-year-old Afro-Caribbean woman attends her antenatal booking appointment with the midwife at 15 weeks' gestation. 4 weeks later she comes in for her booking blood test results. Her haematological, biochemical and virology results were normal and her blood group was 'O' positive with no antibodies. However, her quadruple test for trisomy 21 showed an increased risk (more than 1 in 100). She refuses to have invasive testing.

31. A 29-year-old Asian woman attends the ultrasound department for her dating scan at 13 weeks and 5 days. It reveals a monochorionic diamniotic twin pregnancy and an increased nuchal translucency of both the twins. She is quite anxious because this is her 5th attempt at an IVF pregnancy. After appropriate counselling, she declines invasive testing and leaves the consultation room. 2 weeks later, she returns and decides to have the test.

Questions 32–36

Options for Questions 32–36

A Twin reversed arterial perfusion (TRAP)
B α–Thalassaemia
C β–Thalassaemia
D Congenital toxoplasmosis
E Congenital heart disease
F Congenital adenomatoid malformation of lungs
G Congenital diaphragmatic hernia
H Non-immune hydrops
I Idiopathic hydrops
J Immune hydrops
K Down's syndrome
L Turner's syndrome
M Twin-to-twin transfusion
N Sickle cell disease
O Parvovirus infection
P Placental insufficiency

Instructions: For each clinical scenario described below, choose the single most appropriate diagnosis from the list of options above. Each option may be used once, more than once, or not at all.

32. A 36-year-old white woman attends the obstetric day assessment unit at 28 weeks' gestation with reduced fetal movement for the last 2 days. An ultrasound scan reveals an absence of fetal heart activity and a hydropic fetus. She delivers 24 hours later following induced labour and agrees to be investigated. At her 6-week postnatal follow-up visit, the postmortem results reveal a macerated fetus with ventricular septal defect and oesophageal atresia. Her booking blood tests were normal.

33. A 36-year-old Asian woman attends the obstetric day assessment unit at 37 weeks' gestation with reduced fetal movements for the last 24 hours. A CTG shows fetal tachycardia of more than 200 bpm. An ultrasound scan reveals an obvious scalp oedema and ascites. The fetal heart rate normalised following administration of flecainide to the mother. Subsequently, she was delivered by Caesarean section and the baby was admitted to the neonatal unit. Her booking blood tests were normal.

34. A 36-year-old Asian woman attends the obstetric day assessment unit at 34 weeks' gestation with reduced fetal movements. Clinical examination reveals she is small for dates and has reduced amniotic fluid. Vital signs show raised blood pressure with normal pulse and temperature. She does not have a history of ruptured membranes or any recent illness. A fetal cardiotocograph (CTG) reveals a baseline heart rate of 140 bpm, variability <5 bpm, absence of accelerations and unprovoked shallow decelerations with slow recovery for 40 minutes. A tocograph reveals an absence of uterine activity.

35. A 36-year-old white woman, para 1, attends the obstetric day assessment unit at 32 weeks' gestation with reduced fetal movements. A CTG reveals baseline heart rate of 150 bpm, variability <5 bpm, absence of accelerations and 2 shallow unprovoked decelerations in the last 40 minutes. A repeat CTG 6 hours later shows baseline 150, variability <5, absence of accelerations and occasional repeat decelerations. An ultrasound scan reveals fetal ascites and pleural effusion. Her booking blood tests show her blood group to be 'O' negative with anti-D antibodies (titre 1:16).

36. A 36-year-old white woman attends the obstetric day assessment unit at 30 weeks' gestation with reduced fetal movements. An ultrasound scan revealed fetal ascites and an absence of fetal heart activity. Her booking blood tests and anomaly scan at 20 weeks' gestation were normal. She had a vaginal delivery and attends for her bereavement appointment and postmortem results 6 weeks later. Her haematological, biochemical and infection screen for hydrops was normal. However, postmortem results revealed hydropic changes in the fetus.

Questions 37–41

Options for Questions 37–41

A	Anencephaly	H	Gastroschisis
B	Adenomatoid malformation of the lung	I	Meconium ileus
		J	Microcephaly
C	Choroid plexus cyst	K	Neural tube defect
D	Cardiac echogenic foci	L	Patau's syndrome
E	Diaphragmatic hernia	M	Pelvicaliceal dilatation
F	Down's syndrome	N	Ventriculomegaly
G	Exomphalos	O	Virilisation of fetus

Instructions: For each condition described below, choose the single most appropriate association from the list of options above. Each option may be used once, more than once, or not at all.

37. A 38-year-old white woman attends her antenatal clinic appointment for a review of her booking investigations. Her booking blood tests are normal. The anomaly scan at 20 weeks' gestation reveals a hyperechogenic bowel.

38. A 38-year-old white woman is referred to the fetal medicine unit because her 20-week anomaly scan shows an abnormality of the head. A repeat ultrasound scan by a fetal medicine specialist reveals holoprosencephaly.

39. A 38-year-old Asian woman attends her antenatal clinic appointment at 20 weeks' gestation. The anomaly scan at 20 weeks' gestation reveals pulmonary hypoplasia and mediastial shift to right side. She does not give any history of ruptured membranes.

40. A 38-year-old Afro-Caribbean woman was referred to the day assessment unit by her midwife because her clinical examination revealed a uterine height of 29 cm at 32 weeks' gestation. Because the fetus was fine, a growth scan was arranged and she was discharged home. 1 week later she attends the antenatal clinic with her growth scan report which shows an estimated fetal weight of 1300 g with short long bones.

41. A 38-year-old Asian woman attends her antenatal clinic appointment at 28 weeks' gestation following her growth scan, which showed her to be small for dates. The scan shows normal growth with a double bubble sign.

Questions 42–46

Options for Questions 42–46

A   Angiotensin-converting-enzyme (ACE) inhibitors
B   Amitriptyline
C   Amiodarone
D   Bendroflumethiazide
E   Citalopram
F   Cabergoline
G   Change therapy to oral carbimazole
H   Change therapy to oral propylthiouracil

I   Commence 5 mg folic acid/day
J   Commence 0.4 mg folic acid/day
K   Commence 10 mg oral vitamin K
L   Commence thyroxine
M   Frusemide
N   Increase the dose of thyroxine
O   Propylthiouracil
P   Propranolol

Instructions: For each scenario described below, choose the single most appropriate therapy from the list of options above. Each option may be used once, more than once, or not at all.

42. A 29-year-old primiparous woman presents to the early pregnancy assessment unit at 6 weeks' gestation with mild vaginal bleeding. She has a history of diabetes with well-controlled blood glucose levels. An ultrasound scan reveals a single intrauterine viable pregnancy. Currently, the only medication she is taking is insulin.

43. A 29-year-old primiparous woman presents to the early pregnancy assessment unit at 6 weeks' gestation with mild vaginal bleeding. She has a history of epilepsy controlled by sodium valproate and carbamazepine. An ultrasound scan reveals a single intrauterine viable pregnancy.

44. A 29-year-old primiparous woman attends the antenatal clinic at 16 weeks of pregnancy for review of booking (her first midwife appointment) blood tests. She suffers from hypothyroidism and is currently on 75 µg of thyroxine. Her haematological, biochemical and virology results are normal. Her thyroid-stimulating hormone (TSH) is 6.5 mU/mL and T4 is 14 pmol/L.

45. A 29-year-old primiparous woman attends the obstetric day assessment unit at 34 weeks' gestation with itching. Fetal cardiotocograph is normal. Her blood tests reveal raised alanine aminotransferase (48 U/L) and a normal autoimmune screen. A diagnosis of obstetric cholestasis is made.

46. A 29-year-old primiparous woman attends the antenatal clinic at 18 weeks' gestation for review. She gives a history of Graves' disease prior to pregnancy and had discontinued prophythiouracil because she developed a severe sore throat and agranulocytosis. At present her haematological results are normal. Her TSH is 0.5 mU/L.

Answers: SBAs

1. A Antepartum infections

The risks of having a myocardial infarction during pregnancy are the same as outside pregnancy. The risks identified in the *Confidential Enquiry into Maternal and Child Health* (2016) include:

- Multiparity (>3)
- Age >35 years
- History of hypertension
- History of diabetes
- History of heart disease
- Smoking
- High body mass index or obesity
- Hyperlipidaemia
- History of pre-eclampsia in previous pregnancies
- History of thrombophilia
- History of migraine headaches
- Current post-partum infection
- Blood transfusion

Wuntakal R, Shetty N, Ioannou E, Sharma S, Kurian J. Myocardial infarction and pregnancy. Obstet Gynaecol 2013; 15:247–255.

2. C Peripartum cardiomyopathy

There are three types of cardiomyopathy: peripartum, hypertrophic and dilated. Peripartum cardiomyopathy usually occurs in the first few weeks after giving birth but can occur up to 5 months postpartum. It has a high recurrence rate. It can occur in women who have no risk factors.

The risk factors for this condition include:

- Older age
- Black ethnicity
- Obesity
- Hypertension
- Multiparity

3. D Oxygen

Asthma exacerbations often occur between 24 and 36 weeks of pregnancy. The most common trigger is a viral infection (34%), followed by poor adherence to corticosteroid therapy (29%). In pregnancy, the severity of the illness remains unchanged, worsens or improves (in equal proportions). People with severe asthma are more likely to deteriorate (60%) compared with those who have mild asthma (10%).

In women with an acute exacerbation of asthma, it is very important first to secure the airway, and second to administer oxygen.

Goldie MH, Brightling CE. Asthma in pregnancy. Obstet Gynaecol 2013; 15:241–245.

4.   E Streptomycin

Streptomycin is both ototoxic and nephrotoxic. It is teratogenic as it crosses the placenta and can affect the fetus. The fetal effect includes minor impairment of hearing to severe, irreversible bilateral loss of hearing.

Isoniazid is safe to use during pregnancy. However, there are reports of demyelination in the fetus as it crosses the placenta. Pregnant women taking isoniazid should therefore be advised to take pyridoxine supplements to reduce the risk of demyelination process. There is no known increase in malformation or growth restriction.

The risk to fetus with rifampicin is theoretical and the overall risk of congenital malformations is not increased.

Ethambutol use may theoretically increase the risk of ocular toxicity.

There are no reports of fetal abnormalities from pyrazinamide use.

Mahendru A, Gajjar K, Eddy J. Diagnosis and management if tuberculosis in pregnancy. Obstet Gynaecol 2010; 12:163–171.

5.   E Weekly liver function tests (LFTs), and start ursodeoxycholic acid and antihistamine tablets

This patient has obstetric cholestasis and initially will require weekly liver function tests and ursodeoxycholic acid for symptom relief. This acts by lowering of the concentration of bile acids which contribute to itching. The antihistamine chlorpheniramine maleate 4 mg should be adminstered orally, as and when required or just before sleep. Induction of labour is advised by most obstetricians at 37 weeks' gestation but the evidence is limited regarding its effect on fetal outcome. However, if the liver function tests deteriorate then one must consider delivery of the fetus. Ultrasound and cardiotocography are unlikely to be useful in this situation as they can neither predict nor prevent fetal death.

6.   A Acute fatty liver disease

Acute fatty liver is a rare but life-threatening condition. A multidisciplinary approach to treatment should be taken in view of the complexity of this condition. Fresh frozen plasma and vitamin K are required to manage intravascular coagulopathy, and 50% dextrose to treat hypoglycaemia. If liver function does not improve or if encephalopathy develops, a liver transplant may be required; the woman should then be transferred to a liver unit. Acute fatty liver can be inherited as an autosomal recessive condition. The predicted incidence of acute fatty liver of pregnancy (AFLP) in the UK is 1/21,900 births. Most of these patients are primiparous, white and who are less than 35 years of age. The gestational age at diagnosis and delivery is usually around 36 weeks' gestation (range 27–40 weeks).

Acute fatty liver is aassociated with high mortality if not recognised or treated. Women may present with vomiting, liver dysfunction, fulminant hepatic failure, jaundice, disseminated intravascular coagulopathy, encephalopathy and uterine and gastrointestinal bleeding. A high index of suspicion and early intervention are necessary for a better outcome. The treatment is delivery of the baby and supportive treatment in the intensive care unit. This condition usually resolves after delivery and has a reported recurrence rate of 25% in the next pregnancy.

The Swansea criteria considers symptoms, imaging findings, haematological and biochemical markers and histopathology of liver biopsy to predict the risk of developing AFLP. When six or more of the following criteria are present in a pregnant woman and no other cause is found then it is high likely that this woman has AFLP:

The symptom include:

- Abdominal pain
- Vomiting
- Frequent micturition
- Excessive thirst

The haematological and biochemical markers include:

- Raised bilirubin >14 μmol/L
- Low blood glucose <4 mmol/L
- Markedly raised blood urea levels >340 μmol/L
- Raised serum alanine aminotransferase >42 IU/L
- Raised serum ammonia levels>47 μmol/L
- Elevated creatinine >150 μmol/L
- Elevated white cell count
- Leucocytosis >11 × 10^9/L
- Clotting abnormality and or coagulopathy: prothrombin time >14 seconds or activated partial thromboplastin time >34 seconds

Imaging criteria include:

- Ascites or a bright liver on ultrasound scan

Histopathological criteria include:

- Microvesicular steatosis on liver biopsy

The differential diagnoses obviously will include severe pre-eclampsia with liver involvement, and haemolysis, elevated liver test and low platelets (HELLP syndrome).

James D, Steer PJ, Weiner CP, et al (eds). High risk pregnancy: management options, 4th edn. St Louis: Saunders; 2011.
Kingham JG. Swansea criteria for diagnosis of acute fatty liver of pregnancy. Gut 2010; 60:139-140.
Knight M, Nelson-Piercy C, Kurinczuk JJ, Spark P, Brocklehurst P; UK Obstetric Surveillance System. A prospective national study of acute fatty liver of pregnancy in the UK. Gut 2008; 57:951–956.
Nelson-Piercy C. Handbook of Obstetric Medicine, 4th edn. London: Informa Healthcare; 2010.

7. C Continue with sulfasalazine and prednisolone but stop azithromycin or avoid breastfeeding.

Sulfasalazine can be found in breast milk so caution should be exercised with its use. Prednisolone can also be found in breast milk. Immune modifiers are secreted in breast milk; therefore they should be discontinued or the baby should be bottle-fed.

8. D 36%

This patient has severe appendicitis; the appendix has probably perforated. The severity of appendicitis determines fetal and maternal morbidity. Fetal loss has been quoted to be 1.5% with simple appendicitis, 6% with generalised peritonitis and 36% with a perforated appendix. Also, the risk of preterm delivery is increased 17 times with appendicitis during pregnancy. Because this is a acute surgical emergency, the patient needs a laparotomy which need to be performed jointly by the consultant surgeon and obstetrician.

Moroz P, Weston P. Appendicitis in pregnancy: how to manage and whether to deliver. Obstet Gynaecol 2015; 17:105–110.

9. A Oxygen, antibiotics, analgesia, prophylactic low molecular weight heparin

The diagnosis is sickle cell crises secondary to a chest infection. Therefore the management should be oxygen, antibiotics, analgesia and prophylactic low molecular weight heparin. This is not an acute chest syndrome, and therefore there is no need for an exchange transfusion. Thromboprophylaxis should be provided to all women with sickle cell disease who are admitted to the hospital. These women are also at high risk of thromboembolism. Appropriate advice, including an assessment of work and home conditions, should be given to reduce the risk of sickle cell crises. These women should avoid dehydration, overexertion and exposure to extreme temperatures.

10. B Stop chelation therapy, stop vitamin C, start folic acid 5 mg, continue penicillin

Iron chelation therapy is associated with an increased risk of teratogenicity so the patient should be advised to stop taking it. Vitamin C should be stopped because it is usually given with chelation therapy and the latter is being stopped. Folic acid 5 mg should be started to support haemopoeisis because the patient will have chronic anaemia. Penicillin is safe during pregnancy and should be maintained during the pregnancy because there is a risk of infection in view of the previous splenectomy. Thromboprophylaxis is not required antenatally unless additional risk factors are present, e.g. antiphospholipid syndrome or a history of venous thromboembolism. However, it should be given for 6 weeks after delivery.

Eissa A, Tuck S. Sickle cell disease and β-thalassaemia major in pregnancy. Obstet Gynaecol 2013; 15:71–78.

11. A α-Fetoprotein (α-FP), lactate dehydrogenase (LDH), β-human chorionic gonadotropin (β-hCG)

Some tumour markers can be elevated in pregnancy, and this should be borne in mind when undertaking or interpreting these tests. Lactate dehydrogenase, α-fetoprotein and β-hCG should be measured because these tumour markers are commonly high with ovarian tumours such as germ cell tumours, which are common in young women of reproductive age. CA-125 levels are usually high with epithelial cell tumours, which are commonly seen in postmenopausal women. C-reactive protein is non-specific and is therefore not useful in this situation; it is usually used as a marker of inflammation. CA-19.9 concentration is raised in colon and pancreatic cancer and is therefore not relevant here.

12. E Urgent ultrasound of the breast, and an antenatal clinic appointment with the consultant

The diagnosis of a lump can be difficult in a pregnant woman because of breast tissue proliferation and breast engorgement. If a woman presents with a lump in pregnancy, urgent ultrasound should be arranged to assess the nature of lump. The tissue diagnosis is made by ultrasound-guided biopsy for histology rather than cytology – cytology is usually inconclusive in pregnant women because of the proliferative changes of pregnancy. If a diagnosis of cancer is made, a mammogram should be performed, with fetal lead shielding, to assess the extent of the disease and assess the other breast. The patient should be managed by a multidisciplinary team including a designated breast care specialist nurse.

13. C Do not admit her, give labetolol, measure blood pressure twice a week, test for proteinuria at each visit with no further blood tests if there is no proteinuria

The management of pregnancy-induced hypertension is as follows:

- Mild hypertension (140/90 to 149/99 mmHg) – conservative management with weekly blood pressure measurement, test for proteinuria at each visit, and take routine antenatal bloods
- Moderate hypertension (149/99 to 150/109 mmHg)– outpatient management in the day assessment unit with oral labetolol, twice weekly blood pressure measurement and urine dipstick to check for proteinuria at each visit with no further blood tests if there is no proteinuria
- Severe hypertension (160/110 mmHg or higher) – patient must be admitted. Administer oral labetalol to control her blood pressure, blood pressure measurement four times a day, test for proteinuria daily, pre-eclampsia bloods at presentation and at-least weekly after that. But most of the time this will require early delivery

14. A Admit to hospital, do not treat the hypertension, measure blood pressure 4 times a day, do not repeat quantification for proteinuria, take blood tests twice weekly

The NICE recommendations for the management of pre-eclampsia in pregnancy are:

- Mild hypertension (140/90 to 149/99 mmHg) – admit to hospital, do not treat the hypertension, measure blood pressure 4 times a day, do not repeat quantification for proteinuria, and take blood tests twice weekly
- Moderate hypertension (149/99 to 150/109 mmHg) – admit, give labetolol, measure blood pressure 4 times a day, do not repeat quantification for proteinuria, and take blood tests 3 times a week
- Severe hypertension (160/110 mmHg or higher) – admit, give labetolol, measure blood pressure more than 4 times a day (depending on the clinical situation), do not repeat quantification for proteinuria, and do blood tests 3 times a week

15. A Active disease within 12 months but not within 6 months before conception

Systemic lupus erythematosus (SLE) does not usually affect fertility. The infertility is usually caused by high cumulative doses of cyclophosphamide which is used in treatment of SLE leading to ovarian failure. It can also be caused when there is end-stage renal failure from lupus nephritis. Non-steroidal anti-inflammatory drugs can also contribute to infertility by inhibiting cyclo-oxygenase, which in turn controls ovulation, leading to luteinised unruptured follicle syndrome.

One should also test for anti-Ro and anti-La antibodies as these can cause congenital heart block and neonatal cutaneous lupus syndrome.

Antiphospholipid antibodies are present in 30% of women with SLE and can cause arterial and venous thromboembolism, a small-for-gestational-age baby, fetal loss and premature labour. Women should be counselled regarding association of active disease in the 6 months prior to conception can have adverse effects on the pregnancy.

Cauldwell M, Nelson-Piercy C. Maternal and fetal complications of systemic lupus erythematosus. Obstet Gynaecol 2012; 14:167–174.

16. B Aspirin 75 mg once a day with or without low molecular weight heparin at a low prophylactic dosage

Antiphospholipid syndrome (APS) is an autoimmune condition and is associated with thromboembolic vascular episodes in life. It can affect organs including the heart, skin and central nervous system. With regards to obstetric outcomes, lupus anticoagulant is the most relevant assay to perform.

Treatment is not required when the patient has APS and does not have complications and had a previous normal pregnancy.

Treat with aspirin 75 mg once daily orally, plus low molecular weight heparin (LMWH) prophylactic dose is recommended in a patient with APS with history of recurrent miscarriage (3 or more consecutive miscarriages) or prior fetal death.

Treatment with aspirin 75 mg once daily orally, plus low molecular weight heparin (LMWH) intermediate dose is recommended in a patient with APS with history of thrombotic episode in the past.

Treatment with aspirin 75 mg once daily orally, plus low molecular weight heparin (LMWH) therapeutic dose is recommended in a patient with APS with history of recurrent thrombotic episodes.

Myers. B, Pavord S. Diagnosis and management of antiphospholipid syndrome in pregnancy. Obstet Gynaecol 2011; 13:15–21.

Answers: EMQs

17. G Human papilloma virus

Maternal genital warts are caused by human papilloma virus 6 and 11. The presence of genital warts during vaginal birth can transmit the virus to the baby and can cause laryngeal papillomas which obstruct the airway in the infant.

18. M Rubella

Rubella causes a triad of symptoms:

- Cardiac – patent ductus arteriosus, pulmonary artery stenosis, pulmonary valvular stenosis, coarctation of aorta, atrial septal defect and ventricular septal defect (the last two are rare abnormalities);
- Eye – congenital cataract;
- Ear – sensorineural deafness.

19. O Varicella

Congenital varicella infection causes limb hypoplasia, cutaneous scarring, hypoplastic digits, muscular atrophy, paralysis, seizures, microcephaly, chorioretinitis, chorioretinal scarring, optic disc hypoplasia, Horner's syndrome, cataracts, cerebral cortical atrophy, early childhood zoster and psychomotor retardation.

20. H Cytomegalovirus

Cytomegalovirus infection of the fetus can cause abnormalities which manifest in the early or late neonatal period. These include hepatosplenomegaly, jaundice, haemolytic anaemia, thrombocytopenia, growth restriction, microcephaly, chorioretinitis, optic atrophy, seizures, cerebral atrophy, psychomotor retardation, learning disabilities, dental abnormalities, pneumonitis and intracerebral calcifications.

21. O Varicella

Varicella affects the fetus in less than 2% of cases before 20 weeks' gestation. It causes various defects, including limb defects, but it usually manifests weeks later, before it can be identified on the ultrasound scan. Therefore, an ultrasound scan should be arranged 5 weeks after the date of presentation.

James D, Steer PJ, Weiner CP, Gonik B, Crowther C, Robson S (eds). High Risk Pregnancy: Management Options (4th edn). St Louis: Saunders, 2011.
Nelson-Piercy C. Handbook of Obstetric Medicine (4th edn). London: Informa Healthcare, 2010.

22. O Venlafaxine

If taken in high doses venlafaxine is associated with high blood pressure and an increased risk of withdrawal symptoms.

Tricyclic antidepressants

- Amitriptyline and imipramine are associated with lower risks in pregnancy
- No increase in incidence of miscarriage or malformation
- Associated with neonatal withdrawal syndrome and therefore, if possible, reduce the dose 3–4 weeks prior to delivery
- Can have an adverse synergistic effect if taken with multiple drugs or alcohol

Other drugs

- All antidepressants are associated with neonatal withdrawal symptoms. In most cases these effects are mild and self-limiting.
- Imipramine, nortriptyline and sertraline have lower levels in breast milk than other antidepressants.
- Citalopram and fluoxetine have higher levels in breast milk than other antidepressants

23. K Paroxetine

Selective serotonin reuptake inhibitors (SSRIs)

SSRIs are the most commonly used drugs for the treatment of depression. Data on the safety of SSRIs in human pregnancy are limited, but their use during pregnancy has shown to be associated with congenital heart defects in the fetus.

Important points include:

- Fluoxetine has the lowest risks.
- Paroxetine is associated with heart defects if taken during the first trimester, hence advise women to stop taking this drug.
- SSRIs can be associated with neonatal withdrawal syndrome, which includes convulsions, irritability, tremors, rigidity and feeding problems.
- Persistent pulmonary hypertension in the neonate if taken after 20 weeks' gestation (persistent pulmonary hypertension occurs in 1–2 infants per 1000 live births and is associated with increased morbidity and mortality. Despite treatment, 10–20% of affected infants will not survive. Newborns with this condition are typically full-term or near-term infants who present shortly after birth with severe respiratory failure requiring intubation and mechanical ventilation).
- SSRIs use in the first trimester is associated with an increased risk of anencephaly, craniosynostosis and omphalocele, specifically with use of paroxetine.
- Sertraline use is associated with omphalocele and septal defects.
- Paroxetine is associated with right ventricular outflow tract obstruction.

24. J Olanzapine

Antipsychotic associations

- Risperidone and sulpiride: raise prolactin levels
- Olanzapine: risk of gestational diabetes and weight gain
- Are associated with extra pyramidal symptoms in the neonate especially depot preparations. They are usually self-limiting

25. D Clozapine

The antipsychotic can cause agranulocytosis in the fetus and breastfed infants.

26. B Benzodiazepines

Benzodiazepines are used in anxiety disorders and panic attacks but should be not be used routinely except for the short-term treatment of extreme anxiety and agitation because of the risk of cleft palate and floppy baby syndrome in the neonate.

Louik C, Lin AE, Werler MM, Hernández-Díaz S, Mitchell AA. First-trimester use of selective serotonin-reuptake inhibitors and the risk of birth defects. N Engl J Med 2007; 356:2675–2683.
Alwan S, Reefhuis J, Rasmussen SA, Olney RS, Friedman JM. Use of selective serotonin-reuptake inhibitors in pregnancy and the risk of birth defects. N Engl J Med 2007; 356:2684–2692.
Chambers CD, Hernandez-Diaz S, Van Marter LJ, Werler MM, Louik C, Lyons Jones K, Mitchell AA. Selective serotonin-reuptake inhibitors and risk of persistent pulmonary hypertension of the newborn. N Engl J Med 2006; 354:579–587.

27. A Avoid amniocentesis in the third trimester

In women with HIV, amniocentesis should be avoided, particularly in the third trimester.

If invasive prenatal diagnosis is considered essential in HIV positive women, it should be undertaken under anti-retroviral treatment cover.

Invasive prenatal testing in the first or second trimester can be carried out in women who carry hepatitis B or C. However, the available data are limited and this should be explained to the patient.

The indications for third-trimester amniocentesis include:

- Late karyotyping
- Amniotic fluid optical density assessments for Rhesus disease
- Measure amniotic fluid insulin levels
- Lung maturity studies
- Detection of indices of infection in suspected pre-term labour or rupture of the membranes

The risk of emergency delivery does not appear to be high with third-trimester amniocentesis. However, complications such as multiple attempts and blood stained fluid are more common compared to mid-trimester procedures.

28. N Second-trimester amniocentesis

Amniocentesis

Early: before 14 completed weeks' gestation

Late: after 15 weeks' gestation

One of the main reasons for amniocentesis is to detect whether or not the fetus has a chromosomal disorder (e.g. Down's syndrome). The safest time to do an amniocentesis is after 15 weeks of pregnancy. However, one should counsel the woman about the risks, which include:

- Abdominal discomfort and vaginal spotting
- 1% risk of miscarriage, infection and leakage of amniotic fluid
- Inadequate first sample and need for reinsertion of the needle: about 8 in every 100 women having amniocentesis
- Serious infection: less than 1 in 1000 women who have amniocentesis
- Anti-D immunoglobulin injection is recommended for women who are Rhesus negative to prevent formation of antibodies against fetal red blood cells

It is recommended that early amniocentesis (before 14 weeks) should be avoided because it is associated with greater fetal loss compared with late amniocentesis (after 15 weeks) (7.6% vs. 5.9%).

Also, a 10-fold increase in fetal neonatal talipes is reported with early amniocenteses. However, the RCOG recommends that an early amniocentesis is undertaken in exceptional circumstances after the mother is counselled adequately and fully made aware of the potential complications.

There are two types of laboratory test used for the detection of chromosomal abnormalities:

- A full karyotype: usually takes 2–3 weeks for results
- A rapid test to check for specific chromosomes: usually takes 3 working days for results. This is used to detect Down's syndrome (trisomy 21), Edwards' syndrome (trisomy 18), Patau's syndrome (trisomy 13) and sex chromosome disorders.

29. E Chorionic villus sampling after 10 weeks

Chorionic villus sampling (CVS) is usually performed between 11 and 13 weeks and under ultrasound guidance (performed transvaginally between 11 and 13 weeks and transabdominally from 13 weeks onwards).

CVS before 10 weeks is associated with oromandibular hypoplasia and isolated limb disruption defects (attributed to transient fetal hypoperfusion and vasospastic phenomenon secondary to vascular disruption of the placental circulation). Therefore, CVS is not recommended before 10 completed weeks' gestation.

The risks of CVS include:

- Abdominal discomfort and vaginal bleeding
- Miscarriage: 2%
- A full karyotype may not give a clear result following CVS: about 1 in 100

- Serious infection: less than 1 in 1000 women who have CVS
- Anti-D immunoglobulin injection is recommended for women who are Rhesus negative to prevent formation of antibodies against fetal red blood cells

30. G Detailed fetal anomaly scan and fetal cardiac scan

Women should be appropriately counselled to make an informed choice. Following this, one should respect their decision and support her through the pregnancy. A detailed anomaly scan and fetal cardiac scan is important to check for abnormalities (since trisomy 21 is associated with gut and cardiac abnormalities) to inform and prepare them for delivery. Also, a multidisciplinary team should be involved to treat the child with abnormalities at birth (medical as well as surgical treatment).

31. B Amniocentesis of a single twin sac

Nuchal translucency is the screening test for trisomies performed for women with twin pregnancy. In monochorionic and diamniotic twins, amniocentesis of one twin sac is enough to make the diagnosis.

Royal College of Obstetricians and Gynaecologists (RCOG). Amniocentesis and chorionic villus biopsy. Green-top guideline no 8. London: RCOG; 2005.
Royal College of Obstetricians and Gynaecologists (RCOG). Amniocentesis: what you need to know (patient information leaflet). London: RCOG Press; 2006.
Royal College of Obstetricians and Gynaecologists (RCOG). Chorionic villus biopsy: what you need to know (patient information leaflet). London: RCOG Press; 2006.

32. K Down's syndrome

Oesophageal atresia

- Absence of stomach bubble or poor visualisation of the stomach
- Present after 25 weeks' gestation
- It is associated with chromosomal abnormalities in 20% of cases
- Mostly associated with Down's syndrome
- It is also associated with cardiac anomalies in 50% of cases

33. H Non-immune hydrops

Fetal tachyarrhythmia is one of the causes for non-immune hydrops. The mother should be urgently referred to a fetal medicine specialist for review as well as for a scan to confirm the findings.

Treatment for the fetus can be started in utero with maternal administration of drugs. Also, an urgent fetal echocardiogram should be performed to determine the rate and rhythm, and to rule out any cardiac abnormalities (because a cardiac cause is found in 30% of the cases of non-immune hydrops). The prognosis is better in the absence of structural cardiac abnormalities.

The poor prognosis and risk of intrauterine death if the fetus does not respond to treatment should be explained to the mother.

In this case, she is already at term, therefore delivery can be accomplished.

34. P Placental insufficiency

The clinical findings are suggestive of placental insufficiency. The CTG is pathological because there are recurrent unprovoked decelerations. She needs immediate Caesarean delivery because she is not in labour.

35. J Immune hydrops

The investigation reveals that this woman is Rhesus negative and has antibodies. If the antibody titre is 1:4, it is more likely to be due to administration of an anti-D immunoglobulin injection. However, if the titre is more than this (more than 1 in 4), it indicates rhesus isoimmunisation leading to hydrops fetalis.

36. I Idiopathic hydrops

When no cause is found for hydrops, it is labelled as idiopathic which accounts for one third of the cases of hydrops.

Magowan B. Churchill's Pocketbook of Obstetrics and Gynaecology (3rd edn). London: Churchill Livingstone; 2005.
James D, Steer PJ, Weiner CP, Gonik B, Crowther C, Robson S (eds). High Risk Pregnancy: Management Options (4th edn). Philadelphia: Saunders Elsevier; 2011.

37. I Meconium ileus

Hyperechogenic bowel is associated with cystic fibrosis, meconium ileus, cytomegalovirus infection, trisomy 21, fetal growth restriction and fetal death. Most cases are not clinically significant. However, it is important to screen for the cystic fibrosis gene (ΔF508 mutation), serum IgM for cytomegalovirus and karyotyping for aneuploidy. Because it is also associated with fetal growth restriction (8%) and intrauterine fetal death (23%), serial scans should be arranged.

38. L Patau's syndrome

Holoprosencephaly is a disorder in which the prosencephalon or the forebrain of the embryo fails to develop into two hemispheres. Other features include partially or completely fused thalami or ventricles (single ventricle), absence of cavum septi pellucidi, dysgenesis of the corpus callosum and associated midline facial abnormalities (with a single eye and midline proboscis in the region of the nose). The malformations of the brain are very severe and will lead to miscarriage or stillbirth.

It is usually associated with trisomy 13 and 18, triploidy and warfarin use during early pregnancy.

39. E Diaphragmatic hernia

Diaphragmatic hernia (incidence 1 in 2500) is difficult to diagnose on an ultrasound scan. The stomach in the chest or dextrocardia should raise a high suspicion of this condition. It is commonly associated with trisomy 18. In 85% of cases, it occurs on the left side and may cause mediastinal shift and pulmonary hypoplasia. The prognosis is bad when the liver is involved on the right side.

40. F Down's syndrome

Shortened long bones on ultrasound scan (especially the femur and humerus) are more likely seen in fetuses with Down's syndrome. The risk increases 11-fold if both the bones are short. The fetal growth restriction is symmetrical unlike babies with placental insufficiency which have an asymmetrical growth pattern (head sparing). It is important to consider performing karyotyping in the fetus with symmetrical fetal growth restriction to rule out chromosomal abnormalities.

41. F Down's syndrome

Duodenal atresia

- Double bubble sign is seen in duodenal atresia
- It is present after 25 weeks' gestation
- It is associated with chromosomal abnormalities in 40% of cases
- It is mostly associated with Down's syndrome
- It is also associated with cardiac anomalies in 50% of cases

Soft markers on the ultrasound scan in the fetus are usually transient features which may indicate a risk to the fetus in the form of chromosomal abnormalities. However, if they are found alone they may not pose any major problem or risk to the fetus. The most common soft markers include echogenic focus in the heart, hyperechogenic bowel, pelvicaliceal dilatation, choroid plexus cyst and short femur.

Choroid plexus cyst

- Incidence: 1–2% of fetuses in the second trimester scan
- Echolucent structures found in the choroid plexus of the lateral ventricles
- If it is an isolated finding, it does not have much significance. The majority (90%) of them disappear by 26 weeks' gestation
- If associated with other soft markers, chromosomal abnormalities need to be ruled out
- It is usually associated with trisomy 18, while the risk for trisomy 21 is not increased

Increased nuchal translucency

- It can be simple or septated
- The risk is higher with a septated pattern
- It is associated with increased risk of chromosomal abnormalities
- It is also associated with Turner's syndrome, Noonan's syndrome and Robert's syndrome
- It is associated with fetal cardiac abnormalities
- it is associated with increased perinatal mortality

Cardiac echogenic foci

- Hyperechogenicity is located in the chordate tendineae
- It resolves spontaneously in most cases
- The risk of chromosomal abnormalities is low
- If it is an isolated finding and there are no other risk factors, there is no need for invasive testing

Ventriculomegaly

- Incidence: 1% of pregnancies
- Lateral ventricular dilatation >10 mm
- It can be unilateral or bilateral
- It can be associated with chromosomal or congenital anomalies or may be an acquired condition due to infection and haemorrhage or may be unexplained
- Prognosis depends on associated chromosomal abnormalities or other defects.

James D, Steer PJ, Weiner CP, Gonik B, Crowther C, Robson S (eds). High risk pregnancy: management options (4th edn). St Louis: Saunders, 2011.
Connor JM. Medical Genetics for MRCOG and Beyond. London: RCOG Press, 2005.

42. I Commence 5 mg folic acid/day

Diabetic women during pregnancy are at high risk of congenital anomalies. NICE recommends 5 mg folic acid supplementation for these women during the first trimester instead of 0.4 mg.

43. I Commence 5 mg folic acid/day

Epilepsy and pregnancy

It is the most common neurological disorder in pregnant women with an incidence of 3–4 in 1000 pregnancies. Most women will not have problems with regards to seizures (60%). However, the seizure frequency can either decrease (10%), increase (30%) or remain the same during pregnancy (the risk of seizure is highest during labour and in the first 24 hours postpartum) (1–2%). The increase in seizure frequency is attributed to non-compliance with medication, hyperemesis, weight gain and altered pharmacokinetics.

The risk of congenital anomalies increases due to the antifolate action of anti-convulsants (phenytoin, phenobarbitone, sodium valproate and carbamazepine). Therefore, the principle of treatment during pregnancy is to maintain the lowest possible dose to control the seizures and mono-drug therapy instead of high doses and polydrug therapy. However, routine monitoring of drug levels in pregnancy is not recommended (monitor only if seizure frequency increases).

Sodium valproate particularly increases the risk of neural tube defects, orofacial clefts and congenital heart defects. The newer drugs levetiracetam, gabapentin and tiagabine are not teratogenic in animals. However, human data are sparse. Lamotrigine has a weak antifolate action (it inhibits dihydrofolate reductase) and therefore caries similar risk of teratogenesis to other mono-drug therapies.

Benzodiazepines (clonazepam) as an add-on therapy are not said to be teratogenic if used in monotherapy.

To avoid some of these risks to the fetus, it is recommended that these women take 5 mg folic acid daily during pregnancy. Risks to the fetus are as follows:

- Congenital malformations
- Fetal growth restrictions
- Increased perinatal mortality
- Increased risk of epilepsy (4–5% if one parent affected, 15–20% if both parents affected and 10% if one sibling affected)
- Neurodevelopment delay

Women with epilepsy should have consultant-led care in the hospital and should be seen in specialist clinics (neurology/obstetric joint clinic). Pain and anxiety should be avoided during labour with early recourse to epidural anaesthesia. Vaginal delivery is not contraindicated and a Caesarean section should be offered only for obstetric indications.

Breast feeding is not contraindicated and the baby should receive vitamin K at birth to prevent haemorrhagic disorders.

44. N Increase the dose of thyroxine

Hypothyroidism

- Incidence: affects 1% of pregnancies.
- Aetiology: is more common in women than men, with a positive family history in most women.
- Most cases are due to autoimmune destruction of the thyroid gland (autoimmune thyroiditis and Hashimoto's thyroiditis) indicated by the presence of antimicrosomal antibodies.
- It may be due to radioiodine therapy, surgical thyroidectomy or drug therapy (amiodarone, lithium, iodine and antithyroid drugs).
- Subacute de Quervain's thyroiditis and postpartum thyroiditis are causes of transient hypothyroidism.
- It is also associated with other autoimmune diseases such as type 1 diabetes mellitus, vitiligo and pernicious anaemia.
- Most women are already on treatment before conception.
- The fetus depends on maternal thyroid hormones until 12 weeks' gestation. Hence, adequate thyroid replacement therapy in early pregnancy is important. If pregnant women remain untreated, it increases the risk of miscarriage, fetal loss and low birth weight. Reduced intelligence quotient (IQ) and neurodevelopmental delay have also been reported in the offspring of undertreated mothers (especially in the first and second trimesters).
- Neonatal hypothyroidism is a rare condition (incidence 1 in 80,000) caused by transplacental transfer of TSH receptor-blocking antibodies. It is more commonly seen in women with atrophic rather than Hashimoto's thyroiditis. One should suspect diagnosis in the presence of fetal goitre. The Guthrie heel prick test is used as a screening test to identify the condition in newborn babies.

- In the mother, the disease should be optimised or controlled prior to conception, with dose adjustments in the first trimester to ensure adequate treatment (one should be cautious because TSH levels increase in the first trimester and hence thyroxine should not be increased unless treatment is confirmed by low serum T4 levels). If the woman is already on an adequate dose, thyroid function should be checked at least once in each trimester. However, if the dose is adjusted (increased or decreased) at any time during pregnancy, thyroid function should be checked every 4–6 weeks.
- Overall, women will require an increase in dose by almost 20–30% as the pregnancy progresses. The aim is to achieve a TSH level of 2.5 mU/L or less. If untreated or uncontrolled it can cause anaemia (due to inadequate stimulation of red blood cell development in the bone marrow) and pre-eclampsia.
- Postpartum thyroiditis affects 1% of women and usually presents within 1 year of childbirth. Its aetiology is generally unknown although it is attributed to having an autoimmune origin and is more common in diabetics. These women initially present with hyperthyroidism (lasts for 1–3 months) with one third progressing to hypothyroidism (lasts for about 9–12 months). Also, 20% of these will continue to be hypothyroid. The risk of recurrence is reported to be 20%. The treatment for hypothyroidism is thyroxine and treatment for hyperthyroidism is β-blockers, because this is a temporary phase.

45. K Commence 10 mg oral vitamin K

Daily supplementation of vitamin K until delivery is recommended for women with obstetric cholestasis in view of the theoretical risk of postpartum haemorrhage (PPH) and haemolytic disease in the newborn.

46. G Change therapy to oral carbimazole

Hyperthyroidism

- Incidence: 0.2% of pregnant women.
- Causes: Graves' disease (90%), toxic multinodular goitre, toxic nodule, hyperemesis gravidarum and hydatidiform mole.
- Symptoms: the physiological symptoms of pregnancy (palpitation, heat intolerance and increased metabolic rate) mimic symptoms of hyperthyroidism, making diagnosis difficult. The most sensitive symptoms for diagnosis include failure to gain weight despite adequate appetite, tremor and persistent resting tachycardia.
- Treatment: propylthiouracil or carbimazole block the thyroid hormone synthesis and reduce TSH receptor antibody levels.
- Fetus: both of the above drugs cross the placenta and are secreted in breast milk (propylthiouracil less than carbimazole) and can therefore cause fetal goitre and hypothyroidism in high doses. Neonatal thyrotoxicosis (usually transient) can occur in 1% of babies (if untreated the mortality is 30%) due to stimulation of fetal thyroid by maternal antibodies crossing the placenta. Other risks to the fetus include prematurity, fetal growth restriction and stillbirth.

- Mother: if the condition is not treated or well-controlled, there is an increased risk of pre-eclampsia and heart failure.
- Monitoring: thyroid function should be measured every 4–6 weeks during pregnancy and free T4 levels should be kept at the upper limit of their normal values.
- Role of surgery: surgery is rarely required in pregnancy. It is indicated if there is retrosternal extension of goitre causing pressure symptoms, if women are not responding to medical therapy or if women develop serious adverse effects with medical therapy (surgery should be performed during the second trimester).

Nelson-Piercy C. Handbook of Obstetric Medicine (4th edn). London: Informa Healthcare, 2010.
Anthony K and Nelson-Piercy C. Obstetric cholestatis. Personal assessment in continuing education. Reviews, questions and answers. Volume 3. London: RCOG Press, 2003: 48–49.
Royal College of Obstetricians and Gynaecologists (RCOG). Obstetric cholestasis. Green-top guideline no. 43. London: RCOG; 2006.

Chapter 9

Management of labour

Questions: SBAs

For each question, select the single best answer from the five options listed.

1. A 26-year-old woman attends antenatal clinic at 28 weeks' gestation. She has had one previous pregnancy 2 years ago, which ended in a Caesarean section after failure to progress beyond 6 cm cervical dilatation. Her current body mass index is 30 kg/m^2. She would like know the likelihood of having a successful vaginal delivery should she try for one this time.

    What is the likelihood of her achieving a vaginal birth after having had a Caesarean section?

    A   38%
    B   40%
    C   50%
    D   72%
    E   82%

2. You are the specialist registrar on the labour ward and have been asked to see a patient who appears to have been previously subjected to female genital mutilation. She did not disclose this during antenatal clinic appointments. On examination, you find that there is total removal of the clitoris and labia minora, but no excision of the labia majora.

    According to the RCOG's classification, what type of female genital mutilation is this?

    A   Type 1
    B   Type 2
    C   Type 3
    D   Type 4
    E   Type 5

3. You are the specialist registrar covering the labour ward. A 23-year-old patient had a history of female genital mutilation with a deinfibulation at 25 weeks' gestation. You have just been informed that she is now insisting that you reinfibulate her because otherwise she will not be accepted back into her society.

What action will you take?

A   Do not perform reinfibulation
B   Discuss the situation with the consultant
C   Reinfibulate the woman
D   Ask the midwife to reinfibulate the woman
E   Call the police

4. A 28-year-old woman is pregnant for the second time and is currently at 30 weeks' gestation. She delivered her first child after an obstructed labour and Caesarean section in India. A pelvimetry report from India states that she has a platypelloid pelvis.

In a pelvimetry report, what is the measurement between the sacral promontory and the top of the symphysis pubis called?

A   Biparietal diameter
B   Diagonal conjugate
C   Interspinous diameter
D   Obstetric conjugate
E   True conjugate

5. You are the specialist registrar on the labour ward. An American woman on holiday in the UK has had an emergency admission with contractions. She is 37 weeks pregnant. Her previous labour involved a difficult forceps delivery in the USA. She shows you the results of a pelvimetry scan performed in the USA. These show an oval-shaped pelvis in which the anteroposterior diameter at the pelvic inlet is greater than the transverse diameter. When you examine her, the baby is lying occipitoposterior.

What shape of pelvis does this patient have?

A   Android
B   Anthropoid
C   Platypelloid
D   Androgenous
E   Gynecoid

6. A 40-year-old primiparous woman has attended the labour ward at 40 weeks' gestation. She had a normal vaginal delivery in her last pregnancy, with no concerns over the baby. A vaginal examination reveals her to be 6-cm dilated and whilst she is being examined, the membranes rupture spontaneously. You are called by the midwife because the patient says that she was diagnosed with group B *Streptococcus* (GBS) during her last pregnancy.

   What is the best management plan?

   A   Take a swab to screen for GBS but do not treat until the results are available
   B   Take a swab to screen for GBS and treat anyway
   C   Treat with antibiotics intravenously during labour
   D   Treat with antibiotics orally during labour
   E   Do not screen for GBS and do not give antibiotics

7. You are the specialist registrar on the labour ward and have been asked to review a patient who is 40 weeks pregnant. She is in labour, with cervical dilatation of 5 cm and spontaneous rupture of membranes. She tells you that her previous baby suffered with a neonatal group B streptococcal infection and was admitted to the neonatal unit for antibiotic treatment. When you review the notes, two vaginal swabs during this pregnancy were negative for group B *Streptococcus*.

   How will you manage this patient?

   A   Give intrapartum intravenous antibiotics
   B   Give oral antibiotics
   C   Do not take any action
   D   Take a vaginal swab and await the results
   E   Take a vaginal swab and then start intravenous antibiotics

8. You are the specialist registrar on the labour ward and think one of your patients might benefit from rescue cervical cerclage. She is currently 25 weeks pregnant. Her previous child has cerebral palsy secondary to a hypoxic injury at birth. She asks you how long a pregnancy will be prolonged by cervical cerclage.

   On average, how long is a pregnancy prolonged by the insertation of a rescue cervical cerclage?

   A   1 week
   B   3 weeks
   C   5 weeks
   D   7 weeks
   E   9 weeks

9. A 25-year-old primigravid woman attends the maternity triage unit complaining of mild lower abdominal pain. She is 29 weeks pregnant and has so far been considered to have a low-risk pregnancy. Cardiotocography shows fetal tachycardia of 190 bpm. Observations reveal maternal tachycardia (pulse 110 bpm) and raised temperature (37.7°C). Her respiratory rate and oxygen saturation are normal. The patient gives a history of cough for the previous week, but she has not been concerned by this. Chest examination is clear. Abdominal examination has not revealed contractions or tenderness. Speculum examination reveals 4 cm cervical dilatation with bulging membranes. Blood test results are awaited.

What is the most appropriate next step in management?

A   Expectant management
B   Perform amniocentesis to look for chorioamnionitis
C   Start antibiotics and undertake rescue cerclage
D   Start antibiotics and rupture the fetal membranes
E   Start antibiotics

10. A 25-year-old parous woman attends the labour ward with uterine contractions once every 5 minutes. She is currently 31 weeks pregnant. On examination, the uterine contractions are palpable and the cervix is 2 cm dilated. There are no signs of spontaneous rupture of membranes or vaginal bleeding. The neonatal unit does not have cots and is closed. You are considering transferring her to another hospital's neonatal unit. In the meantime, after a discussion with the on-call consultant, you decide to start tocolysis.

Which of the following will you use?

A   Atosiban
B   Albuterol
C   Magnesium sulphate
D   Nifedipine
E   Ritodrine

11. As the specialist registrar, you have been called to the labour ward to see a patient who is 30 weeks pregnant and is complaining of palpitations, headache, vomiting, chest pain and shortness of breath. She tells you that she was given a tablet 30 minutes ago but does not know its name.

Which one of the following medications has caused these symptoms?

A   Atosiban
B   Albuterol
C   Magnesium sulphate
D   Nifedipine
E   Ritodrine

12. A 35-year-old woman who is 32 weeks pregnant presents with a 3-day history of vaginal leakage of watery fluid. She has no abdominal pain and is otherwise well. She has so far had a low-risk pregnancy, and fetal growth is normal. On examination, the abdomen is soft and non-tender.

What is the best way to confirm that she has spontaneous rupture of membranes?

A   Amniocentesis
B   Microscopic examination of vaginal fluid
C   Nitrazine test
D   Speculum examination
E   Ultrasound

13. A 35-year-old woman who is 32 weeks pregnant presents with a 3-day history of vaginal leakage of watery fluid. She has no abdominal pain and is otherwise well. The pregnancy is low risk, and fetal growth is normal. Observations are normal. On examination, the abdomen is soft and non-tender. You confirm that that the waters have broken.

What is the subsequent management?

A   Antibiotics and steroids
B   Antibiotics, steroids and weekly full blood count, C-reactive protein concentration and weekly high vaginal swabs
C   Antibiotics, steroids and weekly full blood count and C-reactive protein concentration
D   Ultrasound to confirm the diagnosis
E   Weekly full blood count and weekly high vaginal swabs

14. As the labour ward specialist registrar, you have just delivered a baby by Caesarean section at 33 weeks' gestation because the mother has severe pre-eclampsia. The mother is doing well but is upset that her baby has been admitted to the neonatal unit. She asks you what chance there is of developing severe pre-eclampsia in her next pregnancy.

What is the risk of this woman developing pre-eclampsia in her next pregnancy?

A   5%
B   10%
C   15%
D   20%
E   25%

15. Which one of the following conditions should trigger referral of a pregnant woman to a level 3 care unit?

A   Abnormal neurology
B   Eclampsia
C   Evidence of cardiac failure
D   Need for ventilation
E   Severe oliguria

Questions: EMQs

Questions 16–20

Options for Questions 16–20

A   Artificial rupture of membranes
B   Augmentation with oxytocin
C   Acyclovir – oral
D   Acyclovir – intravenous
E   Acyclovir – intravenous followed by oral
F   Consider vaginal delivery
G   Elective Caesarean section at term
H   Emergency Caesarean section
I   Forceps delivery

J   Fetal blood sampling
K   Termination of pregnancy (as long as it is legal in this region)
L   Type specific herpes simplex virus (HSV) antibody testing
M   Symptomatic therapy
N   Swabs for virology
O   Screen for other sexually transmitted infections plus oral acyclovir

Instructions: For each clinical scenario described below, choose the single most appropriate initial management plan from the list of options above. Each option may be used once, more than once or not at all.

16. A 20-year-old pregnant woman presents at 35 weeks' gestation with a primary genital herpes infection. She is generally fit and well. She is worried about the implications for the baby because she has read about neonatal herpes on the internet.

17. A 30-year-old woman presents at 39 weeks' gestation with a primary active genital herpes infection. She gives a history of labour pains for the last 4 hours. Vaginal examination reveals a 2 cm dilated cervix and intact membranes.

18. A 35-year-old pregnant woman presents with a history of recurrent herpes at term. She is contracting twice in 10 minutes on abdominal examination, and vaginal examination reveals a 6 cm dilated cervix with intact membranes.

19. A 32-year-old pregnant woman presents to the labour ward at term with a primary genital herpes infection. She is contracting four times in 10 minutes and is currently 4 cm dilated. She declines Caesarean section.

20. A 29-year-old woman comes to the day assessment unit with painful vesicles on the genital area. She is currently 16 weeks pregnant and clinical examination reveals a primary genital herpes infection.

Questions 21–25

Options for Questions 21–25

A   Apply a fetal scalp electrode
B   Facial oxygen therapy
C   Continue oxytocin
D   Continuous electronic fetal monitoring
E   Fetal scalp electrode application to monitor fetus
F   Fetal blood sampling (FBS) contraindicated

G   Forceps delivery
H   Intravenous 0.5 mg ergometrine
I   Intrauterine fetal blood transfusion
J   Intravenous fluids
K   Left lateral position
L   Perform FBS
M   Repeat FBS in 30 minutes
N   Reduce the rate of oxytocin
O   Subcutaneous 0.25 mg terbutaline

Instructions: For each scenario described below, choose the single most appropriate initial management from the list of options above. Each option may be used once, more than once, or not at all.

21. A 34-year-old woman with three children presents to the labour ward at 40 weeks' gestation with regular contractions. She makes good progress up to 8 cm cervical dilatation but does not progress further. Oxytocin is started at 2 mL/hour for augmentation. A CTG reveals a normal baseline heart rate, variability >5 bpm and with variable decelerations where the baseline drops by 60 bpm, with over 50% of contractions for the last 30 minutes. The tocograph suggests that she is contracting seven times in 10 minutes. The midwife calls you to review the CTG because you are the on-call labour ward registrar for the night.

22. A 34-year-old primigravid woman is admitted to the antenatal ward for induction of labour at 41 weeks' gestation. She has her first prostin at 0800 hours and was reassessed at 1400 hours for artificial rupture of membranes (ARM). A second prostin is inserted due to a poor Bishop score. She is put back on the CTG for fetal monitoring. One hour later CTG shows a fetal heart rate of 160 bpm and variable decelerations. A tocograph shows seven contractions in 10 minutes.

23. A 34-year-old woman with three children attends the labour ward at 40 weeks' gestation with regular contractions. Booking (her first midwife appointment) blood tests reveal she is positive for hepatitis B (low risk for fetal transmission). She was 4 cm at admission but did not progress further. ARM was performed but revealed thick meconium-stained liquor. She was then augmented by oxytocin and 4 hours later, had progressed to 8 cm cervical dilatation. Currently, the CTG reveals a baseline of 170 bpm, variability <5 bpm, for 90 minutes but no accelerations or decelerations.

24. A 34-year-old multiparous woman attends the labour ward at 41 weeks' gestation with regular contractions and spontaneous rupture of membranes (SROM). She is admitted to the high-risk side on the labour ward for continuous fetal monitoring in view of high parity and meconium staining of liquor. 4 hours later she has progressed to 9 cm cervical dilatation. FBS is performed at this stage because her CTG is pathological according to NICE criteria. The FBS results show pH 7.26 and BE –0.3 mEq/L. Thirty minutes later the midwife informs you that the CTG has remained the same.

25. A 34-year-old parous woman attends the labour ward at 40 weeks' gestation with SROM. She was discharged home to return in 24 hours for induction of labour. Twenty-four hours (0800 hours) later she returned contracting with a 4 cm cervical dilatation. She progresses to 8 cm cervical dilatation at next vaginal examination (1200 hours). However, the CTG reveals a baseline FHR of 165 bpm, variability 5 bpm, occasional acceleration and variable decelerations dropping from the baseline by 50 bpm and taking 45 seconds to recover, with more than 50% of contractions, for the last 90 minutes.

Answers: SBAs

1.   B 40%

The success rate of a vaginal birth after Caesarean section (VBAC) is 72–75%. The best predictor of successful VBAC is a previous vaginal delivery, in particular a previous VBAC. The success rate can be as high as 85–90%, but induced labour, no history of a previous vaginal delivery, a BMI greater than 30 and a previous Caesarean for labour dystocia collectively can bring the success rate down to as low as 40%. The advantages of an elective repeat Caesarean section is that the woman can be given a planned delivery date, although this may change according to clinical circumstances.

Royal College of Obstetricians and Gynaecologists (RCOG). Birth after previous Caesarean birth. Green-top guideline no. 45. London: RCOG; 2015.

2. B C Type 3 2

There are 4 types of female genital mutilation:

- Type 1: complete or partial removal of the clitoris and/or prepuce
- Type 2: complete or partial removal of the clitoris and labia minora, with or without removal of the labia majora
- Type 3: narrowing of the vaginal orifice created by a seal. The seal is made by cutting the labia minora, with or without the labia majora, and opposing the sides. The clitoris may or may not be excised
- Type 4: all other procedures on the genitalia for non-medical purposes, including pricking, piercing, scraping, etc.

Royal College of Obstetricians and Gynaecologists (RCOG). Female genital mutilation and its management. Green-top guideline no. 53. London: RCOG; 2015.

3.   A Do not perform reinfibulation

Under the UK Female Genital Mutilation Act 2003 and the Female Genital Mutilation (Scotland) Act 2005, it is illegal to perform or assist with female genital mutilation (FGM). It is also an offence for parents to fail to protect a daughter from FGM. When a woman who has undergone FGM is identified, the health-care professional must explain UK law. In the UK, the professional must also explain that the patient's details will be submitted to the Health and Social Care Information Centre FGM Enhanced Dataset, but this is not mandatory in Scotland. Reinfibulation is illegal and must not be undertaken in any circumstance.

Royal College of Obstetricians and Gynaecologists (RCOG). Female genital mutilation and its management. Green-top guideline no. 53. London: RCOG; 2015.

4.   E True conjugate

There are three anterior–posterior diameters: the true conjugate, the diagonal conjugate and the obstetric conjugate. The true conjugate is measured from the sacral promontory to the top of the symphysis pubis. It usually measures 11 cm or more. The diagonal conjugate runs from the lower border of the symphysis pubis to the sacral promontory and measures 11.5 cm or more. At only 10 cm or more, the obstetric conjugate is the shortest pelvic diameter through which the fetal head must pass during birth. It is measured from the sacral promontory to the thickest part of the pubic bone.

5. B Anthropoid

The gynaecoid pelvis has a round pelvic inlet, a shallow pelvic cavity and short ischial spines. It is the ideal pelvis for delivery. The anthropoid pelvis has an oval-shaped inlet, a large anterior–posterior diameter and a comparatively smaller transverse diameter. The diameters of the inlet favour engagement of the head in an occipitoposterior position, which can slow labour. The android pelvis has a heart-shaped inlet and a narrow transverse outlet diameter. It is more common in Afro-Caribbean women. The inlet of a platypelloid pelvis has a narrow anterior–posterior diameter. The pelvic cavity is shallow and the outlet is favourable for labour.

6. E Do not screen for group B *Streptococcus* (GBS) and do not give antibiotics

If group B *Streptococcus* (GBS) was detected in the previous pregnancy, there is a 38% chance of carriage in the current pregnancy. The risk of neonatal early-onset GBS disease is therefore 0.9 cases/1000 births, compared with a background risk of 0.5 cases/1000 births. As a result, neither screening nor antibiotics are needed. The predictors of repeat colonisation are the time between two pregnancies and the intensity of colonisation.

Royal College of Obstetricians and Gynaecologists (RCOG). The prevention of early onset neonatal group B streptococcal disease. Green-top guideline no. 36. London: RCOG; 2012.

7. A Give intrapartum intravenous antibiotics

This infant is more likely to be infected with GBS disease. The potential increased risk is probably due to the presence of low levels of maternal anti-GBS antibodies. Swabs are not helpful, and intrapartum antibiotics are recommended even if results are negative.

Royal College of Obstetricians and Gynaecologists (RCOG). The prevention of early onset neonatal group B streptococcal disease. Green-top guideline no. 36. London: RCOG; 2012.

8. C 5 weeks

On average, rescue cerclage delays delivery for up to 5 weeks compared with expectant management. There are limited data on whether neonatal morbidity and mortality improve after insertion of a cervical stitch. Evidence shows that insertion of a cervical suture has been associated with a possible twofold reduction in risk of delivery before 34 weeks' gestation. Women should also be informed that cerclage is not associated with prolonged premature rupture of membranes, induction of labour, Caesarean section, preterm delivery or second-trimester loss. However, it is associated with bladder damage, rupture of membranes, and cervical bleeding secondary to cervical trauma.

Royal College of Obstetricians and Gynaecologists (RCOG). Cervical cerclage. Green-top guideline no. 60. London: RCOG; 2011.

9. E Start antibiotics

This woman may have chorioamnionitis, so rescue cerclage is contraindicated. Blood tests will check for raised concentrations of inflammatory markers, which help to confirm the diagnosis. Other contraindications to cerclage include:

- Continuous vaginal bleeding
- Prolonged preterm rupture of membranes
- Cardiotocograph abnormalities
- Intrauterine death
- Fetal abnormality
- Preterm labour

Cerclage is associated with a rise in maternal temperature but no increase in chorioamnionitis. Routinely performing amniocentesis prior to rescue cerclage is not recommended because it does not improve outcome. The prognosis is poor if chorioamnionitis is present.

Royal College of Obstetricians and Gynaecologists (RCOG). Cervical cerclage. Green-top guideline no. 60. London: RCOG; 2011.

10. A Atosiban

Atosiban is the drug of choice for tocolysis for preterm labour. The other drug licensed in the UK is ritodrine. In this case, atosiban is the treatment of choice because it has fewer side effects than ritrodrine. Although nifedipine can be given orally and is more cost-effective, it is not licensed for this use in the UK.

Royal College of Obstetricians and Gynaecologists (RCOG). Tocolysis for women in preterm labour. Green-top guideline no. 1b. London: RCOG; 2011.
National Institute of Clinical Excellence (NICE). Preterm labour and birth [NG 25]. Manchester: NICE; 2015

11. E Ritodrine

β-agonists are associated with an increased frequency of adverse side effects compared with nifedipine, atosiban and cyclo-oxygenase inhibitors. Use of multiple tocolytic drugs also causes even more side effects and should therefore be avoided. The best choice of tocolytic drug is the one with fewest side effects in both the long and the short term. Although ritodrine was widely used in the past, compliance is noted to be poor because of its side effects. It can cause life-threatening pulmonary oedema leading to maternal death. The side effects of nifedipine are flushing, palpitations, vomiting and hypotension .

Royal College of Obstetricians and Gynaecologists (RCOG). Tocolysis for women in preterm labour. Green-top guideline no. 1b. London: RCOG; 2011.

12. D Speculum examination

The diagnosis of spontaneous rupture of membranes is best diagnosed by taking a history and performing a speculum examination. Ultrasound can help to confirm the diagnosis in selected cases. All the other tests, including examination for lanugo hair and fetal epithelial cells, are unnecessary.

Royal College of Obstetricians and Gynaecologists (RCOG). Preterm prelabour rupture of membranes. Green-top guideline no. 44. London: RCOG; 2015.

13. A Antibiotics and steroids

Weekly high vaginal swabs and blood tests do not need to be performed. The mainstay of treatment should be erythromycin for 10 days and steroids.

Royal College of Obstetricians and Gynaecologists (RCOG). Preterm prelabour rupture of membranes. Green-top guideline no. 44. London: RCOG; 2015.

14. E 25%

If the baby was delivered at less than 34 weeks' gestation due to severe pre-eclampsia, there is a 25% risk of severe pre-eclampsia occurring in the next pregnancy. If the birth was before 28 weeks, the chance of severe pre-eclampsia in the next pregnancy is 1 in 2 (55%). The chance of moderate pre-eclampsia during the subsequent pregnancy is 1 in 6 (16%).

National Institute for Health and Care Excellence (NICE). Hypertension in pregnancy: the management of hypertensive disorders during pregnancy [CG107]. London: NICE; 2011.

15. D Need for ventilation

The following require level 1 care:

- Pre-eclampsia with mild or moderate hypertension
- Step-down treatment after the birth
- Continued treatment of severe pre-eclampsia

The following require level 2 care:

- Eclampsia
- Haemolysis, elevated liver enzymes, low platelets (HELLP) syndrome
- Haemorrhage
- Severe oliguria
- Evidence of cardiac failure
- Abnormal neurology
- Stabilisation of severe hypertension
- Coagulation support
- Hyperkalaemia

The following requires level 3 care:

- Severe pre-eclampsia needing ventilation

National Institute for Health and Care Excellence (NICE). Hypertension in pregnancy: the management of hypertensive disorders during pregnancy [CG107]. London: NICE; 2011.

Answers: EMQs

16. O Screen for other sexually transmitted infections plus oral acyclovir

Primary genital herpes infection during pregnancy

Genital herpes is caused by herpes simplex virus (HSV) type 1 and type 2 DNA virus, and is sexually transmitted. The incubation period is 7 days.

Women presenting with primary genital herpes should be referred to the genito-urinary clinic to screen for other sexually transmitted infections (STIs) and should be treated with oral acyclovir for 5 days (200 mg 5 times a day) in order to reduce the severity and duration of symptoms and duration of viral shedding. However, it should be used with caution before 20 weeks.

One can also consider daily suppressive therapy with oral acyclovir from 36 weeks' gestation to reduce the likelihood of recurrent herpes simplex infection (evidence is lacking). Viral cultures can be offered at late gestation to predict the risk of viral shedding if the primary genital herpes infection was reported in the first and second trimesters.

If a woman presents with primary genital herpes within 6 weeks of the expected date of delivery, then maternal intravenous intrapartum acyclovir plus intravenous acyclovir to the newborn baby should be considered to reduce the risk of neonatal herpes.

All women presenting with primary herpes simplex infection within 6 weeks of the expected date of delivery or at delivery should be offered Caesarean section (the highest risk to the fetus is within 6 weeks following primary genital herpes infection). However, there is no need for a Caesarean section for women presenting with primary herpes simplex infection in the first and second trimesters.

The risk of transmission of an STI to the fetus is:

- 30–60% if primary infection is within 6 weeks of delivery
- 3% in recurrent infection
- 1–3% if seropositive for HSV type 1 and HSV type 2
- less than 1% if no visible lesions

Investigation and diagnosis of primary genital herpes include:

- clinical: women characteristically present with painful vesicles or ulcerations on the genitalia and urinary retention
- laboratory: type specific HSV antibody testing with IgG is not recommended during pregnancy because it is not fully evaluated
- viral cultures: direct detection of genital HSV by swabs from the base of the ulcer, fluid sample following de-roofing the vesicle (PCR testing)

17. H Emergency Caesarean section

Neonatal herpes is caused both by HSV type 1 or type 2 and mostly occurs due to direct contact with maternal genital secretions when the baby is passing through the birth canal at delivery. It is a rare condition but is associated with high morbidity and mortality (30% if disseminated infection and 6% with local central nervous system infection). The prognosis is good if only the eyes, mouth and skin are involved.

The following factors influence fetal transmission from mother to baby:

- whether the infection is primary or recurrent
- the presence of maternal neutralising antibodies (antibody transfer to the baby before birth but does not prevent the neurogenic viral spread to the brain of the neonate)
- the duration of the rupture of membranes before delivery (deliver as soon as possible if PROM)
- the use of fetal scalp electrodes or fetal blood sampling; and mode of delivery

The risk to the fetus is high (neonatal infection) if the woman acquires primary genital herpes in the third trimester (<6 weeks of delivery, as viral shedding may persist and the baby is likely to be born before the transfer of passive immunity from the mother). Therefore, if the primary infection occurs at the time of labour, or within 6 weeks of the expected date of delivery, Caesarean section is recommended for all women.

18. F Consider vaginal delivery

Recurrent genital herpes during pregnancy

With recurrent genital herpes, the risk of transmission to the fetus is much lower than with primary genital herpes and therefore Caesarean section is not routinely recommended for such women (Caesarean section is not indicated if episodes of recurrent herpes occur during the antenatal period). However, women should be counselled about the 3% risk of neonatal herpes with recurrent herpes during labour (Caesarean section can be performed if the woman wishes after weighing the risks of Caesarean section versus the risks of fetal transmission of infection). One may consider daily suppressive oral acyclovir from 36 weeks' gestation onwards in anticipation of reducing the recurrent herpetic lesions at term [especially in human immunodeficiency virus (HIV) patients but otherwise not routinely indicated].

There is no need for viral cultures or type-specific HSV antibody testing in women with recurrent herpes. Acyclovir is rarely indicated in the treatment of genital herpes. However, if the woman's partner has active genital herpes, she should be advised to avoid sexual intercourse (the use of condoms is not fully protective against acquiring infection).

19. D Acyclovir – intravenous

Precautions during labour

For women wishing to deliver vaginally the following should be avoided: fetal blood sampling or fetal scalp electrode application during labour, delay or avoid artificial rupture of membranes and the neonatologist should be involved before delivery for neonatal care.

Intravenous administration of acyclovir to the mother during labour and the baby after birth should be considered to reduce the risk of neonatal herpes.

20. M Symptomatic therapy X ⟶ Treat (Oct 2014 RCOG)

Symptomatic and supportive therapy is the main form of treatment (analgesics and sitz baths). Acyclovir should be used with caution before 20 weeks' gestation. Admission to hospital and bladder catheterisation may be required in women presenting with severe pain and retention of urine. One should also be vigilant regarding the symptoms and signs of encephalitis and disseminated infection.

Royal College of Obstetricians and Gynaecologists (RCOG). Management of genital herpes during pregnancy. Green-top guideline no. 30. London: RCOG Press, 2007.

21. N Reduce the rate of oxytocin

In this case, the fetal heart rate (FHR) is suspicious and hyperstimulating on oxytocin. Only four or five contractions are expected for the labour to progress. Therefore, the dose of oxytocin should be reduced.

The NICE recommendations are:

- If the FHR trace is normal, oxytocin may be continued until the woman is experiencing four or five contractions every 10 minutes. Oxytocin should be reduced if contractions occur more frequently than five contractions in 10 minutes.
- If the FHR trace is classified as suspicious, conservative measures should be taken. The left lateral position should be adopted, the syntocin should be stopped to reduce the frequency of the contractions. The patient should be reviewed by an obstetrician and the coordinating midwife.
- If the FHR trace is classified as pathological, oxytocin should be stopped and a full assessment of the fetal condition undertaken by an obstetrician before oxytocin is recommenced.

22. O Subcutaneous 0.25 mg terbutaline

In the presence of abnormal FHR patterns and uterine hypercontractility not secondary to oxytocin infusion, tocolysis should be considered. A suggested regimen is subcutaneous terbutaline 0.25 mg which can be repeated every 15 minutes if necessary.

23. F Fetal blood sampling contraindicated

In this woman, the scenario describes the booking (her first midwife appointment) blood tests results as low risk for infection on hepatitis screening. This means she is negative for hepatitis 'e' antigen and positive for anti-e antibody. Women who are at high risk on hepatitis screening would be positive for e antigen and negative for anti-e antibody.

Contraindications to fetal blood sampling (FBS) include:

- maternal infection: HIV, hepatitis viruses and herpes simplex virus
- fetal bleeding disorders: haemophilia, low platelet disorders
- prematurity: less than 34 weeks

24. M Repeat FBS in 30 minutes

In this case the midwife informs you 30 minutes after the FBS that the CTG has remained the same as before. Therefore, FBS needs to be repeated in 30 minutes and this will be 1 hour from the previous normal FBS.

NICE recommends the results of FBS should be interpreted carefully, taking into account previous pH measurements, the rate of progress in labour and the clinical features of the woman and baby.

The interpretation of a FBS result (pH) is:

- ≥7.25 – normal FBS result
- 7.21–7.24 – borderline FBS result
- ≤7.20 – abnormal FBS result

FBS should be performed when fetal compromise is suspected (which is interpreted on CTG as pathological):

- After a normal FBS result, sampling should be repeated no more than 1 hour later if the FHR trace remains pathological, or sooner if there are further abnormalities
- After a borderline FBS result, sampling should be repeated no more than 30 minutes later if the FHR trace remains pathological, or sooner if there are further abnormalities. The time taken to take a fetal blood sample needs to be considered when planning repeat samples
- If the FHR trace remains unchanged and the FBS result is stable after the second test, a third/further sample may be deferred unless additional abnormalities develop on the trace
- Where a third FBS is considered necessary, a consultant obstetrician's opinion should be sought

25. L Perform FBS

In this case the CTG shows two non-reassuring features (which is by definition considered to be a pathological CTG). Therefore, FBS should be performed.

The NICE definitions of normal, suspicious and pathological FHR traces are:

- Normal – an FHR trace in which all four features are classified as reassuring
- Non-reassuring – an FHR trace with one feature classified as non-reassuring and the remaining features classified as reassuring
- Abnormal – an FHR trace with two or more features classified as non-reassuring or one or more classified as abnormal

National Institute of Health and Clinical Excellence (NICE). Intrapartum care for health women and babies [CG190]. London: NICE; 2016.

Chapter 10

Management of delivery

Questions: SBAs

For each question, select the single best answer from the five options listed.

1. A 40-year-old woman had one previous normal vaginal delivery at the age of 17 years and one maternally requested a Caesarean section at the age of 38 years. She is currently 28 weeks pregnant. She is not sure if she wants to try for a vaginal delivery or have an elective Caesarean section. She wants to know what her chance of death is if she has a Caesarean section.

    What are the chances of this patient dying if she has a Caesarean section?

    A   1/100,000
    B   5/100,000
    C   11/100,000
    D   13/100,000
    E   15/100,000

2. A 35-year-old woman had an elective Caesarean section 4 years ago for a breech presentation. She is now 36 weeks pregnant in her second pregnancy. She would like to try for a vaginal birth after Caesarean section (VBAC). She wants to know what risk her baby has of developing hypoxic ischaemic encephalopathy or brain damage after a VBAC.

    What is the risk of the baby developing hypoxic ischaemic encephalopathy or brain damage after a VBAC?

    A   2/10,000
    B   4/10,000
    C   8/10,000
    D   10/10,000
    E   15/10,000

3. You are the labour ward registrar and have been called to review a woman who is 33 weeks pregnant. She has presented with a history of vaginal bleeding for the previous 2 hours. She has twice attended the maternity day assessment unit with a similar complaint, but the bleeding is heavier this time. Examination reveals uterine contractions occurring every 4 minutes and a cephalic presentation. There is no dizziness or shortness of breath. A review of the notes and obstetric scan findings suggest that the placenta is covering the os. Observations reveal a pulse of 98 bpm, blood pressure 110/62 mmHg, respiratory rate 20 breaths per minute, oxygen saturation of 97% on air and a normal temperature.

    What is the most appropriate course of action?

    A   Caesarean section
    B   Intravenous access, blood tests and give fluids
    C   Tocolysis and steroids
    D   Reassure and observe her
    E   Transfer her to another unit

4. A 32-year-old Afro-Caribbean woman is booked for an elective Caesarean section at 38 weeks' gestation for placenta accreta.

    Which one of the following is not included in the care bundle for placenta praevia accreta?

    A   A consultant obstetrician planning and directly supervising delivery
    B   Blood and blood products available
    C   Multidisciplinary involvement in preoperative planning
    D   Discussion and consent to include possible interventions (e.g. hysterectomy, leaving the placenta in place, cell salvage, interventional radiology)
    E   Local availability of a level 1 critical care bed

5. You are the labour ward on-call registrar for the night. In early hours of the morning, a 33-year-old Asian woman with a body mass index of 43 kg/m² has a vaginal delivery. The baby weighs 4 kg. An emergency buzzer is sounded because the woman is bleeding vaginally. When you enter the room, the midwife tells you she gave the mother 5 IU of Syntocinon intramuscularly after the baby had been delivered but the bleeding has continued. On examination, the uterus is atonic, the placenta is reported to be complete and there is a second-degree perineal tear that is bleeding minimally. You provide all medical treatment as per protocol, taking into account is the patient's asthma. She continues to bleed and has now lost about 1500 mL of blood.

    What is the appropriate management?

    A   Balloon tamponade
    B   Bilateral ligation of the uterine arteries
    C   Bilateral ligation of the internal iliac (hypogastric) arteries
    D   Haemostatic brace suturing (e.g. B-Lynch or modified compression sutures)
    E   Selective arterial embolisation

6. You are the overnight on-call registrar for the labour ward and have been called to review a 34-year-old Afro-Caribbean woman who has failed to progress beyond 7 cm cervical dilatation. She has been induced because of gestational diabetes and her body mass index is 43 kg/m². You obtain her consent and undertake a Caesarean section. After delivery of the baby and placenta, the uterus is atonic. Medical management is given in accordance with the labour ward's protocol, taking into account that she has asthma. You note that when you perform bimanual compression the uterine bleeding reduces, but as soon as you stop the compression the bleeding increases.

    What is the appropriate next step in management?

    A   Balloon tamponade
    B   Bilateral ligation of the uterine arteries
    C   Bilateral ligation of the internal iliac (hypogastric) arteries
    D   Haemostatic brace suturing (e.g. B-Lynch or modified compression sutures)
    E   Selective arterial embolisation

7. A nulliparous woman has progressed well in labour. She is now fully dilated and has only used medical nitrous oxide and oxygen mixture for pain relief. Because the fetal head was felt to be high on vaginal assessment, she was given an hour for the fetal head to descend, after which she was allowed to push. She now has pushed for 2 hours but not yet delivered the baby. You are the labour ward specialist registrar and have been called to review her. On examination, the cervix is 10 cm dilated and the head is in the occipitoanterior position at the level of the ischial spines. There is no moulding or caput.

    What is your management?

    A   Allow her to push for a further 1 hour
    B   Undertake an emergency Caesarean section
    C   Take a fetal blood sample in case the fetus is distressed
    D   Undertake an instrumental delivery in the labour ward room
    E   Try a trial of instrumental delivery in theatre

8. A nulliparous woman has progressed well in labour. She is now fully dilated and has an epidural in situ for pain relief. As the fetal head was high above the spines, she was given 2 hours for the head to descend in the pelvis, after which she was allowed to push. She has now pushed for 1 hour but not yet delivered the baby. You are the labour ward specialist registrar and have been called to review her. Examination reveals 10 cm cervical dilatation. The head is in the occipitoanterior position at the level below the spine. There is no caput or moulding on the fetal head.

    What is your management?

    A   Allow her to push for a further 1 hour
    B   Perform an emergency Caesarean section
    C   Take a fetal blood sample in case the fetus is distressed
    D   Undertake an instrumental delivery in the labour ward
    E   Try a trial of instrumental delivery in theatre

9. You are the labour ward registrar and have been called to the low-risk pregnancy, midwife-led birth centre to review a woman who has been fully dilated for the last 3 hours. She is primigravid and has completed 2 hours of passive stage and 1 hour of pushing. You examine her on the labour ward. The fetal head is at station +2 and in the occipitoanterior position. There has been good descent of the fetal head with pushing.

What is the best course of action?

A   Allow her to push for a further 1 hour
B   Perform an emergency Caesarean section
C   Take a fetal blood sample in case the fetus is distressed
D   Undertake instrumental delivery on the labour ward
E   Try a trial of instrumental delivery in theatre

10. A 30-year-old multiparous woman has been advised to stay on labour ward rather than go to the birth centre because her membranes ruptured more than 24 hours previously. She has been fully dilated for 1 hour, during which she has been pushing. She is using Entonox for pain relief. As the specialist registrar, you have been called to review her because the fetal head is still not visible at the perineum. On examination, the cervix is fully dilated and the fetal head is 1 cm below the ischial spines in the occipitoanterior position. There is no caput or moulding. There has been good descent of the fetal head with pushing.

What is your management?

A   Allow her to push for a further 1 hour
B   Perform an emergency Caesarean section
C   Take a fetal blood sample in case the fetus is distressed
D   Undertake instrumental delivery on the labour ward
E   Try a trial of instrumental delivery in theatre

11. A 29-year-old multiparous woman was admitted in spontaneous labour. The pregnancy so far had been low risk. She wishes to have epidural analgesia so was brought to the labour ward. She was examined by you, the specialist registrar, on admission. Labour assessment revealed cervical dilatation of 10 cm with the fetal head in occipitotransverse position at the level of the ischial spines. There was no caput or moulding. The passive stage was allowed 2 hours to facilitate descent of the fetal head, and oxytocin was given via a drip because of poor contractions. After 2 hours, the fetal head was still at station +1 and still in the occipitotransverse position with no caput or moulding. You ask her to start pushing, but after 1 hour the baby has still not been delivered.

What is your management?

A   Allow her to push for a further 1 hour
B   Perform an emergency Caesarean section
C   Take a fetal blood sample in case the fetus is distressed
D   Undertake instrumental delivery on the labour ward
E   Try a trial of instrumental delivery in theatre

12. A 40-year-old woman gave birth to her fifth child 15 minutes ago. She suddenly complains of shortness of breath, and in the next few minutes after delivery she collapses. The blood pressure is 70/30 mmHg, oxygen saturation is 88% on air and pulse is 75 bpm. Her arms have started to twitch, and there is heavy bleeding vaginally.

What is the likely cause of the collapse?

A   Amniotic fluid embolism
B   Cardiac disease
C   Haemorrhage
D   Pre-eclampsia/eclampsia
E   Sepsis

13. You are the labour ward specialist registrar and hear an emergency buzzer from room 2. The occupant is a 23-year-old primigravida who has so far had a low-risk pregnancy. An epidural cannula is in situ, and the cervix was 5 cm dilated 1 hour ago. You find that the patient has collapsed and the anaesthetist is intubating her. As you are trying to feel a pulse, you are informed that she had an epidural top-up 2 minutes ago.

What is the cause of the collapse?

A   Amniotic fluid embolism
B   Respiratory arrest
C   Haemorrhage
D   Pre-eclampsia/eclampsia
E   Sepsis

14. You are the overnight on-call registrar on the labour ward and have been called to review a 24-year-old South Asian woman who has failed to progress beyond 9 cm cervical dilatation. She has been induced because of gestational diabetes and her body mass index is 47 kg/m². You obtain her consent and undertake a Caesarean section. After delivery of the baby and placenta, the uterus is atonic. You decide to perform a B-Lynch brace suture.

Which suture material is used when placing a B-Lynch brace suture?

A   Poliglecaprone 25 (1.0)
B   Poliglecaprone 25 (2.0)
C   Polypropylene
D   Polyglactin 910 (1.0)
E   Polyglactin 910 (2.0)

15. A 40-year-old primigravid woman who is currently 37 weeks pregnant is in labour. Labour has progressed well, and vaginal examination reveals that her cervix is dilated 10 cm. The fetal head is 2 cm below the ischial spines and in an occipitoanterior position. Her blood pressure is 170/110 mmHg. 50 mg of labetolol is given intravenously and 20 mg of nifedipine is given orally, but the blood pressure remains high at 160/100 mmHg.

How will you manage her?

A　Administer hydralazine
B　Administer more nifedipine and labetolol
C　Continue to check the blood pressure every 5 minutes and perform a urine dipstick examination
D　Continue to monitor the blood pressure every 5 minutes and deliver the baby instrumentally
E　Deliver the baby by Caesarean section

16. A 32-year-old primigravid woman had an emergency Caesarean section at 39 weeks' gestation because of failure to progress in labour at 5-cm cervical dilatation with oxytocin augmentation for 8 hours. During closure of the parietal peritoneum, a 2-cm bladder injury was noted.

When was the bladder most likely to have been injured during this procedure?

A　During closure of the uterine incision
B　During entry into the peritoneal cavity
C　During dissection of the bladder from the lower uterine segment
D　When closing the visceral peritoneum
E　When securing the uterine angles

Questions: EMQs

Questions 17–21

Options for Questions 17–21

A   Break both the clavicles
B   Delivery of the posterior arm
C   Elective Caesarean section
D   Emergency Caesarean section
E   Episiotomy
F   Fundal pressure
G   Lovset manoeuvre
H   McRoberts' position and suprapubic pressure

I   Rubin manoeuvre
J   Reverse Wood screw manoeuvre
K   Get the patient to roll over onto all fours
L   Symphysiotomy
M   Suprapubic pressure
N   Wood screw manoeuvre
O   Zavanelli procedure

Instructions: For each clinical scenario described below, choose the single most appropriate management option from the list of options above. Each option may be used once, more than once, or not at all.

17. A 30-year-old woman with two children attends the antenatal clinic at 37 weeks' gestation to discuss mode of delivery. She had her last delivery 2 years ago and gives a history of a difficult forceps delivery following which her child developed Erb's palsy.

18. A 30-year-old primiparous woman (vaginal delivery), presents to the labour ward at 42 weeks' gestation with regular contractions. Clinically, the baby appears bigger than 4 kg (her previous child weighed 3.9 kg). She progresses quickly until 7 cm cervical dilatation but subsequently takes 8 hours to progress to full dilatation. A vaginal examination reveals an occipito-posterior position of the fetus with presenting part at +1 station. A turtle sign is noted following delivery of the head.

19. A 42-year-old primigravid woman presents to the labour ward with spontaneous labour at 38 weeks' gestation. She is a type 2 diabetic on insulin. Her last scan at 36 weeks' gestation revealed an estimated fetal weight of 3.7 kg. During labour she needed oxytocin augmentation to progress to full dilatation 2 hours after pushing, she had a spontaneous vaginal delivery with the head on the perineum. An emergency buzzer is pulled by the midwife. On entering the room, you observe the patient is in McRoberts' position and the midwife is giving traction to the fetal head.

20. A 30-year-old primiparous woman presents to the labour ward at 40 weeks' gestation with a spontaneous onset of labour. Clinically, it is difficult to assess the size of the baby because her body mass index is 41 kg/m^2 (growth scan at 36 weeks' gestation revealed an estimated fetal weight of 3.8 kg). 10 hours later she starts a vaginal delivery but the midwife puts out an obstetric crash call after noticing a turtle sign. The registrar attends and tries all the possible named rotational manoeuvres following McRoberts' position but fails to deliver the impacted shoulders.

21. A 30-year-old Asian woman presents to the labour ward at 40 weeks' gestation with spontaneous onset of labour. She is unbooked (she has had no prior appointments, scans or blood tests) and clinically the baby appears big. Her blood sugar level is 10.1 mmol/L. She progresses slowly to full dilatation after 18 hours. The registrar is called in anticipation of shoulder dystocia. The head is delivered and there is an obvious turtle sign. An obstetric crash call is put out. All the manoeuvres are tried including removal of the posterior arm but these fail to deliver the impacted shoulder.

Questions 22–26

Options for Questions 22–26

A   Antenatal corticosteroids
B   Antenatal glucocorticoids and antibiotics
C   Antenatal corticosteroids plus antibiotics plus inpatient monitoring for 48–72 hours
D   Emergency cervical cerclage
E   Elective cervical cerclage
F   Immediate induction of labour with the aim of vaginal delivery plus intravenous antibiotics
G   Immediate delivery by Caesarean section plus intravenous antibiotics
H   Prophylactic tocolysis and intravenous antibiotics
I   Prophylactic tocolysis plus antenatal corticosteroids plus intrauterine transfer
J   Reasonable to deliver at 34 weeks' gestation or after
K   Transabdominal amnioinfusion
L   Transvaginal amniocentesis
M   Tocolysis and antenatal corticosteroids
N   Tocolysis

Instructions: For each scenario described below, choose the single most appropriate initial management from the list of options above. Each option may be used once, more than once, or not at all.

22. A 34-year-old multiparous woman presents to the labour ward with a gush of fluid through the vagina at 26 weeks' gestation. A speculum examination by the on-call registrar confirms a spontaneous rupture of membranes. Abdominal examination reveals no uterine activity. Clinically, she feels well and her vital signs are normal.

23. A 40-year-old multiparous woman presents to the labour ward with a history of premature rupture of membranes (PROM) at 29 weeks' gestation. She complains of regular uterine contractions coming every 3 minutes. Speculum examination confirms a rupture of membranes and her cervix appears to be 3 cm dilated. Clinically, there are no signs of chorioamnionitis.

24. A 38-year-old multiparous woman attends her antenatal clinic appointment at 35 weeks' gestation. She gives a history of PROM at 24 weeks' gestation. Abdominal examination reveals cephalic presentation with no signs of chorioamnionitis. An ultrasound scan reveals oligohydramnios. Her inflammatory markers are normal.

25. A 40-year-old multiparous woman attends the obstetric day assessment unit with reduced fetal movements at 32 weeks' gestation. A cardiotocograph (CTG)

reveals a normal baseline, variable deceleration with reduced variability and no acceleration. Abdominal examination reveals a cephalic presentation and vaginal examination reveals a 2 cm cervical dilatation. An ultrasound scan confirms the cephalic presentation but also reveals severe oligohydramnios. She is tachypnoeic and tachycardic with spiking temperatures of 38°C. A review of her notes indicates that she had PROM at 28 weeks' gestation.

26. A 40-year-old multiparous woman attends the obstetric day assessment unit at 35 weeks' gestation. She gives a history of PROM at 30 weeks' gestation following which she received erythromycin for 10 days. She feels well in herself and her vital signs are normal. However, her blood test results reveal a raised white blood cell count (19,000/mm^3) and C-reactive protein (104 mg/L). An ultrasound examination reveals cephalic presentation with some liquor around the baby. A fetal cardiotocograph is normal.

Answers: SBAs

1. D 13/100,000

Caesarean section carries several risks:

- The risk of maternal death with a planned vaginal birth after Caesarean section (VBAC) is 4/100,000
- The risk of maternal death with an elective repeat Caesarean section (ERCS) is 13/100,000
- The risk of uterine rupture with VBAC is 1/200 (0.5%). This is associated with increased maternal morbidity and fetal morbidity/mortality
- The risk of uterine rupture with ERCS (<0.02%) is less than with VBAC
- ERCS also reduces the risk of pelvic organ prolapse and urinary incontinence in comparison with vaginal birth (in the short but not the long term)

Royal College of Obstetricians and Gynaecologists (RCOG). Birth after previous Caesarean birth. Green-top guideline no. 45. London: RCOG; 2015.

2. C 8/10,000

The risk of hypoxic ischaemic encephalopathy with vaginal birth after Caesarean section (VBAC) is 8/10,000, and with elective repeat Caesarean section (ERCS) <1/10,000 . The risk of instrumental delivery increases by 39% with VBAC compared with ERCS.

The risk of fetal transient respiratory morbidity is 2–3% with VBAC and increase to 4–5% with ERCS. Performing the Caesarean section at 38 rather than 39 weeks' gestation increases the risk to 6%, hence the use of antenatal corticosteroids.

With VBAC, the absolute risk of birth-related perinatal death is very low, comparable to the risk for a nulliparous woman in labour (10/10,000, i.e. 0.1%). The risk of delivery-related perinatal death is 4/10,000 (0.04%), again comparable to that for a nulliparous woman in labour.

Royal College of Obstetricians and Gynaecologists (RCOG). Birth after previous Caesarean birth. Green-top guideline no. 45. London: RCOG; 2015.

3. A Caesarean section

This woman has placenta praevia and is actively bleeding. The first line of action should be establishing intravenous access and fluids and taking blood samples for a full blood count, and cross-match 2 units of blood. However, the most appropriate course of action should be a Caesarean section. Tocolysis is useful in selected cases of bleeding caused by placenta praevia, but further research is needed on this. This patient is at high risk of having a postpartum haemorrhage so preparations should be made in theatre to anticipate this.

Royal College of Obstetricians and Gynaecologists (RCOG). Placenta praevia, placenta praevia accreta and vasa praevia: diagnosis and management. Green-top guideline no. 27. London: RCOG; 2011.

4. E Local availability of a level 1 critical care bed

Severe morbidity is associated with a placenta praevia and previous Caesarean section, or an anterior placenta on an old scar. A care bundle has been created to address this situation. It has six aspects that are uncontroversial, practical and achievable:

- A consultant obstetrician present
- A consultant anaesthetist
- Blood and blood products available
- Preoperative multidisciplinary involvement
- Consent to other possible interventions (e.g. hysterectomy)
- Local availability of level 2 critical care bed

Royal College of Obstetricians and Gynaecologists (RCOG). Placenta praevia, placenta praevia accreta and vasa praevia: diagnosis and management. Green-top guideline no. 27. London: RCOG; 2011.

5. A balloon tamponade

A postpartum haemorrhage of 500–1000 mL should promote basic resuscitation. A postpartum haemorrhage of 1000 mL with continued bleeding (or primary signs of shock) should trigger a protocol of measures to achieve haemostasis and resuscitation. If pharmacological measures fail to control the bleeding, a surgical approach should be taken. In this situation, intrauterine balloon tamponade is the appropriate first-line 'surgical' intervention, because atony is the main cause of the bleeding.

Royal College of Obstetricians and Gynaecologists (RCOG). Prevention and management of postpartum haemorrhage. Green-top guideline no. 52. London: RCOG; 2016.

6. D Haemostatic brace suturing (e.g. B-Lynch or modified compression suture)

If pharmacological measures fail to stop the bleeding, surgical measures are required. In this situation, a brace suture is appropriate as the patient has an atonic uterus at the time of the Caesarean section. Haemostatic sutures are effective in controlling a postpartum haemorrhage and help to avoid hysterectomy.

Royal College of Obstetricians and Gynaecologists (RCOG). Prevention and management of postpartum haemorrhage. Green-top guideline no. 52. London: RCOG; 2016.

7. E Try a trial of instrumental delivery in theatre

A nulliparous woman with no epidural in place should deliver within 3 hours of full dilatation. Higher rates of failure are associated with:

- Body mass index >30 kg/m^2
- Estimated fetal weight >4000 g
- Occipitoposterior position
- Mid-cavity delivery or a head that is one fifth palpable abdominally

Therefore only low and outlet instrumental deliveries should be conducted in the labour ward room. A low delivery occurs when the leading point of the skull is at a station of +2 cm or more; an outlet delivery occurs when the fetal scalp is visible without separating the labia.

National Institute for Health and Care Excellence (NICE). Intrapartum care for healthy women and babies. [CG190]. London: NICE; 2017.
Royal College of Obstetricians and Gynaecologists. Operative vaginal delivery. RCOG Green-top guideline no. 26. London: RCOG; 2011.

8. A Allow her to push for a further 1 hour

A nulliparous woman who has an epidural in place is allowed up to 4 hours in the second stage. In this situation, the patient can continue to push for a further 1 hour.

National Institute for Health and Care Excellence (NICE). Intrapartum care for healthy women and babies. [CG190]. London: NICE; 2017.

9. D Undertaken instrumental delivery on the labour ward

Because this woman is a primigravida, she is allowed 3 hours to deliver without an epidural. Because there have been 2 hours of descent of the fetal head and 1 hour of pushing, delivery should be expedited. The head is low so delivery can be performed in the labour ward room.

National Institute for Health and Care Excellence (NICE). Intrapartum care for healthy women and babies. [CG190]. London: NICE; 2017.

10. A Allow her to push for a further 1 hour

A multigravida is allowed 2 hours to deliver after full dilatation. has been identified. Although the fetal head is low in this case, there is no indication for carrying out an instrumental delivery.

National Institute for Health and Care Excellence (NICE). Intrapartum care for healthy women and babies. [CG190]. London: NICE; 2017.

11. E Try a trial of instrumental delivery in theatre

It is recommended that a multigravida who has an epidural in place should deliver within 3 hours of full dilatation being identified. Because the baby's position is occipitotransverse, an instrumental delivery should be undertaken in theatre.

National Institute for Health and Care Excellence (NICE). Intrapartum care for healthy women and babies. [CG190]. London: NICE; 2017.

12. A Amniotic fluid embolism

The incidence of amniotic fluid embolism (AFE) is 2/100,000 and the survival rate is 80%. It is associated with sever neurological morbidity. Perinatal mortality is 135/1000 total births. AFE manifests as maternal collapse during delivery or within

30 minutes. It is associated with hypotension, hypoxia, respiratory distress, seizures and haemorrhage. If an AFE occurs prior to delivery, there is profound acute fetal distress. In non-fatal cases, the diagnosis is made clinically, and there is no accurate pre-mortem test.

Royal College of Obstetricians and Gynaecologists (RCOG). Maternal collapse in pregnancy and puerperium. Green-top guideline no. 56. London: RCOG; 2011.

13. B Respiratory arrest

This patient is having a cardiac arrest secondary to a high-positioned epidural. With an incorrectly place epidural, the mother can develop a respiratory and subsequently a cardiac arrest. Cardiac arrest is rare in pregnancy (1/30,000). More common causes of cardiac disease in pregnancy include myocardial infarction, aortic dissection and cardiomyopathy. The incidence of congenital and rheumatic heart disease is rising in pregnancy, secondary to improved management of congenital heart disease and immigration in the UK.

Royal College of Obstetricians and Gynaecologists (RCOG). Maternal collapse in pregnancy and puerperium. Green-top guideline no. 56. London: RCOG; 2011.

14. A Poliglecaprone 25 (1.0)

Monocryl is the suture of choice for B-Lynch brace sutures.

Royal College of Obstetricians and Gynaecologists (RCOG). Prevention and management of postpartum haemorrhage. Green-top guideline no. 52. London: RCOG; 2016.

15. D Continue to monitor the blood pressure every 5 minutes and deliver the baby instrumentally

Blood pressure should be measured continually. If it has been controlled so that it falls within the target range, delivery need not be expedited and the mother can be allowed to push. If the blood pressure has not been controlled, delivery should be expedited.

National Institute for Health and Care Excellence. Hypertension in pregnancy: the management of hypertensive disorders during pregnancy [CG107]. London: NICE; 2011.

16. B During entry into the peritoneal cavity

In a primary Caesearean section, most bladder injuries occur during peritoneal entry. In a repeat Caesearean section, the majority occur during dissection of the bladder from the lower uterine section (i.e. when creating the bladder flap).

Field A, Haloob R. Complications of Caesarean section. Obstet Gynaecol 2016; 18:265–272.

Answers: EMQs

---

17. C Elective Caesarean section

Shoulder dystocia

- Failure to deliver the shoulders following delivery of the fetal head (>60 seconds)
- Problem: inlet
- Incidence: 0.5–2% of all vaginal deliveries
- Prediction: difficult to predict or prevent

Risk factors for shoulder dystocia are:

- D – Diabetes
- O – Obesity, operative vaginal deliveries
- P – Prolonged labour (although labour progresses normally in 70% of cases)
- E – Estimated fetal weight >4 kg (although 50% occur in babies weighing <4 kg)
- S – Previous shoulder dystocia and prolonged second stage

Epidural analgesia is not associated with an increased risk of shoulder dystocia.

The incidence of recurrent shoulder dystocia is reported as being between 1 and 16%. A Caesarean section may be considered for a previous history of severe shoulder dystocia with a poor outcome. The approach should be individualised and the decision should be made by the woman and her carers.

---

18. H McRoberts position and suprapubic pressure

Delivery is accomplished in 90% of cases by simple measures such as the McRoberts position and suprapubic pressure.

In this procedure the mother is placed in the supine position, the hips are abducted, and the hips and knees are flexed. This straightens the lumbosacral curvature and moves the symphysis superiorly, therefore releasing the anterior shoulder from behind the pubic symphysis. It increases the pelvic anteroposterior diameters by 1 cm.

---

19. M Suprapubic pressure

Suprapubic pressure should be tried following gentle traction and the McRobert position.

This is done with the flat of an assistant's hand behind the anterior shoulder (it is recommended to stand the side of the baby's back or fetal spine). This promotes adduction of the anterior shoulder and releases it from the symphysis pubis. It also reduces the bisacromial diameter. The initial pressure should be continuous and if there is no success after 30 seconds, a rocking motion should be tried. However, either of the two can be used.

20. B Delivery of the posterior arm

Rotational manoeuvres (Rubin, Wood screws and reverse Wood screws) promote the disimpaction of the shoulders from the pelvic inlet. These procedures normally push the shoulders into the oblique diameter of the pelvis (which is the larger diameter) and hence promotes the release of the anterior shoulder. It is recommended to use gentle neck traction and maternal pushing after every attempt of rotation. If the rotational manoeuvres fail, then go for the posterior arm without delay.

21. K Get the patient to roll over onto all fours

Asking the mother to get on all fours may help with delivery. If this fails, the Zavanelli procedure should be used.

The Zavanelli procedure is rarely used in the management of shoulder dystocia. It is used as a last resort following failure of all other measures. The head is replaced with constant pressure (the palm of the hand is used) in order to flex the head and push it into the pelvis. Delivery of the head is then accomplished by Caesarean section.

Royal College of Obstetricians and Gynaecologists (RCOG). Green-top Guideline No. 42. Shoulder dystocia. London: RCOG Press, 2005.
Neill AC, Thornton S. Shoulder dystocia. Pace review No. 2/4 (B). Volume 3. London: Royal College of Obstetricians and Gynaecologists Press, 2003: 55–57.

22. C Antenatal corticosteroids plus antibiotics plus inpatient monitoring for 48–72 hours

Women with PROM are at increased risk of going into labour within 24 hours. Hence, antenatal corticosteroids should be considered. The RCOG recommends erythromycin (250 mg orally 6-hourly) for 10 days for women with a confirmed diagnosis of pre-term premature rupture of membranes (PPROM).

Women with PPROM should be monitored as outpatients only if facilities are available for rigorous monitoring. The risk of uterine infection is increased, especially in the first 3–7 days following PROM, hence the woman would need initial inpatient monitoring followed by outpatient monitoring once infection is ruled out. As part of outpatient monitoring, she should be observed for signs of chorioamnionitis. Also, weekly high vaginal swabs need not be performed. Maternal full blood counts and C-reactive protein have low sensitivity to detecting intrauterine infection and therefore need not be undertaken on a weekly basis. One should make sure that women are educated about the symptoms and signs of chorioamnionitis, so that they can report immediately if they are unwell.

A CTG should be performed because fetal tachycardia is used in the definition of clinical chorioamnionitis. A biophysical profile score and Doppler velocimetry can be carried out but women should be informed that these tests are of limited value in predicting fetal infection.

23. M Tocolysis and antenatal corticosteroids

The risk of respiratory distress syndrome (RDS) is increased at 29 weeks' gestation and decreases with increasing gestational age. The neonatal admission rate is also increased during early gestation. The main aim is to decrease the risk of RDS and this can be achieved by giving antenatal corticosteroids. PPROM in itself is not a contraindication for administering antenatal corticosteroids. Tocolysis may be considered in women with PPROM who have uterine activity and would need either antenatal glucocorticoids or intrauterine transfer.

24. J Reasonable to deliver at 34 weeks' gestation or after

PPROM complicates 2% of pregnancies and is associated with 40% of pre-term deliveries. It can be associated with increased neonatal morbidity and mortality. The main causes of death associated with PPROM include prematurity, sepsis and pulmonary hypoplasia. For the mother, it carries risk of chorioamnionitis. In women with PPROM, about one third of pregnancies have positive amniotic fluid cultures. However, there is insufficient data to recommend amniocentesis as a modality for diagnosing infection.

Women with PPROM should receive erythromycin for 10 days and antenatal corticosteroids should be given to increase fetal lung maturity. Tocolysis is not routinely recommended in these women because this treatment does not significantly improve perinatal outcome.

In women with PPROM, delivery should be considered at 34 weeks' gestation because continuing pregnancy after this point may put women at risk of chorioamnionitis. If expectant management is considered beyond 34 weeks' gestation, one should balance the risk of uterine infection for the mother versus respiratory problems in the neonate, admission to neonatal intensive care and the increased risk of Caesarean section.

25. G Immediate delivery by Caesarean section plus intravenous antibiotics

If neonatal facilities are available the woman can be kept in the same hospital. However, if these facilities are not available she can be delivered and then transferred out to a different unit because the chances of survival at 32 weeks' gestation are high. The CTG findings (atypical variable decelerations) indicate fetal hypoxia and are categorised as pathological. Amnioinfusion is not recommended for such women with PPROM. This woman needs delivery in view of clinical findings of chorioamnionitis. The delivery should be expedited, hence delivery by Caesarean section.

26. F Immediate induction of labour with the aim of vaginal delivery plus intravenous antibiotics

In this case the signs (inflammatory markers are raised) are suggestive of subclinical chorioamnionitis, hence delivery is indicated. If the cervix is favourable, induction of labour and vaginal delivery can be considered.

Royal College of Obstetricians and Gynaecologists (RCOG). Preterm prelabour rupture of membranes. Green-top guideline no 44. London: RCOG Press; 2010.

Chapter 11

Postpartum problems (the puerperium)

Questions: SBAs

For each question, select the single best answer from the five options listed.

1. A 39-year-old woman had a Caesarean section 3 days ago. The oncology team has recommended tamoxifen because she has a previous history of breast cancer. The woman and the baby are doing well, and the baby is being breastfed.

    How should this patient be managed?

    A   The patient should continue breastfeeding and tamoxifen
    B   The doctor should liaise with the oncology team
    C   Tamoxifen should be stopped
    D   Advise the patient to stop breastfeeding
    E   Tamoxifen should be stopped and the patient should be advised to stop breastfeeding

2. A 33-year-old primiparous woman presents to the labour ward at 4 a.m. with heavy vaginal bleeding and some abdominal pain. She had a low-risk pregnancy and gave birth by normal vaginal delivery 5 days ago. On examination, you think you see small amounts of tissue at the cervical os, but you are unsure. The pulse is 130 bpm, respiratory rate 19 per minute, oxygen saturation of 96% on air, blood pressure 80/40 mmHg and temperature 37.1°C.

    What is the next appropriate step in management?

    A   Examination under anaesthesia and evacuation of retained products
    B   Intravenous access, administer intravenous Hartmans fluid, take bloods for a full blood count and cross match 4 units of blood
    C   Inform the consultant on call
    D   Inform the anaesthetic consultant on call
    b   Undertake balloon tamponade

3. A woman on the postnatal ward collapsed early in the morning with a postpartum
    haemorrhage. The previous day, she had an elective Caesarean section because
    she had a Caesarean section in the past. As the specialist registrar and the on-call
    anaesthetist on the labour ward, you are resuscitating her. An urgent point-of-care
    test (haemocure) reveals a haemoglobin concentration of 50 g/L. You have initiated
    an obstetric haemorrhage emergency and asked for urgent cross-matching of 6
    units of blood. In the meantime, you have started a group O-negative (emergency
    blood) transfusion from the labour ward fridge. After assessing the patient, you
    think that the bleeding has been caused by an atonic uterus. You administer
    uterotonics and transfer her to the labour ward high-dependency unit. You are also
    undertaking bimanual compression. The uterus contracts and then becomes atonic
    as soon as you release the compression; the patient continues to bleed. You have
    asked the consultant to come in to help.

    What is the next most appropriate treatment?

    A   Continue with more medical treatment
    B   Transfer to theatre for laparotomy and hysterectomy
    C   Transfer to theatre for laparotomy and insertion of a uterine brace suture
    D   Transfer to theatre for balloon tamponade
    E   Transfer to radiology department for the interventional radiologist to carry out
         uterine artery embolisation

4. A patient attends the emergency department in the early hours of the morning. She
    gives history of a Caesarean section 8 days previously for prolonged second stage
    of labour. She reports soaking four big sanitary pads, amounting to around 500 mL
    of blood loss, at home but is not now actively bleeding. On examination, the
    abdomen is tender with no guarding or rigidity. The pulse is 110 bpm, temperature
    38.1°C, respiratory rate 25 per minute and oxygen saturation of 100% on air. There
    is no significant history of past medical or surgical conditions or allergies.

    Which antibiotics is it appropriate to give?

    A   Ampicillin + metronidazole + gentamicin
    B   Augmentin + metronidazole
    C   Clindamycin + metronidazole
    D   Cefuroxime and metronidazole
    E   Tazocin

5. A 32-year-old woman had an emergency Caesarean section for failure to progress
    at 6 cm cervical dilatation. She had been attempting a vaginal birth after a previous
    Caesarean section. The current Caesarean section was uncomplicated and she had
    an intraoperative blood loss of 400 mL. She was discharged home on the second
    day after her operation. 2 days later, she presents to the maternity day assessment
    unit with complaints of increasing tenderness of the scar and bruising around it.
    She repeatedly felt dizzy on exertion. Her blood pressure is 101/56 mmHg, pulse
    100 bpm and temperature 36.2°C. Haemoglobin concentration is 80 g/L. On
    examination, she is tender at the scar site, particularly on the right side. Ultrasound
    is requested, and reveals a haematoma of 9 cm × 6 cm on the right side in the
    pelvis.

What is the next best step in management?

A Intravenous antibiotics for 24 hours and observe
B Laparotomy and evacuation of the haematoma
C Repeat ultrasound in 1 week to see if the haematoma has resolved
D Ultrasound-guided abdominal removal of the haematoma
E Ultrasound-guided vaginal removal of the haematoma

6. According to *Confidential Enquiry into Maternal Deaths* (2016), which of the following is not a risk factor for sepsis in pregnancy?

A Anaemia
B Impaired immunity or immunosuppressant medication
C Obesity
D Offensive vaginal discharge
E White ethnicity

7. According to *Confidential Enquiry into Maternal Deaths* (2016), which organism is most commonly identified in pregnant women dying from sepsis?

A *Clostridium perfringens*
B Group B *Streptococcus*
C Lancefield group A β-haemolytic *Streptococcus*
D *Staphylococcus aureus*
E *Streptococcus pneumoniae*

8. A 38-year-old woman with three children gave birth by vaginal delivery. During the postpartum period, she developed bladder dysfunction requiring insertion of a catheter. Many risk factors are associated with voiding dysfunction during the postpartum period.

Which of the following is not a risk factor for voiding dysfunction during the postpartum period?

A Epidural anaesthesia
B Instrumental delivery
C Multiparous mother
D Perineal trauma
E Prolonged labour

9. A 28-year-old woman had an instrumental delivery 8 hours ago for fetal distress, with only Entonox for pain relief during labour. She has not able to pass urine since the delivery.

What is the best course of action?

A Ask her to sit on toilet and continuously change positions
B Increase the oral fluid intake
C Insert an in-and-out catheter and measure the volume drained
D Insert an indwelling catheter and measure the volume drained
E Reassure her that she will soon pass urine

10. A 39-year-old primiparous woman underwent a Caesarean section 24 hours ago.

Which of the following is not considered a risk factor for a thromboembolism during the postnatal period?

A   Age 35 years or above
B   Current pre-eclampsia
C   Induction of labour
D   Three children or more
E   Smoker

11. A 30-year-old primigravid woman with a body mass index of 40.5 kg/m^2 gave birth 5 hours ago. Apart from the high body mass index, there was an uncomplicated antenatal history, and there were no complications during labour. She would like to be discharged within 6 hours of delivery and the midwife has asked you to complete the discharge summary.

What is the appropriate management regarding thromboprophylaxis?

A   Mobilisation and adequate hydration
B   No prophylaxis
C   Only TED stockings
D   6 weeks of low molecular weight heparin
E   10 days of low molecular weight heparin

12. A 28-year-old woman underwent an emergency Caesarean section for failure to progress at 6 cm cervical dilatation. She was discharged the day after the Caesarean section. She presents to the hospital 2 days later with a painful swollen right leg, which started that day. She did not have heparin following delivery because she does not like needles. Clinically, you suspect a diagnosis of deep vein thrombosis and therefore start treatment with low dose molecular weight heparin after thorough counseling to ensure she takes the treatment. The result of compression duplex ultrasound is negative.

What management does the RCOG recommended?

A   Continue anticoagulant treatment and repeat ultrasound on day 3 and day 7 of the symptoms starting
B   Continue anticoagulant treatment and review in 6 weeks
C   Stop anticoagulant treatment and repeat ultrasound on day 3 and day 7 of the symptoms starting
D   Stop anticoagulant treatment and discharge from hospital
E   Stop anticoagulant treatment and repeat ultrasound on day 14 of the symptoms starting

13. You are the specialist obstetric and gynaecology registrar on the labour ward, and you hear the emergency buzzer being sounded in room 4. A baby boy has just been born by vaginal delivery. Whilst awaiting the oncall paediatric doctor, you have been asked to resuscitate the baby. At 1 minute after birth, you note that the baby's arms and legs are flexed. His pulse rate is >100 bpm and there is a grimace, but his skin is blue. Respiration is slow and irregular.

What Apgar score at 1 minute does this correspond to?

A   3
B   4
C   5
D   6
E   7

14. A baby boy born at 39 weeks by vaginal delivery 26 days ago has been brought to the neonatal unit with signs of jaundice. The mother has a history of hyperthyroidism. She is rhesus-negative and had the anti-D dose that was required. The baby has so far been breastfed, without top-up feeds. Blood tests reveal that the baby has a conjugated hyperbilirubinaemia. A liver ultrasound is normal.

What is the most likely cause of the jaundice?

A   Breast milk
B   Haemolytic disease
C   Hypothyroidism
D   Infection
E   Neonatal hepatitis syndrome

15. A 40-year-old woman presented 5 days after an emergency Caesarean section with abdominal pain and a temperature of 37.8°C. This was associated with nausea, vomiting and mild abdominal distension. With a provisional diagnosis of postpartum endometritis, antibiotics were started and she was sent home. 3 days later, she presents again with ongoing symptoms and features of paralytic ileus. On examination, a tube-like mass is felt in her abdomen on deep palpation. An ultrasound of the abdomen and pelvis is requested.

What is the most likely cause of this woman's symptoms?

A   Acute pyelonephritis
B   Infected haematoma
C   Torsion of an ovarian cyst
D   Postpartum ovarian vein thrombosis
E   Tubo-ovarian abscess

Questions: EMQs

Questions 16–20

Options for Questions 16–20

A   Assess for mental capacity
B   Admit to the antenatal ward
C   Admit to the high dependency unit
D   Admit to the gynaecology ward
E   Admit to the surgical ward
F   Admit to the mother and baby unit and drug therapy
G   Antidepressant drug therapy
H   Cognitive behavioural therapy
I   Counselling
J   Referral to a bereavement midwife
K   Referral to a general physician
L   Referral to a neurologist
M   Referral to a cardiologist
N   Referral to the perinatal mental health team
O   Section under Mental Health Act

Instructions: For each clinical scenario described below, choose the single most appropriate initial management option from the list above. Each option may be used once, more than once, or not at all.

16. A 20-year-old woman presents to the emergency department on the fourth postnatal day following a Caesarean section. She is tearful and has not felt like breastfeeding her baby for the last couple of days. She has good family support and has not had depression or any other psychiatric problems in the past.

17. A 20-year-old woman is brought to the emergency department by her mother. She had a vaginal delivery 2 weeks ago which she considered quite traumatic because she suffered a massive postpartum haemorrhage. She feels listless, depressed and shows no interest in her child or in things she enjoyed before. She has had thoughts of harming herself for the last few days.

18. A 20-year-old woman is brought to the emergency department by her partner. She tried harming herself with a knife and does not seem to have any insight into it. She does not show any interest in her 3-week-old child or want to breastfeed the baby. Her history suggests she has been on treatment for schizophrenia in the past and had stopped taking tablets. She refuses to have any treatment or be admitted to the hospital.

19. A 20-year-old woman presents to her GP with mild vaginal spotting. She thinks she is 10 weeks pregnant in the light of a positive pregnancy test 4 weeks ago. She gives a history of depression and is currently taking citalopram.

20. A 20-year-old woman presents to the obstetric day assessment unit for symptoms of depression. She is currently 28 weeks pregnant and is under the care of a perinatal mental health team. However, she does not have any psychotic symptoms or suicidal tendencies. Because she was free of symptoms, antidepressant medications were stopped prior to pregnancy.

Questions 21–25

Options to Questions 21–25

A	Aspirin	I	Isoniazid
B	Bromocriptine	J	Lithium
C	Chloramphenicol	K	Nitrofurantoin
D	Cabergoline	L	Nalidixic acid
E	Combined oral contraceptive pill	M	Propylthiouracil
F	Diazepam	N	Sulphonamides
G	Ergotamine	O	Tetracycline
H	Iodine		

Instructions: For each side effect in neonates described below during breastfeeding or the neonatal period, choose the single most likely drug received by the mother in the antenatal or postnatal period from the list of options above. Each option may be used once, more than once, or not at all.

21. A 40-year-old Asian woman had a vaginal delivery 2 days ago. She is multiparous, having had five previous vaginal deliveries. She had a stroke 2 years ago from which she has recovered. She was restarted on her previous medication following delivery. She comes to the paediatric emergency department with her child who has suddenly become lethargic, started vomiting and developed a rash on the palms of his hands and feet. The registrar makes a differential diagnosis of Reye's syndrome.

22. A 40-year-old woman had an emergency Caesarean section 2 days ago under an epidural top-up. She has now developed meningitis and is on treatment with antibiotics. She is breastfeeding and the baby suddenly shows signs of vomiting and becomes lethargic. The blood tests show aplastic anaemia and a diagnosis of grey baby syndrome is made. The mother is asked to stop breastfeeding.

23. A 40-year-old woman attends for the growth scan of her fetus at 32 weeks' gestation. She has been told that the fetus has developed a swelling on the front of her neck which looks like a thyroid goitre. The woman has recently been diagnosed with Graves' disease and is under treatment with drugs. However, her levels of thyroid stimulating antibodies, thyroid stimulating hormone (TSH) and thyroxine (T4) are within normal range.

24. A 40-year-old woman had a forceps delivery 2 days ago. She was diagnosed with malaria 1 week ago and was started on anti-malarial medication. The paediatricians notice severe worsening jaundice in the baby.

25. A 40-year-old woman had a ventouse delivery 24 hours ago. She suffered from a recurrent urinary tract infection during pregnancy and was on long-term antibiotic prophylaxis which she stopped only 1 week ago. The paediatricians have diagnosed her baby as having severe anaemia due to haemolysis.

Answers: SBAs

1.   D Stop breastfeeding

It is not known whether tamoxifen and trastuzumab are excreted in breast milk; therefore their use is not recommended during breastfeeding. Women undergoing chemotherapy should be advised not to breastfeed because there is a risk of neonatal leucopenia. A gap of 14 days between chemotherapy and starting breastfeeding allows drug clearance. However, the ability to breastfeed has been reported to depend on whether the major ducts have been excised from the breast.

2.   B Intravenous access, administer intravenous Hartmanns fluid, take blood for a full blood count and cross match 4 units of blood

Because this patient is tachycardic and hypotensive, it is imperative that she should be resuscitated quickly and adequately (following ABC – airway, breathing, circulation). The most likely cause of postpartum haemorrhage here is retained products of conception. The most appropriate first step of management is to establish intravenous access, give fluids and prepare blood units for transfusion.

3.   C Transfer to theatre for laparotomy and brace suture

Because there has already been a massive postpartum haemorrhage, the patient should be transferred to theatre for laparotomy with the intention of placing a brace suture. If this is not successful, a hysterectomy should be performed. Gaining access via a laparotomy allows the surgeon to explore other possible reasons for the bleeding, e.g. bleeding from uterine angles.

4.   A Ampicillin + metronidazole + gentamicin

This woman has a secondary postpartum haemorrhage. The usual cause is endometritis. If there is uterine tenderness, the cause is usually endomyometritis. The recommended antibiotic combination is ampicillin + metronidazole + gentamicin. If the bleeding continues, surgical management should be considered regardless of ultrasound findings related to the endometrium. Surgery should be performed by a senior obstetrician because there is a very high risk of perforation during the postpartum period if there is uterine infection.

5.   B Laparotomy and evacuation of the haematoma

This patient has a pelvic collection in the form of a large haematoma. This needs to be removed surgically as she is symptomatic. In addition, it could soon become infected and cause sepsis.

6. E White ethnicity

Similar to the previous report (2009–2011), the risk of death was higher in women from black and ethnic minorities compared to people of white ethnicity.

Knight M, Nair M, Tuffnell D, et al. on behalf of MBRRACE-UK. Saving Lives, Improving Mothers' Care. Surveillance of maternal deaths in the UK 2012–14 and lessons learned to inform maternity care from the UK and Ireland Confidential Enquiries into Maternal Deaths and Morbidity 2009–14. Oxford: MBRRACE-UK; 2016.

7. C Lancefield group A β-haemolytic *Streptococcus*

The organisms that most commonly cause sepsis in obstetrics include β-haemolytic streptococcal groups A, B and D, α-haemolytic pneumococcus and *Escherichia coli*.

Royal College of Obstetricians and Gynaecologists (RCOG). Bacterial sepsis following pregnancy. Green-top guidelines no. 64B. London: RCOG; 2012.

8. C Multiparous mother

- Instrumental delivery increases the likelihood of developing urinary retention from 8% to 33%
- A large perineal tear increases the risk of urinary retention from 4% to 42%
- The use of epidural analgesia in labour increases the risk of urinary retention from 11% to 33%
- Primiparous women who have a long labour are more likely than multiparous women to have urinary retention during the postpartum period (78.1% versus 45.8%, respectively)

Kearney R, Cutner A. Postpartum voiding dysfunction. Obstet Gynaecol 2008; 10:71–74.

9. C Insert an in-and-out catheter and measure the volume drained

Postpartum voiding dysfunction occurs in 0.7–4% of all deliveries. It is defined as an inability to pass urine for 6 hours after delivery or after removal of a catheter. If left untreated, it leads to prolonged voiding bladder dysfunction and, as a result, urinary incontinence and urinary tract infections. If the mother has not voided after 6 hours, a catheter should be inserted and the volume drained should be measured. Alternatively, a bladder ultrasound scan can measure this volume before insertion of a catheter.

Kearney R, Cutner A. Postpartum voiding dysfunction. Obset Gynaecol 2008; 10:71–74.

10. C Induction of labour

Prolonged labour (>24 hours) is considered a risk for the development of thromboembolism but not induction of labour. Other risk factors include:

- Obesity (BMI 30 kg/m^2 or more)
- Multiparity (three or more children)
- Thrombophilia (low risk type)

- Prolonged immobility
- Systemic sepsis
- Preeclampsia in the current pregnancy
- Reproductive age group older than 35 years
- Smoker
- Having elective Caesarean section
- Extensive varicose veins
- Venous thromboembolism in the family members
- Current preterm labour
- Multiple pregnancy
- Current stillbirth
- Instrumental or midcavity rotational delivery
- Blood loss 1000 mL or more during delivery
- Needing blood transfusion for bleeding

When women have two or more above risk factors, it is recommended that they should be prescribed at least 10 days of prophylactic low molecular weight heparin.

11. E 10 days of low molecular weight heparin

A patient with a body mass index >40 kg/m² should receive 10 days of low molecular weight heparin as she has a high risk of developing a thromoboembolism during the postnatal period.

Other indications for 10 days of thromboprophylaxis include:

- Caesarean section
- Readmission or prolonged admission (3 or more days) during the puerperium
- Any surgical procedure in the postpartum period except for immediate repair of the perineum

12. C Stop anticoagulant treatment and repeat ultrasound on day 3 and day 7 of the symptoms starting

If there is a suspicion of a deep vein thrombosis, compression duplex ultrasound should be performed. If the result is negative and the likelihood of a deep vein thrombosis is low, treatment should be stopped and the patient discharged. If, however, the result is negative but suspicion is high, the scan should be repeated on days 3 and 7 of the symptoms, but treatment should be stopped.

13. C 5

Although the Apgar score is in fact named after Virginia Apgar, the components of the Apgar score can be remembered by:

- **A**ctivity (muscle tone)
- **P**ulse rate
- **G**rimace (reflex irritability)
- **A**ppearance (skin colour)
- **R**espiration

Table 11.1 shows the Apgar scoring system. The baby is scored at birth, 5 minutes and 10 minutes of age, and is given a score of 0, 1 or 2.

Table 11.1 Apgar scoring system			
	0	1	2
Activity	Absent	Flexed arms and legs	Active movements
Pulse (bpm)	Absent	<100	>100
Grimace	No response	Grimace	Sneeze, cry
Appearance	Blue or pale	Blue extremities but pink body	Pink all over
Respiration	Absent	Slow and irregular	Regular

14. E Neonatal hepatitis syndrome

The causes of jaundice are shown in **Table 11.2**.

Table 11.2 Causes of jaundice	
Prolonged jaundice (lasting >14 days)	**Early onset jaundice (onset <24 hours)**
Conjugated bilirubin: • Neonatal hepatitis syndrome • Biliary atresia Unconjugated bilirubin: • Breast milk • Hypothyroidism	Physiological Breast milk jaundice Haemolysis, secondary to ABO incompatibility Infection Glucose-6-phosphate dehydrogenase deficiency Liver enzyme defects – Crigler–Najjar syndrome

15. D Postpartum ovarian vein thrombosis

Postpartum ovarian vein thrombosis presents with abdominal pain, pyrexia, nausea, vomiting, malaise and ileus with fever persisting in spite of antibiotics. Upon deep palpation, there is a tube-like mass in the adnexa. This is the thrombosed vein surrounded by an inflammatory mass, and is found in approximately 50% of women. Most cases present within 10 days postnatally. Differential diagnoses include appendicitis, peritonitis, adnexal torsion, tuboovarian disease, infected haematoma and pyelonephritis.

Dougan C, Phillips R, Harley I, et al. Postpartum ovarian vein thrombosis. Obstet Gynaecol 2016; 18:291–299.

Answers: EMQs

16. I Counselling

The diagnosis in this case is postpartum blues. This woman has insight into her symptoms and is seeking advice. Postpartum blues are mild and temporary mood symptoms seen in up to 80% of women during the postpartum period. They typically last for a few hours to several days. The symptoms include tearfulness, sleeplessness, irritability, anxiety, low mood, feelings of isolation and lack of interest in her child.

At 10–14 days after birth, women should be asked about the resolution of symptoms of baby blues. If symptoms have not resolved, the woman should be assessed for postnatal depression, and if symptoms persist, evaluated further (urgent action).

17. N Referral to the perinatal mental health team

Mental diseases have been identified as the leading indirect cause of maternal morbidity and mortality in the UK [according to *Confidential Enquiry into Maternal and Child Health* (2016), there were 42 psychiatric deaths and of these 68% were from suicide].

During pregnancy and the postnatal period, perinatal mental health problems can have serious consequences for the mother, her infant and other family members. The mother and baby unit provides specialist inpatient care to women suffering from such problems including postnatal depression, related postnatal illnesses or a recurrence of pre-existing mental health diseases. The aim is to keep the woman and the baby together to promote bonding whenever possible.

The diagnosis in this case is severe depression with suicidal tendencies. She should be referred urgently to the perinatal mental health team, followed by admission to the mother and baby unit before initiating treatment.

18. N Referral to the perinatal mental health team

Patients with mental health problems have the right to accept or decline life-threatening treatment while people without capacity cannot make such decisions, and therefore the Mental Health Act (2005) allows someone else (a professional) to make decisions for them. This patient does not have insight or capacity and is refusing treatment. Therefore, she needs to be urgently referred to the perinatal mental health team before sectioning under the Mental Health Act to initiate treatment.

19. N Referral to the perinatal mental health team

Women with a history of depression should be referred to the perinatal mental health team for assessment at their first antenatal visit during pregnancy.

To identify possible depression, all women should be asked at least 2 questions during the first contact with primary care during pregnancy, at her booking visit (her first midwife appointment) and postnatally (usually at 4–6 weeks and 3–4 months) by healthcare professionals (midwives, obstetricians, health visitors and GPs). For example:

- during the past month, have you often been bothered by feeling down, depressed or hopeless?
- during the past month, have you often been bothered by having little interest or pleasure in doing things?

A third question should be considered if the woman answers 'yes' to either of the initial questions:

- is this something you feel you need or want help with?

Also, at first contact all women should be asked about:

- past and present severe mental illness including schizophrenia, bipolar disorder, psychosis in the postnatal period and severe depression
- previous treatment by a psychiatrist/specialist mental health team including inpatient care
- a family history of perinatal mental illness

20. G Antidepressant drug therapy

This woman has insight because she is seeking medical advice. Because she does not have any psychotic symptoms or suicidal tendencies, admission to hospital is not required. She is depressed and therefore needs antidepressant therapy.

Antidepressant drugs

While choosing an antidepressant medication for pregnant and breastfeeding women, one should bear in mind that the safety of these drugs is not well understood:

- Tricyclic antidepressants (amitriptyline, imipramine and nortriptyline) have fewer known risks during pregnancy than other antidepressants.
- Little is known about the potential risks of the use of fluoxetine [a selective serotonin reuptake inhibitor (SSRI)] in pregnancy.
- Imipramine, nortriptyline and sertraline are present at relatively low levels in breast milk.
- Citalopram and fluoxetine are present at relatively high levels in breast milk.
- SSRIs taken after 20 weeks' gestation may be associated with an increased risk of persistent pulmonary hypertension in the neonate.

- Paroxetine taken in the first trimester may be associated with fetal heart defects.
- Venlafaxine may be associated with an increased risk of high blood pressure at high doses, higher toxicity in overdose than SSRIs and some tricyclic antidepressants, and increased difficulty in withdrawal.
- All antidepressants carry the risk of withdrawal or toxicity in neonates; in most cases the effects are mild and self-limiting.

National Institute of Health and Clinical Excellence. NICE guideline on antenatal and postnatal mental health: clinical management and service management (CG45). NICE, 2007 (revised 2010).
Nicholas N and Nicholas S. Understanding the Mental Capacity Act 2005: a guide to clinicians. Obstet Gynaecol 2010; 12:29–34.

21. A Aspirin

Aspirin is secreted in breast milk and Reye's syndrome is a side effect of aspirin use.

Reye's syndrome is a fatal disease which mainly affects the brain and liver but can affect any organ in the body. It is commonly seen in children following consumption of aspirin with viral illness. In the UK, the use of aspirin is not recommended in children under 16 years of age unless there is a specific indication (recommendation by the Committee on Safety of Medicines). Similar recommendations are given elsewhere, for example the US Food and Drug Administration (FDA) does not approve its use in children under the age of 19 years.

The disease itself can cause a fatty liver and severe encephalopathy. Jaundice is not a feature of Reye's syndrome. Most children will recover with conservative supportive therapy. Brain injury and death are potential complications.

22. C Chloramphenicol

Chloramphenicol is an antimicrobial drug effective against gram-positive and gram-negative bacteria, including most anaerobic organisms. It is no longer a first line treatment due to the development of resistance and safety issues. The most common and serious side effect is bone marrow suppression which is usually reversible. The less common side effect is aplastic anaemia which is idiosyncratic and generally fatal (unpredictable and unrelated to the dose).

Oral chloramphenicol crosses the placenta and is also excreted in the breast milk. When used in late pregnancy or during puerperium it is known to cause grey baby syndrome in the neonate. Therefore, its use near term and during breastfeeding is not recommended.

23. M Propylthiouracil

Hyperthyroidism (50% of affected women have a family history of autoimmune thyroid disease) is more common in women than men and 95% of cases in pregnancy are due to Graves' disease. Such women are usually treated with antithyroid drugs: carbimazole and propylthiouracil are the most commonly used drugs in the UK. Both of these drugs cross the placenta, propylthiouracil less easily than carbimazole, and are generally safe to use in pregnancy using the minimum effective dose to maximise the therapeutic effect. However, reports of aplasia cutis (scalp defect) have been noted with the use of carbimazole, and fetal hypothyroidism and goitre have been noted with both drugs when used in high doses.

Propylthiouracil is preferred during puerperium because very little is excreted in the breast milk (0.07% of the dose taken by the mother).

Fetal hypothyroidism may be caused by placental passage of maternal thyroid stimulating hormone (TSH) inhibitory immunoglobulins or high doses of propylthiouracil, more often the latter. The risk can be minimised by using vigorous antithyroid treatment before conception and by the use of lower doses of these drugs during pregnancy. However, fetal hyperthyroidism can be caused by transplacental passage of thyroid stimulating antibodies and is reported in 1% of the babies born to mothers with a past or current history of Graves' disease. If it develops in utero and is left untreated the mortality is 50%, while if it develops at birth and is left untreated the mortality is 15%. In utero, the fetus may present with fetal tachycardia, fetal growth restriction and fetal goitre. The risk of the fetus being affected with hyperthyroidism is higher if the TSH-binding inhibiting immunoglobulin (TBI) index is >30% (predictive) and increases further if the TBI index is >70% (strongly predictive).

24. N Sulphonamides

Long acting sulphonamides should be avoided in the last few weeks of pregnancy because they increase the risk of neonatal kernicterus (bilirubin binds with albumin but sulphonamides interfere with bilirubin binding with albumin by competitively binding to albumin).

25. K Nitrofurantoin

Urinary tract infection (UTI): the antibiotic choice depends on the sensitivity of the organism. 3 days of antibiotics are sufficient to treat asymptomatic bacteriuria. It is recommended that regular urine cultures are done to ensure eradication of the organism because 15% of women will have recurrent bacteriuria during their pregnancy, thus needing a second course of antibiotics.

Amoxicillin, ampicillin and cephalosporins are safe to use in pregnancy. Nitrofurantoin (50–100 mg 4 times daily for 7 days, if using a long-acting preparation, the dose would be 100 mg twice daily) is a safe alternative to treat UTI but should be avoided in the third trimester as it can precipitate neonatal haemolytic anaemia. Trimethoprim should be avoided in the first trimester due to its antifolate action.

Nelson-Piercy C. Handbook of Obstetric Medicine (4th edn). London: Informa Healthcare, 2010.

Chapter 12

Gynaecological problems

Questions: SBAs

For each question, select the single best answer from the five options listed.

1. A 48-year-old woman underwent the insertion of a levonorgestrel-releasing intrauterine system (Mirena coil) 2 years ago for menorrhagia. 2 weeks ago, she attended the gynaecology clinic because of heavy bleeding for the previous 2 months. You performed an endometrial pipelle biopsy at that visit. You are now seeing her to discuss the histology result, which shows complex endometrial hyperplasia with atypia. She has no other significant past medical history and is not currently taking any medication.

    What is the most appropriate management?

    A   Repeat the endometrial pipelle biopsy in 3 months
    B   Remove the current levonorgestrel-releasing intrauterine system and insert a new one
    C   Start tranexamic acid
    D   Start the combined oral contraceptive pill
    E   Refer for total abdominal hysterectomy and bilateral salpingo-oophorectomy

2. A 57-year-old woman attended the gynaecology clinic with a history of postmenopausal bleeding that began 1 month ago. An ultrasound of the pelvis revealed an endometrial thickness of 7 mm, so you undertook an endometrial pipelle biopsy. The report shows endometrial hyperplasia without atypia. The patient is anxious because she has read on the internet that this condition may lead to cancer.

    What is the chance of the patient developing endometrial cancer over the next 20 years?

    A   1–5%
    B   6–10%
    C   11–15%
    D   16–20%
    E   More than 20%

3. A 39-year-old woman has come to the gynaecology clinic with a history of amenorrhoea for the past 6 months. She has noticed an increase in weight, hot flushes and decreased concentration over the same period. There have been no other changes in her physical condition. A home pregnancy test was negative.

    Which single laboratory investigation is most likely to establish a diagnosis in this woman?

    A   Karyotyping
    B   Levels of follicle-stimulating hormone, luteinising hormone and oestradiol in plasma
    C   Prolactin concentration in plasma
    D   Thyroid function tests
    E   Ultrasound

4. Which one of the following is not a cardiovascular benefit of taking oestrogen in the form of hormone replacement therapy?

    A   It prevents platelet aggregation
    B   It promotes coronary artery vasodilatation
    C   It reduces high-density lipoprotein cholesterol
    D   It reduces atherosclerosis
    E   It reduces low-density lipoprotein cholesterol

5. A 17-year-old girl comes to the clinic accompanied by her mother. She reports that she has not yet attained menarche. On examination, secondary sexual characteristics have not fully developed. The girl is upset and also says she is being bullied at school for being short.

    What is the most appropriate investigation?

    A   Karyotyping
    B   Pelvic ultrasound
    C   Levels of follicle-stimulating hormone, luteinising hormone and oestradiol in plasma
    D   Prolactin concentration in plasma
    E   Thyroid function tests

6. A 50-year-old woman attends the gynaecology clinic because she would like to take hormone replacement therapy. She is complaining of hot flushes and night sweats, and has infrequent periods. Her pelvic ultrasound reveals a normal uterus and ovaries.

    Which type of hormone replacement therapy would you advise?

    A   Continuous combined
    B   Sequential combined
    C   Tibolone
    D   Vaginal oestrogen
    E   Unopposed oestrogen

7. Polycystic ovarian syndrome is a common condition with many long-term consequences.

    Which of the following is not one of the risks of polycystic ovarian syndrome?

    A   Endometrial cancer
    B   Hypertension
    C   Ovarian cancer
    D   Sleep apnoea
    E   Type 2 diabetes

8. An 18-year-old girl has been referred to the gynaecology clinic because she has not yet attained menarche. Examination reveals normal development of secondary sexual characteristics but a short vagina. Plasma concentrations of follicle-stimulating hormone, luteinising hormone and oestrogen are normal. She is 1.68 m (5 ft 6 in) tall and has a normal body mass index. She has just been accepted into medical school and is anxious that she has not attained menarche although her friends have.

    What is the diagnosis?

    A   Androgen insensitivity syndrome
    B   Congenital adrenal hyperplasia
    C   Imperforate hymen
    D   Mayer–Rokitansky–Küster–Hauser syndrome
    E   Turner's syndrome

9. A 32-year-old lawyer attends the gynaecology clinic with complaints of irritability, depression and feeling out of control. Other symptoms include breast tenderness, bloating and headaches. These occur premenstrually and improve as each period starts; symptoms resolve by the end of menstruation. She has kept a menstrual diary for the last 3 months. She is anxious because this is causing her to take time off work and is affecting her quality of life. She has started drinking heavily because of this.

    What is the best initial management?

    A   Advice on diet, exercise and stress reduction
    B   Gonadotropin-releasing hormone analogue and add-back therapy
    C   A combined oral contraceptive
    D   Continuous or luteal-phase low-dose selective serotonin reuptake inhibitor
    E   Oestradiol patch and oral progesterone

10. A 40-year-old multiparous woman with a history of menorrhagia attends the gynaecology clinic. She gives a history of previous 2 Caesarean sections. Her blood test reveals that her haemogolobin level has dropped from 120 g/L to 100 g/L over the last 4 months. She has no significant past medical history and is not taking any medication. An ultrasound of the pelvis shows an enlarged uterus with multiple fibroids measuring 3–5 cm. She is known to have fibroids and she previously underwent a myomectomy at the age of 21 years. She does not wish to have more children.

What is the best management plan?

A   Levonorgestrel-releasing intrauterine system (Mirena coil)
B   Myomectomy
C   Hysterectomy
D   Ulipristal acetate 5 mg once a day (up to four courses)
E   Uterine artery embolisation

11. A 21-year-old woman with a body mass index of 32 kg/m^2 has been referred to the gynaecology clinic. She gives history of non-cyclical pelvic pain and dyschezia. She is virgo intacta and therefore declines vaginal examination. On general examination, there is no obvious palpable abdominal mass or tenderness. An abdominal ultrasound report reads: 'Anterverted uterus, measuring 86.6 mm × 49.6 mm × 40.6 mm. The right ovary measures 12 mm × 13 mm × 10 mm. The left ovary contains a mass measuring 50 mm × 60 mm. The mass appears to be of ground-glass echogenicity with three compartments, with detectable blood flow and no papillary structures.'

What is the next best step in her management?

A   Undertake diagnostic laparoscopy and cystectomy
B   Order transvaginal ultrasound
C   Arrange blood tests for tumour markers
D   Start the combined oral contraceptive pill
E   Start progestogen therapy

12. You are the on-call gynaecology registrar and have been asked to review a 22-year-old woman admitted by the surgical team with possible appendicitis. She describes a sudden onset of right iliac fossa pain, which radiates to the groin. This occurs intermittently and varies in severity. She has vomited six times that day and is exhausted. Abdominal examination reveals tenderness in the right iliac fossa, and pelvic examination reveals cervical excitation. Observations reveal tachycardia (pulse 101 bpm), raised temperature (37.7° C) and a normal respiratory rate. An ultrasound revealed a 5 cm cyst on the right ovary with stromal oedema and follicles pushed to the periphery of the ovary. The left ovary appears normal. There is a moderate degree of free fluid in the rectouterine pouch (pouch of Douglas). The uterus appears normal. A pregnancy test has proved negative.

What is the most likely diagnosis?

A   Adnexal torsion
B   Fibroid torsion
C   Functional ovarian cyst
D   Pelvic inflammatory disease
E   Renal infection

13. When a woman has been sexually assaulted, it is imperative to take samples from the correct sites to assist the investigation. The sites depend on the type of assault.

How long is the DNA present if a patient has been vaginally assaulted but a condom has been used?

A   50 hours
B   105 hours
C   128 hours
D   140 hours
E   168 hours

Questions: EMQs

Questions 14–18

Options for Questions 14–18

A	Aphthous ulcers	I	Lichen sclerosus
B	Behcet disease	J	Pemphigoid
C	Group B *Streptococcus*	K	Pemphigus
D	Candidial vulvovaginits	L	Syphilis
E	Chanchroid	M	Lymphogranuloma venereum
F	Eczema	N	Molluscum contagiosum
G	Genital herpes simplex	O	Acanthosis nigricans
H	Lichen planus		

Instructions: For each scenario described below, choose the single most appropriate diagnosis from the list of options above. Each option may be used once, more than once, or not at all.

14. A 55-year-old woman presents with redness and itching in the vulval region. Clinical examination reveals an inflamed labia associated with oedema, scaling and fissuring. She expresses that this has been an ongoing symptom for the last 6 months. She also gives a recent history of a flare-up of systemic lupus for which she is receiving treatment. She is worried that this could be cancer because her sister died of liposarcoma of the thigh.

15. A 20-year-old woman went to Amsterdam for summer vacation. She attends a sexual health clinic after her return to UK with complaints of a small ulcer on her vulva. Clinical examination reveals a solitary ulcer on the left labia, with a well-defined margin and indurated base. It is non-tender to touch and is associated with painless inguinal lymphadenopathy.

16. A 58-year-old woman is referred to the vulval clinic by her GP. She complains of vulval itching and pain for the last 2 years. Examination reveals a labial fusion, pale atrophic vulva and lichenification in the vulval and perineal region. She is diabetic and has been on 40 units of insulin per day for the last 20 years.

17. A 55-year-old woman is referred to a joint vulval/dermatology clinic with blisters and erosions on the vulval region. Examination reveals subepidermal blisters, vulval scarring and introital narrowing. Immunofluorescence studies on biopsies showed antibody deposits at the dermoepidermal junction. She was prescribed steroids following her consultation.

18. A 22-year-old woman presents to a sexual health clinic with a painful vulval ulcer. It is tender on touch and is associated with inguinal lymphadenopathy.

Questions 19–23

Options for Questions 19–23

A Combined oral contraceptive pill (COCP)
B Cimetidine
C Ciprofloxacin
D Cyproterone acetate
E Dexamethasone
F Depot medroxyprogesterone acetate
G Desmopressin
H Gonadotropin-releasing hormone analogues
I Eflornithine
J Finasteride
K Flutamide
L Ketoconazole
M Progesterone only pill (POP)
N Spironolactone
O Spiramycin

Instructions: For each mechanism of action described below, choose the single most appropriate drug used in the treatment of hirsutism from the list of options above. Each option may be used once, more than once, or not at all.

19. A 28-year-old woman is referred to an endocrinologist for an increase in facial hair and acne with bloating during her periods. She has been prescribed an aldosterone antagonist which also has a diuretic action.

20. A 30-year-old woman is referred to an endocrinologist for an increase in facial hair which she describes as embarrassing because she has to shave almost every week. Investigations so far have been normal. She has been prescribed a drug which reduces 5α-reductase enzyme activity.

21. A 40-year-old woman is referred to an endocrinologist for an increase in facial hair. She has been prescribed a non-steroidal anti-androgen which acts directly on the hair follicles.

22. A 20-year-old woman is referred to an endocrinologist for an increase in facial hair and acne. She has been prescribed an anti-androgenic which has weak progestational activity.

23. A 20-year-old woman presents to her GP with an increase in facial hair. Clinical examination reveals a mild increase in facial hair with no major concerns. The GP prescribes her a facial cream which inhibits ornithine decarboxylase.

Questions 24–28

Options for Questions 24–28

A   Aromatase inhibitor
B   Anti-glucocorticoid and anti-progestogenic
C   Anti-progestogen, anti-oestrogen and weak androgen
D   Endometrial atrophy
E   Endometrial proliferation
F   Endometritis
G   Pituitary down regulation
H   Pituitary up regulation
I   Prostaglandin inhibitor
J   Progestogenic and anti-androgenic
K   Reduces endometrial tissue plasminogen activator
L   Reduces endometrial thromboplastin
M   Reduces and blocks oestrogen receptors at pituitary level
N   Stimulates endothelial growth factor
O   Vasopressin analogue

Instructions: For each drug used in management in gynaecology, choose the single most appropriate mechanism of action for the following drugs from the list of options above. Each option may be used once, more than once, or not at all.

24. Danazol

25. Gestrinone

26. Luteal phase progestogens (days 15–25)

27. Tranexamic acid

28. Combined oral contraceptive pill (COCP)

Questions 29–33

Options for Questions 29–33

A	Cryotherapy	I	Microwave ablation of endometrium
B	Cold knife conisation of cervix	J	Radio frequency endometrial ablation
C	Electrode ablation	K	Roller ball ablation of endometrium
D	Endometrial laser ablation	L	Transcervical resection of endometrium
E	Hydrothermal endometrial ablation		
F	Laparoscopic uterine artery clipping	M	Transcervical resection of fibroid
G	Laparoscopic myolysis	N	Transcervical resection of polyp
H	Laparoscopic internal artery ligation	O	Uterine artery embolisation

Instructions: For each action described below, choose the single most appropriate method of treatment for menorrhagia from the list of options above. Each option may be used once, more than once, or not at all.

29. This reduces menstrual blood loss, pressure effects, size of fibroids and dysmenorrhoea.

30. This burns the endometrial lining following introduction of hot fluid into the endometrial cavity.

31. It causes collagen denaturation and programmed cell death by heating.

32. A procedure where the endometrium is available for histopathological analysis.

33. It causes severe postoperative adhesions and sepsis.

Questions 34–38

Options for Questions 34–38

A Continuous oestrogens and progestogens (oral) hormone replacement therapy (HRT)
B Desogestrel
C HRT not recommended
D Levonorgestrel-releasing intrauterine system (Mirena coil)
E Norgestimate
F Oestrogens plus progestogens plus testosterone (oral)
G Testosterone only (oral) HRT
H Oestrogen-only (oral) HRT
I Oestrogen transdermal patch and vaginal progesterone cream HRT
J Oestrogen transdermal patch only HRT
K Oestrogen cream or pessaries vaginally HRT
L Oestrogen cream for vaginal application and oral progestogens HRT
M Progestogen-only (oral) HRT
N Sequential oestrogens and progestogens (oral) HRT
O Cyproterone acetate

Instructions: For each scenario described below, choose the single most appropriate hormonal drug therapy from the list of options above. Each option may be used once, more than once, or not at all.

34. A 50-year-old Asian woman presents to her GP with one episode of postmenopausal minimal vaginal bleeding which lasted for 2 days but has now stopped. Clinical examination reveals atrophic vagina and cervix. A transvaginal scan shows an endometrial thickness of 4 mm. She gives a history of breast cancer in her first cousin who is 69 years old.

35. A 50-year-old white woman presents to her GP with severe menopausal symptoms (hot flushes and night sweats). She gives a past history of total abdominal hysterectomy and bilateral salpingo-oophorectomy 10 years ago for menorrhagia. Currently, she is on citalopram and levothyroxine for depression and hypothyroidism respectively. She is receiving dermatological treatment for psoriasis.

36. A 50-year-old Asian woman presents with severe hot flushes and night sweats. Her periods have been very irregular for the last 8 months and she has not had any periods for the last 4 months. Her follicle-stimulating hormone (FSH) level is 45 IU/mL. She is very religious and wishes to have regular menstrual periods every month. She is happy to take tablets.

37. A 50-year-old Afro-Caribbean woman presents to her GP with severe menopausal symptoms. She gives a past history of menorrhagia and myomectomy 5 years ago. A recent cervical smear is negative. She does not like to have cyclical vaginal bleeding.

38. A 50-year-old white woman presents to her GP with severe menopausal symptoms (hot flushes and night sweats). She had a vaginal hysterectomy for genital organ prolapse 2 years ago. However, she is epileptic and is taking 600 mg carbamazepine twice a day.

Answers: SBAs

---

1. E Refer for total abdominal hysterectomy and bilateral salpingo-oophorectomy

The indications for endometrial biopsy include persistent intermenstrual bleeding, ineffective treatment and failed treatment in women aged over 45 years. Around 29% of cases of complex hyperplasia with atypia progress to cancer within 4.1 years, and on hysterectomy 43% of women will have an associated underlying malignancy. Therefore abdominal hysterectomy and bilateral salpingo-oophrectomy should be carried out.

National Institute for Health and Care Excellence (NICE). Heavy menstrual bleeding [CG44]. Manchester: NICE; 2007.

---

2. A 1–5%

In this case, the risk of endometrial cancer is <5% over the next 20 years. Most endometrial hyperplasia without atypia regresses spontaneously. Hormone replacement therapy and obesity are reversible factors that should be addressed, and the patient should be counselled on these. The management options are (1) follow-up with endometrial biopsies to ensure disease regression, and (2) treatment with progestogens, which leads to a higher rate of disease regression than observation alone. The levonorgestrel-releasing intrauterine system (Mirena coil) is the first choice for treatment. Oral progestogens should be used only if the levonorgestrel releasing intrauterine system is declined.

---

3. B Levels of follicle-stimulating hormone, luteinising hormone and oestradiol in plasma

The mean age of menopause is 50–52 years in the UK. As a woman approaches this age, ovarian function decreases, oestrogen levels fall and gonadotropin levels increase. The gonadotropins surges are associated with hot flushes. There is also reduced fertility with increasing age.

Menopause that occurs before the age of 40 years is known as premature ovarian failure (POF), primary ovarian insufficiency or premature ovarian dysfunction. It is defined as 4 months of amenorrhoea, with two blood tests for follicle-stimulating hormone, conducted at least 1 month apart, showing concentrations >30 IU/mL.

The incidence of POF is around 0.9%. In most cases, the cause is unknown. It is not necessarily permanent: 50% of women have fluctuating ovarian follicular function with sporadic ovulation, and 5–10% of women with POF conceive.

Arora P, Polson D. Diagnosis and management of premature ovarian failure. Obstet Gynaecol 2011; 13:67–72.

4.   C It reduces high-density lipoprotein cholesterol

Hormone replacement therapy (HRT) leads to an increase in high-density lipoprotein cholesterol and can be cardioprotective. Epidemiological studies have shown that men suffer from cardiovascular disease (CVD) at an earlier age than women. It is also reported that women who attain menopause earlier have an increased risk of CVD. This suggests that oestrogen protects against cardiovascular disease.

The US Women's Health Initiative study found in 2007 that giving HRT to women within 10 years of menopause reduced the risk of CVD (by 6/10,000 women–years). However, giving HRT 20 years after menopause was associated with an increased risk of CVD (by 17/10,000 women–years). The 10-year period after menopause is called the 'window of opportunity', during which HRT is reported to be beneficial.

Bakour S, Williamson J. Latest evidence on using hormone replacement therapy in the menopause. Obstet Gynaecol 2015; 17:20–28.

5.   A Karyotyping

This girl probably has Turner's syndrome, which can be confirmed by karyotyping. Turner's syndrome is usually associated with short stature, poor development of secondary sexual characteristics and amenorrhoea. If there is an 45XO genotype, primordial follicles undergo atresia at an accelerated pace; the ovarian follicle pool is therefore low at the time of puberty, which leads to primary amenorrhoea. With a mosaic 45XO/46XX genotype, in which the X chromosome is missing from some but not all cells, the atresia is slower so these women present later with secondary amenorrhoea.

Arora P, Polson D. Diagnosis and management of premature ovarian failure. Obstet Gynaecol 2011; 13:67–72.

6.   B Sequential combined

The average age of the menopause in the UK is 51.4 years. Women usually complain of vasomotor symptoms, which respond well to oestrogen therapy. If the woman does not have a uterus, unopposed oestrogen can be given. If the uterus is in situ, there are two options:

- If there has been <12 months of amenorrhoea, continuous combined hormone replacement therapy or tibolone can be given
- If there are infrequent periods, sequential combined oestrogen and progestogens should be given. Progestogen or micronised progesterone is recommended to prevent endometrial cancer. It is usually taken orally, but it can also be delivered in the form of the levonorgestrel-releasing intrauterine system (Mirena coil)
- Vaginal oestrogen should be given if the patient has urogenital symptoms

Bakour S, Williamson J. Latest evidence on using hormone replacement therapy in the menopause. Obstet Gynecol 2015; 17:20–28.

7.   C Ovarian cancer

Polycystic ovarian syndrome (PCOS) is associated with a higher prevalence of type 2 diabetes, sleep apnoea, hypertension, dyslipidaemia, visceral obesity and hyperinsulinaemia. Oligomenorrhoea and amenorrhoea can cause endometrial hyperplasia, which can then lead to endometrial carcinoma. It is therefore recommended that progestogens should be prescribed to initiate withdrawal bleeds every 3–4 months to help shed the endometrium. An endometrial thickness of <7 mm in PCOS is unlikely to be hyperplasia. If, however, there is a thickened endometrium or an endometrial polyp, an endometrial pipelle biopsy should be undertaken with or without hysteroscopy. PCOS is not associated with breast or ovarian cancer.

8.   D Mayer–Rokitansky–Küster–Hauser syndrome

In Mayer–Rokitansky–Küster–Hauser syndrome, the secondary sexual characteristics are generally well developed because ovarian function is normal. However, the vagina is short because mullerian hypoplasia or aplasia can occur. Musculoskeletal and renal abnormalities can also be associated with this condition.

The incidence of Mayer–Rokitansky–Küster–Hauser syndrome is 1/4000 – 1/5000, and 70–80% of women present with primary amenorrhoea. It is caused by agenesis or hypoplasia of the paramesonephric ducts. The karyotype is normal (46XX).

Turner's syndrome is usually associated with short stature and a 45XO karyotype. Congenital adrenal hyperplasia is associated with abnormal external genitalia, and androgen insensitivity usually with tall stature.

Valappil S, Chetan U, Wood N, Garden A. Mayer–Rokitansky–Küster–Hauser syndrome: diagnosis and management. Obstet Gynaecol 2012; 14:93–98.

9.   A Advice one diet, exercise and stress reduction

Women with possible premenstrual syndrome (PMS) should be asked to record their symptoms in a diary, prospectively, over 2 months – a daily record of severity of problems. It is simple to record.

PMS is often associated with:

- Psychological symptoms: mood swings, low mood and feeling out of control
- Physical symptoms: breast tenderness, bloating and headaches
- Behavioural symptoms: an increase in accidents

Mild symptoms may not interfere with the woman's personal and professional life. However, severe symptoms can lead to poor quality of life from social withdrawal.

The initial management is lifestyle modification, including dietary changes, regular exercise and stress management and reduction. Non-randomised trials have shown that exercise alone helps to improve the symptoms of PMS.

10. D Ulipristal acetate 5 mg once a day (up to four courses)

Ulipristal acetate 5 mg once a day should be offered if fibroids are 3 cm or more in diameter and haemoglobin concentration is 102 g/L or less. It should also be considered if the haemoglobin is >102 g/L and the fibroids are 3 cm or more in diameter.

For large fibroids, heavy menstrual bleeding and other symptoms such as pressure symptoms or dysmenorrhoea, first-line treatment is surgery or uterine artery embolisation.

National Institute for Health and Care Excellence (NICE). Heavy menstrual bleeding [CG44]. Manchester: NICE; 2007.

11. A Undertake diagnostic laparoscopy and cystectomy

This patient has endometriosis. Around 39% of women with endometriosis complain of non-cyclical pain. Ultrasound has revealed an endometrioma. Laparoscopy and removal of the cyst is necessary to confirm the diagnosis. More areas in the pelvis and intestine tend to infiltrated by endometriosis in women with ovarian endometriosis than in women without ovarian endometriosis.

European Society of Human Reproduction and Embryology (ESHRE). Management of women with endometriosis. Guideline of the European Society of Human Reproduction and Embryology. Belgium: ESHRE; 2013.

12. A Adnexal torsion

Ovarian torsion accounts for around 2.7–7.4% of gynaecological emergencies. It is most common in women of reproductive age but also occurs in prepubertal girls and postmenopausal women. The presentation is typically acute (or acute-on-chronic), intermittent, colicky pain. Nausea and vomiting are present in 85% of patients. There may be tachycardic and/or low-grade pyrexia.

It is often difficult to diagnose ovarian torsion, the resulting delay in diagnosis leading to necrosis and loss of the ovary. As a result, reproductive capacity can be diminished. The data on cyst size and torsion are conflicting. Some authors suggest that an ovarian cyst >5 cm is likely to undergo torsion, whereas others suggest that cysts >5 cm are, conversely, less likely to cause torsion. Torsion is less likely to occur with endometriomas and malignancies, owing to the presence of adhesions.

Damigos E, Johns J, Ross J. An update on the diagnosis and management of ovarian torsion. Obste Gynaecol 2012; 14:229–236.

13. E 168 hours

The different time frames for the persistence of DNA in different types of assault are:

- Oral penetration: 48 hours
- Vaginal penetration: 168 hours
- Anal penetration: 72 hours
- Digital penetration of any orifice: 48 hours
- Skin: 48 hours to 168 hours

Answers: EMQs

14. D Candidal vulvovaginitis

Candidal vulvovaginitis typically presents with vulval redness, oedema and scaling with scratch marks and fissuring on the vulva. It is also associated with an erythematous vagina and thick white non-offensive discharge. Microscopy of the vaginal discharge will reveal hyphae.

Imidazoles are the drugs of choice for treating this condition.

15. L Syphilis

Syphilis is rare in the UK.

Primary chancre: a macule forms at the site of entry (cervix, vagina, vulva and anal canal) of the organism into the body and is followed by ulceration (which is single, indurated and painless). It is often associated with painless inguinal lymphadenopathy. If not treated, secondary syphilis occurs 3–8 weeks later and manifests with genital mucosal ulceration, rash, malaise and condylomata lata. The drug of choice is penicillin. Erythromycin is recommended during pregnancy if the woman is allergic to penicillin.

16. I Lichen sclerosus

Vulval disorders typically involve the perineal area in an hourglass pattern.

Lichen sclerosus is a common, inflammatory condition of the vulval region which is associated with pale atrophic vulva. It is also associated with scratch marks and lichenification on the vulval and perineal region. An underlying malignancy should be ruled out if this is suspected, although this is an uncommon finding.

Highly potent short-term local steroid application (0.05% clobetasol propionate) is recommended for treatment. Local emollients are also prescribed to prevent dryness.

17. J Pemphigoid

Pemphigoid and pemphigus rarely affect the vulva. Their differences are summarised in **Table 12.1**.

Systemic immunosuppressive therapy and oral corticosteroids are usually required to prevent scarring.

Table 12.1 Differences between pemphigoid and pemphigus	
Pemphigoid	Pemphigus
Occurs in older women	Occurs in younger women
Subepidermal blistering	Intraepidermal blistering
Lesions heal with scarring	Lesions heal without scarring
Immunofluorescence studies on biopsies of lesions show antibody deposits at dermoepidermal junction	Immunofluorescence studies on biopsies of lesions show antibody deposits at intercellular spaces of the epidermis

18. E Chanchroid

Chanchroid is caused by *Haemophilus ducreyi*. The ulcer is typically painful, unlike the ulcers in syphilis which are painless. Both are associated with inguinal lymphadenopathy.

Nunns D, Scott IV. Ulcers and erosions of the vulva. Personal assessment in continuing education. Reviews, questions and answers. Volume 3. London: Royal College of Obstetricians and Gynaecologists Press, 2003.

19. N Spironolactone

Spironolactone is a potassium-sparing diuretic. It has a variable effect on the ovaries and adrenal glands by mainly reducing androstenedione levels. It causes competitive inhibition of the 5α-reductase enzyme. The side effects include fatigue, increased frequency of micturition due to diuresis and hyperkalaemia due to the potassium-sparing effect. However, it should be used with caution because it can cause demasculinisation of a male fetus if the woman is pregnant.

20. J Finasteride

Finasteride is an anti-androgen which is rarely used in the management of hirsutism. It inhibits 5α-reductase enzyme activity, and therefore blocks the conversion of testosterone to dihydrotestosterone. However, it should be used with caution because it can cause demasculinisation of a male fetus if the woman is pregnant.

21. K Flutamide

Flutamide is an anti-androgen which acts at the receptor level. It acts directly on the hair follicles and has few side effects. These include hepatotoxicity and dry skin. Like finasteride, it should be used with caution because it can cause demasculinisation of a male fetus.

22. D Cyproterone acetate

Cyproterone acetate is a synthetic derivative of 17-hydroxyprogesterone which is an androgen receptor antagonist with weak progestational and glucocorticoid activity. It suppresses actions of both testosterone and its metabolite dihydrotestosterone on tissues by blocking androgen receptors. It also suppresses luteinising hormone which in turn reduces testosterone levels. The pharmacological actions of this drug are mainly attributed to the acetate form (cyproterone acetate has three times the anti-androgenic activity of cyproterone).

The side effects include mastalgia, weight gain and fluid retention causing oedema and fatigue. In high doses (200–300 mg/day) it can cause liver toxicity and hence should be monitored with liver enzymes. However, the low doses (2 mg) used in gynaecology are unlikely to cause any major problems.

23. I Eflornithine

Eflornithine hydrochloride inhibits ornithine decarboxylase, an enzyme that is present in the dermal papillae and is required for hair growth. It slows hair growth and softens it when applied as a topical cream twice daily. It is recommended for facial hair but can cause acne because it blocks the glands.

Barth J. Chapter 26: Hirsutism and virilisation. In: Shaw RW, Luesley D, Monga A (eds). Gynaecology (4th edn). Edinburgh: Churchill Livingstone, 2011.

24. C Anti-progestogen, anti-oestrogen and weak androgen

Danazol has various actions. These include:

- anti-gonadotrophin
- anti-oestrogen
- anti-progestogen
- also a weak androgen

It is effective in the treatment of menorrhagia (it reduces menstrual blood loss by 85%) but the side effects preclude its use. Contraception should be used when using this drug as it can cause masculinisation of a female fetus. The dose used is 200 mg once daily.

The side effects are mainly androgenic and include:

- irreversible voice change
- terminal hair growth
- frontal baldness
- increase in muscular mass
- osteoporosis due to anti-oestrogen action
- weight gain

25. C Anti-progestogen, anti-oestrogen and weak androgen

Gestrinone has similar actions to danazol but with better compliance. Contraception should be used during its use as it can cause masculinisation of a female fetus.

26. D Endometrial atrophy

Luteal phase (days 15–25) progestogens are not effective in reducing menstrual blood loss and therefore should be avoided in the management of menorrhagia.

27. K Tranexamic acid

Tranexamic acid is an antifibrinolytic agent (it reduces endometrial tissue plasminogen activator) which reduces menstrual blood loss by 54%. It is used as second line therapy for menorrhagia and is considered safe, effective and less expensive. Side effects include headache, nausea and dizziness. It should be avoided in women with a previous history of thromboembolism because there is small risk of venous thromboembolism (VTE).

28. D Endometrial atrophy

The COCP reduces menstrual blood loss by 50%. It is effective in treating menorrhagia and also provides contraception for women who want it. It inhibits luteinising hormone and therefore ovarian hormones, thus causing endometrial atrophy. Side effects can be minor (nausea, headache, mastalgia) or major (thromboembolism).

National Institute of Health and Clinical Excellence (NICE). Heavy menstrual bleeding: assessment and management [CG44]. Manchester: NICE; 2007.
Sen S and Lumsden MA. Chapter 31: Menstruation and menstrual disorder. In: Shaw RW, Luesley D, Monga A (eds). Gynaecology (4th edn). Edinburgh: Churchill Livingstone, 2011.
Letsky E, Murphy MF, Ramsay JE, Walker I. Haemorrhagic Disease and Hereditary Bleeding Disorders. London: Royal College of Obstetricians and Gynaecologists Press, 2005.

29. O Uterine artery embolisation

Uterine artery embolisation (UAE) requires interventional radiology and needs to be done in specialist centres. The main purpose of this method is to obliterate the blood flow in both uterine arteries by using a substance (polyvinyl alcohol) which causes emboli in these arteries until flow ceases. This is done by passing a catheter through the femoral vessels in a retrograde fashion to reach the uterine vessels to facilitate the introduction of these substances to block the vessels.

UAE causes shrinkage of the fibroids and reduces menstrual blood loss by 80–96%. Side effects include post-embolisation syndrome (seen in 8–10% and manifests with fever, chills and pain abdomen), sepsis (due to infection in the necrotic fibroid), bowel perforation and fibroid expulsion. Some women may need a hysterectomy in view of the ongoing complications. It rarely causes death.

There is risk of ovarian failure in 1% of cases and therefore its use is not suggested for women who wish to preserve their fertility. Reports have suggested an increased risk of miscarriage and pre-term labour in women who have had uterine artery embolisation in the past.

30. E Hydrothermal endometrial ablation

Hydrothermal endometrial ablation reduces menstrual blood loss by 75% (it burns the endometrium after introduction of hot fluid into the uterine cavity).

Other ablative methods include:

- Fluid balloon reduces menstrual blood loss by 73–88%.

- Radiofrequency ablation of the endometrium reduces menstrual blood loss by 84%. In this procedure, a sheath with a bipolar radiofrequency electrode is introduced into the uterine cavity. On pulling the sheath back, the electrode conforms to the shape of the uterine cavity and then emits radiofrequencies. The electrode is subsequently withdrawn into the sheath and removed from the uterus. The disadvantage is there is no specimen for histopathological examination.
- Microwave ablation of the endometrium reduces menstrual blood loss by 83%. It involves insertion of a probe into the endometrial cavity to heat the endometrium. During the procedure the temperature is maintained between 75 and 80°C to destroy the endometrium. Lack of histopathological specimens for examination is one of its disadvantages.

31. G Laparoscopic myolysis

Myolysis: the evidence is limited to anecdotal reports. It may be useful in a selected group of women (fibroid <8 cm). Heating at 40–60°C causes programmed cell death and at 60–65°C causes collagen denaturation. It causes shrinkage of fibroids by 30–50% and causes no postoperative pain or regrowth of fibroids.

32. L Transcervical resection of endometrium

Transcervical resection of the endometrium (TCRE) is the resection of the endometrial lining up to a depth of 5 mm (including stratum basalis which normally regenerates endometrium). This leads to amenorrhoea. The most common fluid medium used is glycine. It is a non-conducting fluid but can cause dilutional hyponatraemia and glycine emboli. One also needs to be cautious due to the increased risk of uterine perforation with this procedure.

33. G Laparoscopic myolysis

Myolysis may cause extensive postoperative adhesions and sepsis.

De Souza N and Cosgrove D. Chapter 5: Imaging techniques in gynaecology. In: Shaw RW, Luesley D, Monga A (eds). Gynaecology (4th edn). Edinburgh: Churchill Livingstone, 2011.
National Institute of Health and Clinical Excellence. Excellence (NICE). Heavy menstrual bleeding: assessment and management [CG44]. Manchester: NICE; 2007.

34. K Oestrogen cream or pessaries vaginally HRT

Oestrogen deficiency during the menopause causes atrophy of the genital organs. This makes the tissues in the genital organs fragile (especially the epithelium of the vagina and the cervix) and thus can result in bleeding with minimal trauma (e.g. sexual intercourse) or even without. The treatment is local oestrogens (oestrogen vaginal cream or tablets). This may be required in the long term to revert the symptoms of urogenital atrophy (late manifestation of oestrogen deficiency). It appears to be more effective than systemic therapy.

Low-dose vaginal oestrogens can be used in the management of recurrent urinary tract infection in postmenopausal women once underlying pathology has been excluded. There is no evidence that local vaginal oestrogen is associated with any significant risks.

35. H Oestrogen-only (oral) HRT

HRT is beneficial in relieving symptoms for women with severe menopausal symptoms that adversely affect quality of life. The standard preparation contains oestrogen and progestogen. In women with a uterus, progestogens are given along with oestrogens for endometrial protection because unopposed oestrogens given alone can cause endometrial hyperplasia, which can even lead to endometrial cancer. In women who have undergone a hysterectomy, preparations containing only oestrogen can be used because there is no uterus.

The minimum effective dose should to be used for the shortest duration of time and then should be reviewed on a yearly basis. An individualised approach is necessary and HRT should be started with the informed consent of the woman after appropriate counselling of the risks (breast cancer, thromboembolism and stroke) and benefits. If symptoms return after stopping HRT, it can be restarted.

A short duration of HRT can be used for up to 5 years for symptom relief in menopausal woman in their early 50s.

Younger women with premature menopause can be treated with HRT for their menopausal symptoms and for preventing osteoporosis until the age of normal menopause, following which the therapy should be reviewed.

HRT can be used as an 'add-back' therapy to avoid menopausal symptoms in women on gonadotrophin-releasing hormone (GnRH) agonist therapy.

36. N Sequential oestrogens and progestogens (oral) HRT

Sequential oestrogens and progestogens cause cyclical monthly bleeding. Women who wish to have a monthly withdrawal bleed should be prescribed a sequential regimen of HRT. However, they should be warned about the slightly increased risk of endometrial cancer.

37. A Continuous oestrogens and progestogens (oral) HRT

Women who do not like to have cyclical bleeding should be prescribed a continuous regimen of oestrogen and progestogen.

38. J Oestrogen transdermal patch only HRT

This woman needs only oestrogens since she has had a hysterectomy in the past. She is on a liver enzyme inducing drug (carbamazepine) and therefore would benefit from a transdermal oestrogen patch rather than oral oestrogens to avoid first bypass metabolism.

Cartwright B, Robinson J, Rymer J. Treatment of premature ovarian failure trial: description of an ongoing clinical trial. Post Reproductive Health 2010; 16:18–22.
Royal College of Obstetricians and Gynaecologists (RCOG). Scientific Advisory Committee Opinion Paper 6 (2nd edn). Alternatives to HRT for the management of symptoms of the menopause. London: RCOG Press; 2010.

Chapter 13

Subfertility

Questions: SBAs

For each question, select the single best answer from the five options listed.

1. You are the registrar in the fertility clinic and are about to see a couple who have been having trying to conceive for the last 18 months.

   What is the most likely cause of infertility in this couple?

   A   Male factors
   B   Ovarian factors
   C   Tubal factors
   D   Unexplained causes
   E   Uterine factors

2. A 34-year-old woman attends the infertility clinic with her husband. She has been in this relationship for 10 years and has been trying to conceive for the last 2 years. Her periods were normal up until 2 years ago while she was on the combined oral contraceptive pill; they are now once every 6 months. Her body mass index is $35\,\text{kg/m}^2$. General and pelvic examination is normal.

   What investigation should be requested next?

   A   Blood tests to measure luteinising hormone, follicle-stimulating hormone, sex hormone-binding globulin, testosterone, prolactin and thyroid function
   B   Hysterosalpingogram
   C   Pelvic ultrasound
   D   17-hydroxyprogesterone
   E   Semen tests

3. A 34-year old woman has been referred to the infertility clinic because she has been trying to conceive for 2 years with her current partner. She has regular normal periods. She became pregnant twice 10 years ago with her previous partner but both pregnancies ended in miscarriage. There is no past medical history. Her body mass index is 26 kg/m². The results of the semen analysis are normal. An ultrasound reveals a bulky uterus with multiple intramural fibroids. The endometrial thickness could not be measured because the fibroids were compressing the uterine cavity.

    What initial investigation will you request?

    A   Blood tests – full blood count, urea and creatinine, and clotting factors
    B   Diagnostic hysteroscopy
    C   MRI of the pelvis
    D   Pipelle biopsy
    E   Repeat ultrasound

4. A 25-year-old woman and her partner have been referred to the fertility clinic because she has been trying to conceive for the last 2 years. There is no significant past medical history and she is not taking any medication. Her body mass index is 24 kg/m². The results of blood hormone measurement, pelvic ultrasound and hysterosalpingography results are normal. The partner, who is a teacher and exercises regularly has a normal body mass index, is not taking any medication and has no past medical history. The results of the semen analysis are:

- Volume 3 mL
- Total sperm count 55 million per ejaculate
- Sperm concentration 20 million/mL
- pH >7.2
- Overall motility 25%
- Normal forms 6%
- Vitality 68%

    What does the semen analysis show?

    A   Asthenozoospermia
    B   Oligozoospermia
    C   Oligoteratozoospermia
    D   Oligoasthenoteratozoospermia
    E   Teratozoospermia

5. A 25-year-old woman and her partner have attended the infertility clinic because she has been trying to conceive for the last 12 months. They have had unprotected sexual intercourse 3 times a week over that time. The woman has no significant past medical history and is not taking any medication. Her body mass index is 23 kg/m^2. Her periods are regular. The results of blood hormone concentrations, pelvic ultrasound and hysterosalpingography are normal, as are the results of semen analysis .

    What management will you advise?

    A   Clomifene citrate for 12 months
    B   Clomifene citrate for 6 months
    C   Continue unprotected intercourse for 12 months
    D   Intrauterine insemination
    E   In vitro fertilisation

6. A 31-year-old woman and her partner are attending the infertility clinic because she has been trying to trying to conceive for the last 2 years despite regular unprotected sexual intercourse. She had a normal vaginal delivery 10 years ago, with the same partner. The woman has no past medical history and is not taking any medication. Her body mass index is 23 kg/m^2 and her periods are regular. The results of blood tests, ultrasound and hysterosalpingography are normal, as are the results of semen analysis .

    What management will you advise?

    A   Clomifene citrate for 12 months
    B   Clomifene citrate for 6 months
    C   Continue unprotected intercourse for 12 months
    D   Intrauterine fertilisation
    E   In vitro fertilisation

7. A 39-year-old woman has been trying to conceive for the last 2 years. She has no past medical history and is not taking any regular medication. Her body mass index is 23 kg/m^2. The results of blood hormone measurement and pelvic ultrasound and hysterosalpingography are normal. Her partner's semen analysis is also normal.

    What is the most appropriate management plan?

    A   Clomifene citrate for 12 months
    B   Clomifene citrate for 6 months
    C   Continue unprotected intercourse for 12 months
    D   Intrauterine fertilisation
    E   In vitro fertilisation

8. A 25-year-old woman presents to the infertility clinic because she has been trying to conceive for the last 2 years. She does not have any children at present. An ultrasound shows bilateral hydrosalpinges and blocked fallopian tubes. The results of her partner's semen are normal.

What is your advice for the management of this woman?

A   Antibiotics
B   Intrauterine insemination
C   In vitro fertilisation
D   Laparoscopic salpingectomy and then in vitro fertilisation
E   Tubal aspiration

9. A 44-year-old woman and her partner attend the infertility clinic because despite regular unprotected sexual intercourse over the last 2 years, she has not conceived. The woman has no significant past medical history and is not taking any medication. She has no children. Her body mass index is 23 kg/m². She has regular menstrual periods. The results of blood hormone measurement, pelvic ultrasound and hysterosalpingography are normal. Semen analysis also shows normal results.

What is the most appropriate management plan?

A   Clomifene citrate for 12 months
B   Clomifene citrate for 6 months
C   Intrauterine insemination
D   Continue unprotected intercourse for 12 months
E   In vitro fertilisation

10. A 25-year-old woman and her partner attend the infertility clinic because she has been trying to conceive for the last 2 years. She has no past significant medical history and is not taking any medication. Her body mass index is 24 kg/m². The results of blood hormone measurement, hysterosalpingography and pelvic ultrasound are normal. Her partner, who is an accountant and exercises regularly, has a normal body mass index, is not on any medication and has no past medical problems. The results of his semen analysis are:

- Volume ≥1.5 mL
- Total sperm count 2 million per ejaculate
- Sperm concentration <15 million/mL
- pH ≥7.2
- Overall motility ≥40%
- Progressive motility ≥32%
- Normal forms ≥4%
- Vitality ≥58%

What is the initial plan of management?

A   In vitro fertilisation
B   Repeat semen analysis as soon as possible
C   Repeat semen analysis in 3 months

D   Start intrauterine insemination treatment

E   Clomifene treatment

11. A 35-year-old woman and her partner attend the infertility clinic because they want to start a family. They have been using condoms for protection during intercourse. The woman's partner is HIV positive and is taking highly active antiretroviral therapy. The plasma viral load has been <50 copies/mL for more than 6 months, and there are no other infections. The woman is HIV-negative.

What is your advice to the couple?

A   Not to attempt pregnancy

B   In vitro fertilisation

C   Timed intercourse without sperm washing

D   Timed intercourse with sperm washing

E   Timed intercourse with pre-exposure prophylaxis

12. A 25-year-old woman attends the infertility clinic because she has been trying to conceive with her current partner for the last 3 years. Her periods are irregular and occur every 6 months. Blood tests results are normal, as are pelvic ultrasound and hysterosalpingography. There is no significant past medical history and she is not taking any medication. She does not smoke or drink. She works as a secretary and has run marathons several times; her body mass index (BMI) is 17 kg/m². Her partner is also a fitness instructor and is healthy. Semen analysis is normal.

What is your advice to this couple?

A   Clomifene treatment

B   Intrauterine insemination treatment

C   In vitro fertilisation

D   Putting on weight to increase BMI to >19 kg/m²

E   Putting on weight to increase BMI to >22 kg/m²

13. A 33-year-old woman who is known to have polycystic ovarian syndrome presents to the fertility clinic because of an inability to conceive for the last 2 years. There is no significant past medical history apart from a severe phobia of general anaesthesia. She has no children at present. Her body mass index is 27 kg/m². Her pelvic ultrasound and hysterosalpingography are normal which shows that her Fallopian tubes are patent. The results of semen analysis are normal. The woman has been taking clomifene citrate and metformin for the last 6 months but has still not become pregnant.

How will you best manage her?

A   Continue clomifene citrate only for a further 6 months

B   Continue clomifene citrate and metformin for a further 6 months

C   Gonadotropin treatment

D   Laparoscopic ovarian drilling

E   Advise her to lose weight

14. A 35-year-old woman and her partner are attending the infertility clinic as she has been trying to conceive for the past 2 years. Her last period was 8 months ago. There is no significant past medical history and she is not taking any medication. Blood tests results are normal apart from a follicle-stimulating hormone concentration of 72 IU/L and luteinising hormone of 32 IU/L. The results of a pelvic ultrasound and hysterosalpingography are normal. The semen analysis results are also normal.

What is the correct management?

A   Check the antimüllerian hormone level
B   Clomifene citrate induction
C   Donor oocyte
D   Gonadotropin treatment
E   Repeat blood tests in 3 months

Questions: EMQs

Questions 15–19

Options for Questions 15–19

A Androgen insensitivity syndrome	I Hypogonadotrophic hypogonadism
B Androgen secreting tumour	J Granulosa cell tumour of the ovary
C Adenomyosis	K Ovarian remnant syndrome
D Autoimmune disease	L Ovarian resistant syndrome
E Cushing's syndrome	M Residual ovary syndrome
F Endometriosis	N Parovarian cyst
G Fibroid uterus	O Premature ovarian failure
H Fitz–Hugh–Curtis syndrome	P Unexplained infertility

Instructions: For each clinical scenario described below, choose the single most appropriate diagnosis from the list of options above. Each option may be used once, more than once, or not at all.

15. A 38-year-old Asian woman attends the infertility clinic with her partner. She has been trying to conceive for the last 3 years without success. She gives a history of regular periods associated with dysmenorrhoea which outlasts the periods. She is 1.52 m (5 ft) tall and is a normal weight for her height. Pelvic examination reveals thickened, tender uterosacral ligaments. Hormonal tests reveal normal luteinising hormone (LH), follice-stimulating hormone (FSH), testosterone, prolactin and ovulatory day 21 progesterone. Her partner's semen analysis is normal.

16. A 20-year-old Asian woman attends the infertility clinic with her husband. She has been trying to conceive for the last 2 years without any success. She is very anxious because her mother-in-law is pressuring her and abusing her for not conceiving. Clinically, she has a blind vagina with small breasts and scant pubic hair. Investigations reveal grossly elevated testosterone levels above the normal range and relatively elevated oestrogen levels.

17. A 38-year-old white woman attends the infertility clinic with her partner. She has been trying to conceive for the last 2.5 years. She has a normal body mass index (BMI) and gives a history of regular menstrual cycles. Hormonal tests reveal normal FSH, LH, testosterone, prolactin and ovulatory day 21 progesterone. Her partner's semen analysis is normal. A hysterosalpingogram (HSG) confirms bilateral patent fallopian tubes.

18. A 40-year-old white woman attends the infertility clinic. She has been trying to conceive for the last year and had noticed very scant periods over the last 6 months. She gives a history of rapid hair growth on the face, chin and chest in the last 4 months. Her voice has deepened and she has noticed an increase in muscle bulk. The rest of the physical examination is normal. Her partner's semen analysis is normal.

19. A 30-year-old white woman attends the day surgery unit for a diagnostic laparoscopy. She has been trying to conceive for the last 3 years and has some

pelvic pain on the right side. She is a normal weight and gives a history of regular menstrual cycles. Hormonal tests reveal normal LH, FSH, prolactin, thyroid function tests (TFTs) and ovulatory day 21 progesterone. Laparoscopy reveals absence of spill in both Fallopian tubes and perihepatic adhesions. Her partner's semen analysis is normal.

Questions 20–24

Options for Questions 20–24

A	Admit to the ward	I	Laparotomy and salpingectomy
B	Arrange in vitro fertilisation (IVF)	J	Laparoscopy and ovarian cystectomy
C	Bilateral ovarian drilling	K	Offer medical termination of pregnancy
D	Counsel and offer support	L	Perform suction evacuation
E	Do serial β-hCG blood tests	M	Perform laparoscopy and dye test
F	Explain and offer laparoscopic salpingectomy	N	Refer to the recurrent miscarriage clinic
G	Intramuscular methotrexate	O	Repeat scan in 1 week
H	Intramuscular tranexamic acid		

Instructions: For each clinical scenario described below, choose the single most appropriate management from the list of options above. Each option may be used once, more than once, or not at all.

20. A 36-year-old Asian woman attends the early pregnancy assessment unit with mild vaginal bleeding. She gives a history of an embryo transfer 2.5 weeks ago at a fertility centre, hence she is anxious. She is under a lot of family pressure to have children. A pregnancy test performed today is negative.

21. A 36-year-old white woman attends the early pregnancy assessment unit with abdominal pain. She had an embryo transfer 5 weeks ago at a fertility centre and has come for a routine scan. A transvaginal scan reveals a single viable intrauterine pregnancy and a 3.5 cm echogenic mass seen adjacent to the left ovary suggestive of an ectopic pregnancy. There is no free fluid in the rectouterine pouch (pouch of Douglas) and both ovaries appear normal.

22. A 36-year-old Asian woman attends the infertility clinic with her husband. She has been trying to conceive for the last 2 years. She is overweight and gives a history of irregular periods over the last 2 years. Her history and investigations are suggestive of polycystic ovary syndrome (PCOS). She has been using clomiphene citrate for the last 6 months with day 21 progesterone of 30 nmol/L. Her husband's semen analysis is normal.

23. A 36-year-old white woman attends the infertility clinic with her partner. She is a normal weight and gives a history of regular menstrual cycles. However, her periods are heavy and are associated with severe pain that outlasts her periods. Hormonal tests reveal normal LH, FSH, prolactin and ovulatory day 21 progesterone levels. She recently had a laparoscopy and a dye test that showed pelvic adhesions with an absence of dye spill in both fallopian tubes. Her partner's semen analysis is normal.

24. A 36-year-old white woman attends the infertility clinic with her husband. She has been trying to conceive for the last 2 years. She is overweight and gives a history of irregular cycles for the last 2 years. Her history and investigations are suggestive of PCOS. She has been using clomiphene citrate for the last 8 months. Hysterosalpingogram reveals patent fallopian tubes. Her husband's semen analysis is normal.

Answers: SBAs

1. A Male factors

The causes of infertility are:

- Male factors (30%)
- Ovarian factors (25%)
- Unexplained causes (25%)
- Tubal disorders (20%)
- Uterine or peritoneal disorders (10%)

2. A Blood tests to measure luteinising hormone, follicle-stimulating hormone, sex hormone-binding globulin, testosterone, prolactin and thyroid function

The history is suggestive of polycystic ovarian syndrome (PCOS). The blood tests listed in the answer aid in diagnosing this.

Approximately 90–95% of women who attend an infertility clinic with anovulation have PCOS. PCOS is characterised by:

- Anovulatory infertility
- Oligomenorrhoea
- Hyperandrogenism – hirsutism and/or acne

The diagnosis of PCOS is made by the presence of polycystic ovaries on an ultrasound plus signs and symptoms of hyperandrogenism and/or menstrual problems. 20% of women of reproductive age demonstrate ultrasound evidence of PCOS, and 10% of women have biochemical or clinical signs of anovulation or hyperandrogenism.

Obese women with PCOS have greater resistance to insulin, which causes increased insulin secretion. This in turn increases ovarian androgen production, which aggravates menstrual disturbances and infertility. By the age of 40 years, 40% of women with PCOS have diabetes, osteoporosis and increased cardiovascular risk. There is also an increased risk of endometrial hyperplasia and cancer.

The following differential diagnoses should be excluded:

- Congenital adrenal hyperplasia
- Adrenal gland tumours
- Cushing's syndrome

Other causes which can contribute to anovulatory dysfunction, such as thyroid dysfunction and hyperprolactinaemia, should be ruled out.

The European Society of Human Reproduction and Embryology criteria require 2 of the following for diagnosis:

- Oligo-ovulation or anovulation
- Clinical and/or biochemical signs of hyperandrogenism
- Polycystic ovaries and exclusion of other aetiologies (congenital adrenal hyperplasia, androgen-secreting tumours, Cushing's syndrome)

In women with PCOS, follicle-stimulating hormone (FSH) levels and the ratio of luteinising hormone (LH) levels to FSH levels are raised. Increased LH levels are found in only 60% of women, whereas LH:FSH ratios are increased in 95%. Investigation of the effect of LH on fertility has suggested that high LH concentrations impair oocyte maturity and fertilisation, reduce fertility and increase risk of miscarriage. However, some studies disagree, so LH levels are not currently considered necessary for the diagnosis of PCOS.

Antimüllerian hormone (AMH) is released by cells involved in the monthly growth of the ovum. Levels correlate with the number of antral follicles found on the ovary every month: the higher the antral follicle count, the higher serum AMH levels are. Women with PCOS typically have more antral follicles and therefore higher AMH levels. AMH is used in many clinics as a potential diagnostic marker for PCOS and as an indicator of ovarian reserve in older women.

The main problems in diagnosing PCOS are:

- Biochemical abnormalities are seen in women with regular cycles and normal ultrasound results who present with hirsutism or acne
- Women with normal body mass index who present with oligomenorrhoea often have abnormal biochemical and ultrasound results
- There is a significant variation in clinical and biochemical pictures
- It is important that patients are diagnosed properly in order to treat the metabolic complications of PCOS

Although PCOS affects women with a normal body index, an association between PCOS and obesity has been found, and there is evidence that exercise and weight control increase fertility in a significant number of obese anovulatory PCOS patients (the loss of 5–10% of body weight can lead to normal periods and pregnancy). There is no evidence of an improvement with exercise and diet in women with a normal body mass index, but adverse lipid profiles are seen in normal-weight PCOS patients, and screening fasting blood glucose, lipids and triglyceride concentrations helps to indicate long-term risk

Treatment for PCOS involves:

- Lifestyle modifications (exercise and weight loss)
- Symptomatic management, e.g. regulate periods, treat hirsutism and acne
- Ovulation induction agents for women who want to conceive (e.g. clomifene citrate, which results in an ovulation rate of 70–85% and a pregnancy rate of 40–50%). The limitation is short-term use because there is a possible risk of ovarian cancer when used for more than 12 months
- Metformin (promotes resumption of menstruation, increases rate of spontaneous ovulation, enhances ovulatory response to clomifene citrate)
- Laparoscopic ovarian drilling
- In vitro fertilisation if other methods of fertility treatment fail

Regarding laparoscopic ovarian drilling as a treatment for PCOS:

- It is used in clomifene-resistant PCOS
- It is as effective as gonadotropin therapy
- Ovulation occurs in 80% of patients, and 40–69% become pregnant
- Serum levels of LH, androgens and sex hormone-binding globulin normalise in >60% of women
- It is associated with a low miscarriage rate (14%)
- There is no risk of multiple pregnancy or ovarian hyperstimulation syndrome
- There is no need for intensive monitoring
- However, the effect of treatment is short term (6–12 months), the treatment is expensive, and operative and anaesthetic complications may develop

Proven PCOS is associated with complications in pregnancy:

- Gestational diabetes (13% versus 5% in normal individuals)
- Pregnancy-induced hypertension
- Increased risk of miscarriage (30–40%)

Clark AM, Ledger WL, Galletly C, et al. Weight loss results in significant improvement in pregnancy and ovulation rates in anovulatory obese women. Hum Reprod 1995; 10:2705–2712.
Rotterdam ESHRE/ASRM-Sponsored PCOS Consensus Workshop Group. Revised 2003 consensus on diagnostic criteria and long-term health risks related to polycystic ovary syndrome. Fertil Steril 2004; 81:19–25.

3.   B Diagnostic hysteroscopy

Hysteroscopy is necessary here to exclude submucous fibroids or fibroids compressing the uterine cavity because these can be removed. If one of the answer options had been sonohysterography or saline sonography, this would have been correct because submucous fibroids can be visualised by this modality, which is also less invasive for diagnosis than diagnostic hysteroscopy. Large fibroids that protrude into or compress the uterine cavity interfere with implantation by secretion of vasoactive substances, vascular compromise, endometrial inflammation or disordered placentation. There is increasing evidence that even intramural fibroids that do not impinge on the uterine cavity can still affect pregnancy rates after assisted conception.

4.   A Asthenozoospermia

The World Health Organization defines a normal result for semen analysis as:

- Volume ≥1.5 mL
- Total sperm count ≥39 million per ejaculate
- Sperm concentration ≥15 million/mL
- pH ≥7.2
- Overall motility ≥40%
- Progressive motility ≥32%
- Normal forms ≥4%
- Vitality ≥58%

A low sperm count is called oligozoospermia. Reduced morphology and increased abnormal form are called teratozoospermia. Asthenospermia, as is the case here, refers to reduced motility. The combination of low sperm count, reduced motility and reduced morphology with abnormal forms is called oligoasthenoteratozoospermia.

World Health Organization (WHO). WHO laboratory manual for the examination and processing of human semen (5th edn). Geneva: WHO; 2010.

5. C Continue unprotected intercourse for 12 months

The diagnosis is unexplained infertility. The NICE recommends that women with this diagnosis try to conceive for 2 years (which can include up to 1 year before their fertility investigations) before fertility treatment is given.

National Institute for Health and Care Excellence (NICE). Fertility: assessment and treatment for people with fertility problems [CG156]. London: NICE; 2013. Updated 2016.

6. E In vitro fertilisation

In this situation, in vitro fertilisation is needed. Because there is unexplained infertility, ovarian stimulation agents such as clomifene citrate, anastrozole and letrozole have no role because they do not improve clinical pregnancy or live birth rates.

National Institute for Health and Care Excellence (NICE). Fertility: assessment and treatment for people with fertility problems [CG156]. London: NICE; 2013. Updated 2016.

7. D Intrauterine fertilisation

This patient has unexplained infertility, so in vitro fertilisation (IVF) is the first-line option. IVF as opposed to intrauterine insemination is the best option because of the patient's age and the higher success per cycle.

National Institute for Health and Care Excellence (NICE). Fertility: assessment and treatment for people with fertility problems [CG156]. London: NICE; 2013.

8. D Laparoscopic salpingectomy and then in vitro fertilisation

In vitro fertilisation (IVF) is the best treatment for moderate to severe bilateral tubal disease. Evidence shows that laparoscopic salpingectomy for hydrosalpinges increases the likelihood of successful IVF treatment, from 24% without salpingectomy to 72% with salpingectomy. Therefore, laparoscopic salpingectomy followed by IVF is the appropriate management.

9. E In vitro fertilisation

In vitro fertilisation should be advised. Because there is unexplained infertility, ovarian stimulation agents such as clomifene citrate, anastrozole and letrozole do not have a role because they do not improve the likelihood of clinical pregnancy or live birth. As this patient is 44 years of age, she will not qualify for treatment funded by the NHS.

National Institute for Health and Care Excellence (NICE). Fertility: assessment and treatment for people with fertility problems [CG156]. London: NICE; 2013.

10. B Repeat semen sample analysis as soon as possible

This patient's partner has oligozoospermia. In this situation, and with azoospermia, the semen sample should be repeated as soon as possible. Other abnormalities identified by the semen analysis warrant a repeat sample in 3 months to allow the spermatozoal cycle to be completed.

National Institute for Health and Care Excellence (NICE). Fertility problems: assessment and treatment for people with fertility problems [CG156]. London: NICE; 2013.
National Institute for Health and Care Excellence (NICE). Fertility problems. Quality standard 73. London: NICE; 2014.

11. C Timed intercourse without sperm washing

The couple should be informed that the chance of HIV transmission following unprotected sexual intercourse is very low if:

- The man is taking highly active antiretroviral therapy
- He has had a viral load of <50 copies/mL for more than 6 months
- There are no other infections
- Unprotected intercourse is limited to the time of ovulation

If these criteria are met, sperm washing is unlikely to reduce the likelihood of HIV transmission, although it may affect the chance of successful pregnancy. If these criteria are not met, couples should be offered sperm washing and informed that sperm washing does not completely eliminate the risk of HIV transmission. There is insufficient evidence to advise women to take pre-exposure prophylaxis if the above criteria have been met.

National Institute for Health and Care Excellence (NICE). Fertility: assessment and treatment for people with fertility problems [CG156]. London: NICE; 2013.

12. D Putting on weight to increase body mass index (BMI) to >19 kg/m^2

This patient has anovulatory infertility. Increasing body mass index to >19 kg/m^2 and moderating exercise levels provides the best chance of regulating her periods, improving the likelihood of conception and leading to an uncomplicated pregnancy. If the desired body mass index is reached but the woman still does not conceive, pulsatile of gonadotropin-releasing hormone or gonadotropins with luteinising hormone activity should be administered.

National Institute for Health and Care Excellence (NICE). Fertility: assessment and treatment for people with fertility problems [CG156]. London: NICE; 2013.

13. C Gonadotropin treatment

If a woman's body mass index is >30 kg/m^2, she should first be advised to lose weight because this is likely to initiate ovulation. The first-line pharmacological treatment is clomifene citrate, metformin or a combination of the two, but she has already received this. Clomifene citrate treatment should not last longer than 6 months. If the patient has still not conceived after 6 months of medical treatment, laparoscopic ovarian drilling or gonadotropins are the next step. Because this woman has a severe phobia of general anaesthesia, gonadotropins are the correct treatment.

National Institute for Health and Care Excellence (NICE). Fertility: assessment and treatment for people with fertility problems [CG156]. London: NICE; 2013.

14. C Donor oocyte

This patient has premature ovarian failure. The best treatment is oocyte donation.

National Institute for Health and Care Excellence (NICE). Fertility: assessment and treatment for people with fertility problems [CG156]. London: NICE; 2013.

Answers: EMQs

15. F Endometriosis

Endometriosis has symptoms which include deep dyspareunia, severe dysmenorrhoea, chronic pelvic pain, ovulation pain, cyclical or premenstrual bowel or bladder symptoms, infertility and dyschezia (painful defaecation).

When performed during menstruation, clinical examination may reveal deeply infiltrating nodules. The gold standard for diagnosing endometriosis is by visual inspection of the pelvis at laparoscopy. However, ultrasonography is a useful tool to diagnose ovarian endometrioma.

Serum CA-125 may be elevated in this condition but has no value as a diagnostic tool compared to laparoscopy.

Medical therapy

A therapeutic trial of hormone drug therapy to reduce menstrual flow is appropriate if the woman has symptoms suggestive of endometriosis and wants treatment. It has been shown that suppression of ovarian function can reduce endometriosis-associated pain. The use of a levonorgestrel-releasing intrauterine system is also known to reduce endometriosis-related pain. However, recurrence of symptoms is common following medical treatment of endometriosis. The duration of therapy depends on the drug choice, response to therapy and side effect profile.

There is not enough evidence to suggest non-steroidal anti-inflammatory drugs (NSAIDs) are effective in reducing endometriosis-associated pain.

A gonadotropin-releasing hormone (GnRH) agonist with 'add back' therapy with oestrogen and progesterone can be used for treatment. 'Add back' therapy protects against bone mineral density loss during GnRH therapy and for a further 6 months after.

Surgical treatment

Endometriosis-related pain can be reduced by removing the entire lesions in severe deeply infiltrating lesions. However, before undertaking such extensive surgery planning is important and this should be done in a multidisciplinary context.

The involvement of the bladder, bowel and ureters should be assessed to plan the extent of surgery. Therefore, consider performing an MRI scan or ultrasound (transrectal or renal) scan with or without intravenous urogram and barium enema studies to map the disease.

The ideal treatment is removal of endometriosis. However, ablation of endometriotic lesions has been shown to reduce endometriosis-related pain compared to diagnostic laparoscopy alone.

Laparoscopic uterine nerve ablation has not been shown to reduce endometriosis-associated pain.

There is not sufficient evidence to justify the use of hormonal therapy prior to or after surgical treatment.

Infertility treatment

Ovarian hormone suppression to improve fertility in minimal to mild endometriosis is not effective and there is no evidence that it is effective in more severe disease. However, ablation of endometriotic spots with adhesiolysis is effective for improving fertility in minimal to mild endometriosis compared to diagnostic laparoscopy alone. Also, in women with endometriosis-related infertility, tubal flushing appears to improve pregnancy rates while treatment with intrauterine insemination also improves fertility. One should offer IVF treatment especially if there is a contributing tubal factor or male factor, or if other treatments have failed.

GnRH agonist use for 3–6 months before IVF in women with endometriosis increases the rate of clinical pregnancy.

The role of surgery in improving pregnancy rates in moderate to severe endometriosis is not certain.

Laparoscopic ovarian cystectomy for ovarian endometrioma is better than drainage and coagulation. It is recommended for lesions ≥4 cm.

Hormonal therapy following surgery does not improve pregnancy rates.

The role of complementary therapies is uncertain.

16. A Androgen insensitivity syndrome

Androgen insensitivity syndrome (46XY) is an X-linked recessive condition where testicular function is normal but cell receptors are unable to respond to androgens. This can impair or prevent the masculinisation of male genitalia in a developing fetus and also the development of male secondary sexual characteristics at puberty. Most of the affected women present at puberty as adolescents with primary amenorrhoea.

The defect may be due to 5α-reductase enzyme deficiency, or partial or complete androgen insensitivity (**Table 13.1**).

Table 13.1 Androgen insensitivity syndrome

5α-reductase enzyme deficiency

- Autosomal recessive trait
- Normal levels of testosterone
- Low dihydrotestosterone
- Internal genitalia male
- External genitalia ambiguous or female
- Male phenotype at puberty

Complete androgen insensitivity

- X-linked recessive disorder
- Normal female external genitalia
- Male internal genitalia
- Blind vaginal pouch
- Absent uterus and ovaries
- Absent Wolffian structures
- Breast growth at puberty
- Sparse pubic and axillary hair
- Testes are found in the labial folds, inguinal canal or intra-abdominal
- Gonads should be removed at puberty because of risk of malignancy
- Elevated testosterone levels
- Relatively elevated oestradiol levels which are testicular in origin and are also derived from peripheral conversion of testosterone to oestradiol

Partial androgen insensitivity

- X-linked recessive disorder
- Mainly caused due to the reduced binding affinity of dihydrotestosterone or a receptor defect in the transcription of the nucleus
- Most common presentation is hypospadias during infancy
- Ambiguous genitalia
- Male internal genitalia
- Blind vaginal pouch
- Phallic enlargement
- Absent uterus and ovaries
- Rudimentary or normal Wolffian ducts
- Testes are azoospermic
- Poor development of secondary sexual characteristics at puberty
- Breast development at puberty
- Gonadectomy and hormone replacement therapy is indicated if assigned as a female

17. P Unexplained infertility

The chance of conceiving following 1 year of regular unprotected intercourse is 80% and after 18 months is 90%. In a couple seeking help to conceive, investigations should be performed only if there is at least a 1-year history of infertility.

Couples are said to have unexplained infertility when there is failure to conceive when basic infertility investigations are normal. It is reported in 10–20% of cases and the chances of conception depend on the age of the female partner, duration of the infertility and whether the infertility is primary or secondary. The pregnancy rate within 3 years of follow-up is reported to be 60–70% with no specific treatment. Counselling is an important aspect of management but may be frustrating for couples.

18. B Androgen secreting tumour

Androgen secreting tumours may arise in the adrenal gland or the ovary.

Adrenal adenomas and late onset congenital adrenal hyperplasia can give rise to such symptoms. The onset is usually sudden and of a short duration. The symptoms are that of virilisation. If the woman is pregnant, it may cause masculinisation of the fetus.

One should differentiate this from Cushing's syndrome.

Cushing's syndrome

Cushing's syndrome is due to an excess of glucocorticoids in the blood [glucocorticoid therapy and tumours that produce cortisol or adrenocorticotropic hormone (ACTH)]. In this condition, there will be other symptoms in addition to hirsutism. These include typical weight gain in the trunk and face, buffalo hump, excessive sweating, telangiectasia and easy bruising due to thinning of the skin, purple skin stria, hyperpigmentation, insulin resistance and diabetes, proximal muscle weakness, baldness, hirsutism, hypertension, hypercalcaemia, osteoporosis, euphoria or psychosis, amenorrhoea and infertility.

ACTH-induced Cushing's syndrome causes hypokalaemic alkalosis and hypertension together with glucose intolerance, while there is no hypokalaemia with increased glucocorticoid excess due to a pituitary cause.

Types

- Pituitary Cushing's or Cushing's disease: it is responsible for 70% of endogenous Cushing's syndrome and is caused by increased ACTH secretion from a benign pituitary adenoma.
- Adrenal Cushing's disease: it is caused by excessive cortisol secretion by adrenal gland tumours or hyperplasia.
- Ectopic or paraneoplastic Cushing's disease: ectopic secretion of ACTH can have an influence on the adrenal gland, e.g. ACTH production from small cell lung cancer.

Diagnosis

- 24-hour urinary cortisol measurement will be high
- Dexamethasone suppression test (normally the administration of dexamethasone would suppress the ACTH production by negative feedback and thereby reduce cortisol secretion. If cortisol levels are high, it would be indicative of Cushing's syndrome because there is an ectopic source of cortisol or ACTH that is not inhibited by dexamethasone)

Ovarian tumours which are androgen secreting include arrhenoblastoma, luteoma, Leydig cell tumour and gynandroblastoma.

19. H Fitz–Hugh–Curtis syndrome

The presence of perihepatic adhesions in women with previous pelvic inflammatory disease is known as Fitz–Hugh–Curtis syndrome.

Royal College of Obstetricians and Gynaecologists (RCOG). The investigation and management of endometriosis. Green-top guideline no 24. London: RCOG Press, 2008.
Keith Edmonds D. Chapter 13: Sexual differentiation – normal and abnormal. In: Shaw RW, Luesley D, Monga A (eds). Gynaecology (4th edn). Edinburgh: Churchill Livingstone, 2011.

20. D Counsel and offer support

A pregnancy test is usually positive at 2 weeks after an embryo transfer. If the pregnancy test is negative it means that the IVF cycle has failed. Hence, this woman needs counsel and support.

21. F Explain and offer laparoscopic salpingectomy

This woman has heterotopic pregnancy (the incidence is 1 in 30,000 pregnancies). She will need a laparoscopic salpingectomy for removal of the ectopic pregnancy (in the UK, most ectopic pregnancies are managed laparoscopically). She cannot be offered medical management with methotrexate because she also has a viable intrauterine pregnancy.

The small risk of miscarriage with surgery and anaesthesia performed in early pregnancy should be explained to her.

22. M Perform laparoscopy and dye test

Midluteal progesterone levels of >30 nmol/L is suggestive of ovulation.

This woman is responding to clomiphene citrate with serum progesterone levels showing ovulation, hence her tubes should be checked for patency before offering other forms of fertility treatment.

23. B Arrange IVF

This woman has endometriosis and both tubes are damaged. Hence, one should offer IVF treatment especially if there is a contributing tubal factor or male factor or if other treatments have failed.

24. C Bilateral ovarian drilling

Ovarian drilling should be offered to women with clomiphene resistant PCOS.

Hamilton M. Chapter 20: Disorders and investigation of female reproduction. In: Shaw RW, Luesley D, Monga A (eds). Gynaecology (4th edn). Edinburgh: Churchill Livingstone; 2011.
Vogiatzi M and Shaw RW. Chapter 17: Ovulation induction. Gynaecology (4th edn). In: Shaw RW, Luesley D, Monga A (eds). Gynaecology (4th edn). Edinburgh: Churchill Livingstone; 2011.

Chapter 14

Sexual and reproductive health

Questions: SBAs

For each question, select the single best answer from the five options listed.

1. While a 24-year-old woman and her husband are having intercourse, the condom tears. The woman attends the family planning clinic 3 days later. She is worried that she will get pregnant because she does not want children for at least 5 years. She is asking for emergency contraception. She is otherwise medically fit and well.

   Which one of the following emergency contraceptive methods will you recommend?

   A   Copper coil
   B   Copper coil and start a combined oral contraceptive
   C   Levonorgestrel 1.5 mg
   D   Levonorgestrel 3 mg
   E   Ulipristal acetate

2. An 18-year-old woman attends the family planning clinic. She had unprotected sexual intercourse with a stranger 5 days ago and is very worried she will get pregnant. She was not able to come to the clinic for advice before this. She has no significant past medical history and is not taking any medication.

   Which one of the following emergency contraceptive methods is appropriate?

   A   Copper coil
   B   Copper coil and start a combined oral contraceptive
   C   Levonorgestrel 1.5 mg
   D   Levonorgestrel 3 mg
   E   Ulipristal acetate

3. An 18-year-old woman attends the family planning clinic. She is very anxious because she had unprotected sexual intercourse with a stranger 3 days ago. She is worried that she will get pregnant but was not able to come to the clinic before this. She has epilepsy, which is well controlled with phenytoin.

   Which contraceptive method will you recommend?

   A   Copper coil
   B   Copper coil and start a combined oral contraceptive

    C   Levonorgestrel 1.5 mg
    D   Levonorgestrel 3 mg
    E   Ulipristal acetate

4. A 20-year-old woman attends the early pregnancy assessment unit at 6 weeks' gestation with vaginal bleeding. Examination confirms mild vaginal bleeding and an ultrasound shows a viable intrauterine pregnancy. She wishes to have a termination of pregnancy. She is not in a relationship, is halfway through her university degree, lives in Scotland and does not want this pregnancy.

Which statutory ground should be chosen on the termination form?

    A   Statutory ground A
    B   Statutory ground B
    C   Statutory ground C
    D   Statutory ground D
    E   Statutory ground E

5. A 32-year-old woman with two children who is 20 weeks pregnant attends her antenatal clinic in South London. The consultant has just told her that earlier investigations have confirmed that the fetus has Down's syndrome. She already has one child with Down's syndrome and one with autism. She is not sure whether she is mentally, physically or financially able to look after another child with Down's syndrome. She is thinking of having a termination of pregnancy.

On which statutory ground should she be offered a termination of pregnancy?

    A   Statutory ground A
    B   Statutory ground B
    C   Statutory ground C
    D   Statutory ground D
    E   Statutory ground E

6. A 14-year-old girl visits her GP in Oxford at 8 weeks' gestation to request termination of pregnancy. She understands the risks and benefits.

Which one of the following should be part of your consultation?

    A   Assessing her Gillick competence
    B   Calling her parents to check if she has any medical conditions
    C   Checking her serum platelet level
    D   Speaking to her school to make sure that they are aware of the pregnancy
    E   Performing an ultrasound in clinic

7. A 21-year-old woman presents to the emergency department because she has not been able to pass urine for the last 8 hours. She reports malaise, a temperature and myalgia a few days ago. When you examine her to insert a catheter, you see multiple blisters on the labia bilaterally.

What is the diagnosis?

    A   *Chlamydia trachomatis*

   B   Herpes simplex virus
   C   Human papillomavirus
   D   *Treponema pallidum*
   E   Varicella zoster virus

8. A 21-year-old woman attends the emergency department with a genital ulcer. She
    is very anxious that this could be a sexually transmitted disease. A few weeks ago,
    she visited friends in South-East Asia and had sexual intercourse with one of them.
    Examination reveals a single painless ulcer on the labia.

    What is the most likely infection?

    A   *Chlamydia trachomatis*
    B   Herpes simplex virus
    C   Human papillomavirus
    D   *Treponema pallidum*
    E   Varicella zoster virus

9. A 21-year-old woman attends the emergency department. She has recently
    changed partners. She complains of pelvic pain and vaginal discharge. Speculum
    and pelvic examination reveal discharge at the cervix and vagina, with pelvic
    tenderness and cervical excitation. As the on-call registrar who examined her, you
    suspect *Chlamydia* infection.

    What is the best test to confirm your suspicion?

    A   Endocervical swab for a nucleic acid amplification test (NAAT)
    B   Low vaginal swab for a NAAT
    C   Low vaginal swab for enzyme immunoassay
    D   Urine test for enzyme immunoassay
    E   Urine test for a NAAT

10. A 21-year-old woman attends the family planning clinic for advice on
    contraception. She gave birth 2 weeks ago by vaginal delivery and is exclusively
    breastfeeding. There is no significant past medical history. She is not taking or
    allergic to any medication.

    Which one of the following represents an unacceptable health risk if used in this
    case?

    A   Combined hormonal contraception
    B   Copper intrauterine device
    C   Depot medroxyprogesterone acetate
    D   Progesterone-only implant
    E   Progestogen-only pill

11. An 18-year-old woman attends the emergency department feeling unwell and complaining of an offensive vaginal discharge. She underwent a medical termination of pregnancy 1 week ago. On admission to the emergency department, her observations are: temperature 38.9°C, pulse 120 bpm, blood pressure 120/80 mmHg and respiratory rate 24 breaths per minute.

A pelvic ultrasound shows retained products of conception (size 54 mm × 45 mm). Intravenous antibiotics are given for 24 hours, followed by an evacuation of retained products of conception. After this, you, as the specialist registrar, review events with her. During this review, she asks for advice because she wants to start contraception as soon as possible to avoid getting pregnant again.

Which one of the following represents an unacceptable health risk if used in this case?

A   Combined hormonal contraception
B   Copper intrauterine device
C   Depot medroxyprogesterone acetate
D   Progesterone-only implant
E   Progestogen-only pill

12. A 36-year-old woman and her husband have come to the family planning clinic for advice on contraception. They have four children and do not want any more. As the registrar, you discuss with them permanent (vasectomy and sterilisation) and long-term reversible forms of contraception. They prefer permanent contraception and understand that permanent methods are irreversible. They would like to know the first-year failure rate for female (laparoscopic tubal occlusion) and male sterilisation procedures.

Which of the following are the correct rates?

A   Female sterilisation 0.5%, male sterilisation 0.10%
B   Female sterilisation 0.5%, male sterilisation 0.20%
C   Female sterilisation 0.5%, male sterilisation 0.30%
D   Female sterilisation 0.10%, male sterilisation 0.5%
E   Female sterilisation 0.20%, male sterilisation 0.10%

13. As the registrar, you are seeing a 21-year-old woman and her partner in the clinic. They have known each other for 6 months but have not yet achieved vaginal penetration despite repeat attempts. The woman has never had sex before this and describes her vagina as a 'brick wall'. There is no significant past medical history and she is not taking any medication. On examination, she appears to be healthy, with a body mass index of 23 kg/m². Vaginal examination reveals involuntary spasm of the pubococcygeal and other perineal muscles.

What is the diagnosis?

A   Endometriosis
B   Hypoactive sexual desire disorder
C   Primary vaginismus
D   Secondary vaginismus
E   Vulvodynia

14. A 25-year-old woman has come to your registrar-led clinic with vaginal discharge. This started 3 years ago after a surgical termination of pregnancy. The GP has repeatedly arranged investigations, including swabs and pelvic ultrasound, but no cause has been identified for the discharge. The woman does not believe the investigation results are normal. She feels that the discharge has been caused by an instrument left behind during the termination of pregnancy.

How should she be managed?

A Check for *Candida*
B Arrange a psychosocial intervention
C Re-examine the pelvis to rule any other cause
D Repeat the check for sexually transmitted infections
E Repeat ultrasound

15. A 21-year-old woman tells you, as the clinic registrar, that one area in her labia continuously feels as if it is burning. She finds that massaging the area helps, especially when she uses olive oil. There is no significant past medical history and she is not taking any medication. On examination, the vagina and vulva appear normal. However, when you touch a certain point on the labia, she jumps up in pain.

What is the diagnosis?

A Hypoactive sexual desire disorder
B Lichen planus
C Primary vaginismus
D Secondary vaginismus
E Vulvodynia

Questions: EMQs

Questions 16–20

Options for Questions 16–20

A Condoms	**I** Mifepristone
B Copper intrauterine device	**J** Levonorgestrel-releasing intrauterine
C Danazol	system (Mirena coil)
D Medroxyprogesterone acetate	**K** Norethisterone
E Co-cyprindiol (Dianette)	**L** Progestogen only pill
F Levonorgestrel 1.5 mg	**M** Sterilisation
G Ethinylestradiol/drospirenone	**N** Gestrinone
(Yasmin)	**O** GnRH analogues
H Ethinylestradiol/levonorgestrel	
(Microgynon)	

Instructions: For each scenario described below, select the single most appropriate method of contraception from the list of options above. Each option may be used once, more than once, or not at all.

16. A 42-year-old woman presents to the labour ward at 34 weeks' gestation in preterm labour. She progress very quickly and proceeds to have an emergency Caesarean section for fetal distress. She was discharged home after 1 week as her baby was admitted to the special care baby unit. Two weeks later, she attends the GP centre seeking contraception. She wants to continue to breastfeed her baby.

17. A 20-year-old woman presents to the emergency gynaecology services at a hospital at midnight for advice. She gives a history of condom rupture while having sexual intercourse 3 hours ago. She is worried that she will get pregnant and her parents will abandon her.

18. A 28-year-old happily married woman presents to the family planning clinic for advice. She gives a history of unprotected intercourse 3 days ago and does not want to get pregnant. She is also looking for long-term contraception. She has two children who are primary school age.

19. A 20-year-old Asian woman is about to start a new relationship. She had previously used progestogen only pills for contraception but became pregnant after the delayed intake of two consecutive pills. The pregnancy was terminated because it was unwanted. She is still keen to take pills. She has suffered from acne for the last 6 months and is worried that her boyfriend will leave her because of this problem.

20. A 28-year-old woman with two children attends the family planning centre for contraceptive advice. She is keen to take long-term contraception. However, she suffers from menorrhagia for which she is currently taking tranexamic acid.

Answers: SBAs

1. A Copper coil

A copper coil can be inserted up to 120 hours from the time of unprotected sexual intercourse or within 5 days of expected ovulation. It has a low failure rate and can be continued as a contraceptive in this case.

Clinical Effectiveness Unit. Faculty of Sexual and Reproductive Healthcare (FSRH) guideline: Emergency contraception. London: FSRH; 2012.

2. E Ulipristal acetate

Ulipristal acetate is effective for up to 120 hours from the time of unprotected intercourse. It is the only emergency contraception that is licensed to be used between 72 and 120 hours after unprotected intercourse. However, it is not recommended if the patient is taking medication that increases gastric pH, e.g. antacids, histamine H_2 antagonists or proton pump inhibitors.

Clinical Effectiveness Unit. Faculty of Sexual and Reproductive Healthcare (FSRH) guideline: Emergency contraception. London: FSRH; 2012.

3. D Levonorgestrel 3 mg

Levonorgestrel is effective for up to 96 hours after unprotected sexual intercourse. It is not licensed for use after 72 hours. Because phenytoin induces liver enzymes, a double dose of levonorgestrel (two tablets) is required and should be given as soon as possible. The copper coil is the only form of contraception that is not affected by enzyme-inducing drugs but it is not the best emergency contraceptive method for an 18-year-old woman because it may cause menorrhagia. Ulipristal acetate should not be given to women taking enzyme-inducing drugs.

Clinical Effectiveness Unit. Faculty of Sexual and Reproductive Healthcare (FSRH) guideline: Emergency contraception. London: FSRH; 2012.

4 C Statutory ground C

Statutory ground C states that the risk associated with the continuation of a pregnancy is greater than termination of pregnancy, and that the continuation of pregnancy can cause injury to the physical or mental health of the pregnant woman.

5. D Statutory ground D

The Abortion Act (1967; England, Wales and Scotland) mandates that:

- Terminations of pregnancy should be performed by a registered medical practitioner
- They must be performed in an approved place or, in the UK, in a NHS hospital

- Two medical practitioners should certify the termination before it is carried out; it must be justified under one or more of the statutory grounds (**Table 14.1**)

Table 14.1 Statutory grounds for termination of pregnancy in England, Scotland and Wales						
Statutory A	**Statutory B**	**Statutory C**	**Statutory D**	**Statutory E**	**Statutory F**	**Statutory G**
Continuation of pregnancy likely to involve risk to life of pregnant woman which is greater than if pregnancy were terminated	Termination needs to be offered otherwise pregnancy would cause grave permanent injury to physical or mental health of pregnant woman	Risk of continuation of pregnancy is greater than termination, and continuation would cause injury to physical or mental health of pregnant woman	Continuation of pregnancy would involve greater risk than termination, and continuation would cause injury to physical or mental health of any existing children in family	Significant risk that child would suffer from such physical or mental abnormalities as to be seriously handicapped; or, in an emergency, it is certified by the operating practitioner as immediately necessary.	To save the life of the pregnant woman	To prevent grave permanent injury to physical or mental health of the pregnant woman

In England and Wales, abortion is legal when it is certified by two medical practitioners according to one or more of the seven grounds described in **Table 14.1**.

Grounds C and D can only be considered in pregnancies less than 24 weeks' gestation. 98% of all abortions are undertaken on the basis of ground C. This means that the continuation of the pregnancy involves more risk compared to when it is terminated, in terms of damage to the mental and/or physical health of the pregnant women.

An abortion can be carried out according to ground D if the pregnancy does not exceed 24 weeks' gestation and the continuation of pregnancy involves more risk that terminating the pregnancy and can cause injury to the mental health of her children or family of the pregnant woman. Only 1% of the abortions fall into this category, as per 2011 statistics.

An abortion can be carried out according to Ground E in pregnancies that extend up to full term. This is valid generally when there are cases of severe fetal abnormalties.

Grounds A, B, F and G apply to pregnancies that extend up to full term. These may only be considered if the continuation of pregnancy involves severe risk to the woman's life or serious injury to her mental or physical health. These situations are rare and these grounds are rarely used. Only 1% of the abortions fall into this category.

The Abortion Act 1967 does not apply to Northern Ireland, where the termination of a pregnancy is illegal.

6.   A Assessing her Gillick competence

This girl is Gillick competent. Gillick competence is a child's competence to consent to any type of treatment. Fraser guidelines are specifically about prescribing contraceptives without parental advise. This girl satisfies the criteria laid down in the Fraser guidelines because she is able to fully understand the procedure that will be undertaken and its risks and benefits. If she is able to make an informed decision using the information given to her, she is legally competent to give consent to treatment. The decision on competence is made by the doctor reviewing the patient. In this case, the girl can consent to a termination without her parents' or school's knowledge or approval; therefore her parents should not be called without her consent.

7.   B Herpes simplex virus

Herpes simplex virus type 1 usually causes oral lesions, whereas herpes simplex virus type 2 causes genital lesions. However, an increase in the number of genital lesions caused by herpes simplex virus type 1 has been noted.

The blisters tend to occur 3–4 days after the initial skin-to-skin contact with the infected person. Patients can occasionally be asymptomatic and therefore unable to be diagnosed. The usual presentation is painful ulcerations. These make the passage of urine painful and women can present in urinary retention. Some present with vaginal discharge. These women can have raised temperature and myalgia when it is a primary infection.

A swab sample is taken from the vase of the ulcer and is required to type the virus. Typing is especially important in a primary herpes infection.

Treatment is symptomatic and includes saline baths and analgesia. Antiviral treatment, aciclovir, should be started within 5 days of presentation of the primary infection and also if systemic symptoms persist.

Patel R, Green J, Clarke E, et al. 2014 UK national guideline for the management of anogenital herpes. Int J STD AIDS 2014; 0:1–14.

8.   D *Treponema pallidum*

Treponema pallidum is sexually transmitted and causes syphilis. The disease is categorised into early and late disease. Early syphilis is infectious and is seen in the first 2 years of the infection. It includes primary, secondary and 'early latent' syphilis. The incubation period is 9–90 days once the infection occurs.

A papule develops at the site of infection. This ulcerates to become a chancre, which is a painless ulcer, usually 1–2 cm in diameter, that has a moist base and does not bleed. It can present anywhere on the genital region but the usual site is towards the mucosal surface of the labia. Lesions are usually solitary but can be multiple in immunocompromised (e.g. HIV-positive) women. Lesions occasionally develop in extragenital regions such as the mouth, nipple, eyelid or finger. These lesions usually resolve in 3–8 weeks.

Syphilis is described as late syphilis after 2 years of infection. Late latent syphilis is asymptomatic syphilis that is detected only on serum testing or screening.

9. B Low vaginal swab for a nucleic acid amplification test (NAAT)

The nucleic acid amplification test has a sensitivity of 90–95% and a specificity of 97–99%. It can be used on self-obtained specimens, such as urine or vaginal discharge. A sample can be easily swabbed from the lower vagina and vulvovaginal region. Swabs from both these sites are more sensitive than endocervical swabs or urine samples and are more acceptable to women. In men, a 'first-catch' urine sample is taken.

Women with vaginal discharge, unexpected bleeding, an inflamed cervix or pelvic inflammatory disease should be tested for *Chlamydia* infection. Men or women who are sexually active and have lower abdominal pain or reactive arthritis should also be tested.

Scottish Intercollegiate Guideline Network. Management of genital *Chlamydia trachomatis* infection. Clinical guideline 109. Edinburgh: SIGN; 2009.

10. A Combined hormonal contraception

In women who are fewer than 6 weeks' postpartum and are exclusively breastfeeding, combined hormonal contraception is contraindicated but all other methods are acceptable. The combined contraceptive pill does not pose an unacceptable health risk in women who are not breastfeeding and have no other risk factors. **Table 14.2** and **14.3** contain the UK Medical Eligibility Criteria (UKMEC) guidance for several contraceptive methods in breast-feeding and non-breastfeeding women according to the age of the neonate.

Table 14.2 UK Medical Eligibility Criteria (UKMEC) guidance categories for contraceptive methods in breast-feeding women according to the age of the neonate.				
	IMP	DMPA	POP	CHC
0–6 weeks	1	2	1	4
≥6 weeks to < 6 months (primarily breastfeeding)	1	1	1	2
≥6 months	1	1	1	1
Category 1: there is no restriction for the use of this method. Category 2: the advantages of using this method outweigh the theoretical risks of this method. Category 3: the theoretical risks of this method outweigh the advantages of using this method. Category 4: using this method poses an unacceptable risk. CHC, combined hormonal contraception; DMPA, progestogen-only injectable; IMP, progestogen-only implant; POP, progestogen-only pill.				

Table 14.3 UK Medical Eligibility Criteria (UKMEC) guidance categories for contraceptive methods in non-breast-feeding women according to the age of the neonate.		
	Cu-IUD	**LNG-IUS**
0 to <48 hours after birth	1	1
48 hours to <4 weeks after delivery	3	3
≥4 weeks post delivery	1	1
Category 1: there is no restriction for the use of this method. Category 2: the advantages of using this method outweigh the theoretical risks of this method. Category 3: the theoretical risks of this method outweigh the advantages of using this method. Category 4: using this method poses an unacceptable risk. Cu-IUD, copper-bearing intrauterine device; LNG-IUS, levonorgestrel-releasing intrauterine system.		

11. B Copper intrauterine device

All intrauterine devices are contraindicated for women with sepsis after a termination of pregnancy. All other methods of contraception are acceptable.

12. A Female sterilisation 0.5%, male sterilisation 0.10%

Couples should be thoroughly counselled before making an informed decision on long-term contraception.

Clinical Effectiveness Unit. Faculty of Sexual and Reproductive Healthcare (FSRH) guidance: Male and female sterilisation. London: FSRH, 2014.

13. C Primary vaginismus

Involuntary spasm of the pubococcygeal muscle implies vaginismus. It makes sexual intercourse very painful and usually results from fear of having sex or giving birth. Because this woman has never experienced vaginal penetration, this is primary vaginismus. It is the most common form of vaginismus.

Secondary vaginismus occurs when a woman has previously experienced successful vaginal penetration but later develops vaginismus. It can occur after a previous traumatic experience, e.g. childbirth or sexual abuse, and has both psychological and physical elements.

Cowan F, Frodsham L. Common disorders in psychosexual medicine. Obstet Gynaecol 2015; 17:47–53.

14. B Arrange a psychosocial intervention

Organic causes such as sexually transmitted infections, cervical ectropion and candidiasis should be ruled out when a woman presents with recurrent vaginal discharge. If no organic cause is found, psychological causes must be explored. This woman's symptoms started following termination of pregnancy but the results of investigations have been normal. Psychosocial treatment is the correct management here; it includes exploring her beliefs and excluding depression.

Cowan F, Frodsham L. Common disorders in psychosexual medicine. Obstet Gynaecol 2015; 17:47–53.

15. E Vulvodynia

Vulvodynia is defined as vulval discomfort, particularly a burning sensation, for which no obvious cause can be identified on examination. It can be provoked and can affect any age. Vulvodynia is a clinical diagnosis, based on a thorough history including psychological conditions such as anxiety, depression and a hypochondriac state of mind.

Treatment includes:

- Neuromodulators such as amitryptiline
- Perineal massage, particularly with an oil
- Pelvic floor exercises
- Acupuncture
- Topical agents such as lidocaine gel

Cowan F, Frodsham L. Common disorders in psychosexual medicine. Obstet Gynaecol 2015; 17:47–53.

Answers: EMQs

16. L Progestogen only pill

In women who are willing to breastfeed, the progestogen only pill is recommended because it does not affect lactation. It can be started as early as 3 weeks post delivery in such women. The combined oral contraceptive pill should not be used if women are continuing to breastfeed because this can affect both quantity and quality of the breast milk.

17. F Levonorgestrel 1.5 mg

Levonorgestrel 1.5 mg (Levonelle) can be taken up to 72 hours after unprotected intercourse, although the efficacy decreases with time. Women should be advised to take a further dose if vomiting occurs within 2 hours.

18. B Copper intrauterine device

The levonorgestrel-releasing intrauterine system (Mirena coil) is not recommended or licensed for emergency contraception. A copper intrauterine device can be inserted up to 5 days after unprotected intercourse or from ovulation. It is important to consider antibacterial prophylaxis and infection screening (for possible sexually transmitted infections) at the same time.

19. G Ethinylestradiol/drospirenone (Yasmin)

This is a monophasic combined oral contraceptive pill which contains 30 µg of ethinyl oestradiol and 3 mg of drospirenone. The anti-mineralocorticoid properties of drospirenone help to counteract the salt and fluid retaining properties of oestrogen and helps women who have symptoms of bloating, while its anti-androgenic properties make it useful to prescribe for women with acne and polycystic ovary syndrome. It can be used as an alternative to co-cyprindiol in the latter condition.

20. J Levonorgestrel-releasing intrauterine system (Mirena coil)

Either a levonorgestrel-releasing intrauterine system or endometrial ablation should be offered before discussing hysterectomy.

Guillebaud J. Your questions answered: contraception (5th edn). Edinburgh: Churchill Livingstone; 2008.

Chapter 15

Early pregnancy care

Questions: SBAs

For each question, select the single best answer from the five options listed.

1. Regarding a molar pregnancy, which one of the following statements is incorrect?

    A   Although an ultrasound is useful in diagnosing a molar pregnancy, the definite diagnosis is made from histopathology results

    B   Anti-D prophylaxis should be given to all women with a molar pregnancy after surgical evacuation of the uterus

    C   It is safe to prime the cervix with prostaglandins before surgical evacuation of the uterus

    D   If the size of the pregnancy allows, a suction catheter is the choice of instrument to remove a partial molar pregnancy

    E   One of the clinical presentations of a molar pregnancy is hypothroidism

2. Ultrasound in a 38-year-old woman revealed a complete hydatidiform mole and she was managed by surgical evacuation of the uterus. Serial β-human chorionic gonadotropin concentrations, used for monitoring, reverted to normal 4 weeks after the procedure. She would like to know how long she should wait before conceiving.

    What should your advice be for this patient?

    A   She may try to conceive now

    B   She should wait another 5 months before trying to conceive

    C   She should wait another 6 months before trying to conceive

    D   She should wait another 56 days before trying to conceive

    E   She should wait 1 year before trying to conceive

3. You are the specialist registrar on call for gynaecology. A nurse from the early pregnancy assessment unit asks you to review a set of ultrasounds and blood test results and give appropriate advice so she can call the patient, via the telephone clinic, with a management plan. The patient is 28 years old and 5 weeks pregnant by dates. A urine pregnancy test is positive. The results the nurse shows you are as follows:

    'Uterus anteverted and normal. Gestation sac not seen in the uterine cavity. Both ovaries are normal with no adnexal masses. Minimal free fluid in the recto-uterine pouch. No cervical excitation or adnexal tenderness.'

    The β-hCG concentration was measured on the day of the scan and repeated 48 hours later. Concentrations were 500 IU/L and 300 IU/L, respectively.

    What is the most appropriate management plan?

    A   Repeat the urinary pregnancy test in 2 weeks
    B   Repeat ultrasound scan in 7 days
    C   Repeat β-hCG measurement when it is expected to be >1000 IU/L
    D   Repeat serum β-hCG measurement on day 7
    E   Seek senior advice

4. You are the specialist registrar on call for gynaecology and have been asked for advice on a patient who underwent investigations earlier today. She is a 28-year-old woman who is 6 weeks pregnant by dates. A urine pregnancy test is positive. Ultrasound and blood test results are as follows:

    'Uterus retroverted and normal. No gestation sac or yolk sac seen within the uterine cavity. Both ovaries visualised and normal with no adnexal masses. Minimal free fluid in the rectouterine pouch. No cervical excitation or adnexal tenderness.'

    The β-hCG concentration was measured on the day of the scan and then repeated 48 hours later. The results were 500 IU/L and 48 IU/L, respectively.

    How will you manage this woman?

    A   Repeat urinary pregnancy test in 2 weeks
    B   Repeat ultrasound in 7 days
    C   Repeat β-hCG measurement when it is expected to be >1000 IU/L
    D   Repeat serum β-hCG measurement on day 7
    E   Seek senior advice

5. Which of the following statements regarding abdominal ectopic pregnancies is correct?

    A   Abdominal ectopic pregnancies constitute 1% of all ectopic pregnancies
    B   An early abdominal pregnancy will never occur after in vitro fertilisation if both tubes are absent
    C   The combination of ultrasound and clinical evaluation provides only 40% accuracy in diagnosis

D   The mortality rate for abdominal ectopic pregnancies is 10 times higher than with tubal pregnancies

E   The treatment for an abdominal ectopic pregnancy may be performed via laparoscopy or laparotomy

6.   What is the risk of dying from an ectopic pregnancy?

   A   0.2 in 1000
   B   0.4 in 1000
   C   0.6 in 1000
   D   0.8 in 1000
   E   1 in 1000

7.   As the on-call gynaecology registrar, you have been asked by the second-year specialist trainee to review a 23-year-old woman who has presented with lower abdominal pain and mild vaginal bleeding. She is 6 weeks pregnant and a urine pregnancy test is positive. The ultrasound report reads:

'Uterus anteverted and measures 10 cm × 8 cm × 5 cm. Mixed echogenic material seen within the uterine cavity with positive Doppler flow, measuring 20 mm × 15 mm × 15 mm. Both ovaries are normal. Minimal free fluid, measuring 5 mm, seen in the recto-uterine pouch'.

What is the most appropriate management?

   A   Diagnostic laparoscopy
   B   Repeat scan in 7 days if the bleeding continues
   C   Repeat scan in 21 days if the bleeding continues
   D   Take a blood sample to quantify β-human chorionic gonadotropin
   E   Take a blood sample to quantify β-human chorionic gonadotropin + progesterone

8.   You are the on-call gynaecology registrar. The sonographer from the early pregnancy assessment unit wants to discuss a patient's result with you. She has just performed trans-abdominal ultrasound on a 28-year-old woman who is 6 weeks pregnant by dates. The scan has shown a fetal pole with a 7 mm crown–rump length and no fetal heartbeat. The patient has declined a transvaginal scan. The sonographer wants to know when she should book this woman for a repeat trans-abdominal scan.

When would you recommend that this patient has a repeat trans-abdominal ultrasound scan?

   A   In 5 days
   B   In 7 days
   C   In 14 days
   D   The next day, performed by a consultant gynaecologist
   E   On the same day but with a second sonographer

9. As the on-call gynaecology registrar on a Friday night, you have performed an ultrasound for a 28-year-old woman who presented with vaginal bleeding. A urine pregnancy test is positive. There is a 25.2 mm gestational sac in the uterus but no yolk sac or fetal pole. The sonographer and on-call consultant have already left for the weekend.

    What is your best subsequent management plan?

    A   Ask the on-call consultant to return that night to rescan this woman
    B   Book a repeat scan for 7 days' time
    C   Book a repeat scan for 14 days' time
    D   Book a repeat scan with the sonographer on Monday
    E   Reassure the patient and discharge her

10. A 39-year-old woman has attended the early pregnancy assessment unit (EPAU) in tears because the dating scan from the fetal medicine unit has shown a fetal pole (crown–rump length consistent with 8 weeks pregnancy) but no heartbeat. She has a child already which was delivered by Caesarean section. You are the specialist registrar covering EPAU and have been asked to review her. You discuss various options with her for the medical management of her miscarriage.

    What is the correct sequence and regimen of the medical management?

    A   A single 800 µg dose of misoprostol administered vaginally
    B   A single 400 µg dose of misoprostol administered vaginally
    C   Oral mifepristone 50 mg followed by oral misoprostol 24 hours later (200 µg every 4 hours until she passes the products of conception)
    D   Oral mifepristone 50 mg followed by oral misoprostol 24 hours later (400 µg, 3 doses only)
    E   200 µg vaginal misoprostol every 4 hours until she passes the products of conception

11. You are the on-call gynaecology registrar and have been asked to review a 28-year-old nulliparous woman with a positive pregnancy test who has just undergone ultrasound. The sonographer's report reads: 'Uterus anteverted and normal. No gestational sac seen within the uterine cavity. Left ovary is normal and measures 12 mm × 10 mm × 8 mm. Right ovary is normal and measures 13 mm × 9 mm × 5 mm. There is a doughnut-shaped mass measuring 10 mm × 12 mm × 20 mm adjacent to the right ovary consistent with an ectopic pregnancy. No free fluid in the recto-uterine pouch. No adnexal tenderness or cervical excitation.' The plasma β-hCG concentration is 1300 IU/L.

    How should she be managed?

    A   Ask the consultant on call to repeat the ultrasound
    B   Diagnostic laparoscopy
    C   Laparoscopy + salpingectomy
    D   Methotrexate
    E   Repeat the β-hCG measurement in 48 hours

12. Which one of the following statements is correct regarding anti-D immunoglobulin prophylaxis?

  A Anti-D immunoglobulin prophylaxis should be offered to all rhesus-negative women who have had medical management for ectopic pregnancy and miscarriage

  B Anti-D immunoglobulin prophylaxis should be offered to all rhesus-negative women who have had surgical management for an ectopic pregnancy or miscarriage

  C The dose of anti-D immunoglobulin prophylaxis should be 1500 IU

  D A Kleihauer test should be done before giving anti-D immunoglobulin prophylaxis to a rhesus-negative patient who is less than 12 weeks pregnant and has significant vaginal bleeding

  E Anti-D immunoglobulin prophylaxis should be offered to all rhesus-negative women who have had a complete spontaneous miscarriage

13. Regarding hyperemesis gravidarum, which of the following is incorrect?

  A Acupressure does not improve the symptoms of nausea and vomiting

  B Ginger can be used instead of antiemetics for mild and moderate nausea and vomiting

  C Hyperemesis gravidarum is diagnosed only once other causes of nausea and vomiting have been excluded

  D Hypnotic therapies should not be used to treat nausea and vomiting

  E It is diagnosed when there is nausea and vomiting plus a triad of <5% loss of prepregnancy weight, dehydration and electrolyte imbalance.

14. A 39-year-old nulliparous woman has been admitted to the gynaecology ward with hyperemesis gravidarum. She is currently 8 weeks pregnant after in vitro fertilisation and this is her fifth admission with hyperemesis. Oral corticosteroids have not helped the vomiting. A nasogastric tube has been inserted for feeding, and an intravenous line has been inserted for fluid and electrolyte replacement. A significant amount of her pre-pregnancy body weight has been lost.

What is the recommended management?

  A Change to a nasojejunal tube

  B Continue with steroids and a nasogastric tube, and monitor weight

  C Hold a multidisciplinary team meeting with a dietitian, nutritionist, pharmacist, endocrinologist, nurse, gastroenterologist and psychiatrist to discuss management

  D Seek advice from the specialist lead of the early pregnancy assessment unit

  E Do none of the above

Questions: EMQs

Questions 15–19

Options for Questions 15–19

A   Abdominal cerclage
B   Cerclage for women with a multiple pregnancy
C   Cerclage for women with cervical trauma
D   Cervical cerclage contraindicated
E   Cervical cerclage plus progesterone vaginal pessaries
F   Cut the suture through posterior colpotomy
G   Elective cerclage not indicated
H   Elective cerclage at 12–14 weeks
I   Elective Caesarean section
J   Emergency Caesarean section
K   Emergency cerclage not recommended
L   History indicated cerclage
M   Hysterotomy
N   Suction evacuation through the suture
O   Rescue cerclage

Instructions: For each clinical scenario described below, choose the single most appropriate initial management from the above list of options. Each option may be used once, more than once, or not at all.

15. A 28-year-old woman, para 0+3 (second trimester miscarriage), attends the miscarriage clinic in view of her poor obstetric history. She also gives a history of cervical cerclage in her last pregnancy.

16. A 28-year-old woman presents to the labour ward with a premature rupture of membranes at 24 weeks' gestation. Abdominal examination reveals an absence of contractions and a speculum examination reveals a 2 cm dilated posterior cervix with intact forewaters.

17. A 28-year-old woman attends the early pregnancy assessment unit with vaginal bleeding at 8 weeks' gestation. She gives a history of abdominal cerclage prior to pregnancy in view of two previous mid-trimester miscarriages following vaginal cervical cerclage. An ultrasound scan reveals an absence of fetal heart activity.

18. A 28-year-old woman attends the obstetric day assessment unit with reduced fetal movements at 23 weeks and 3 days of gestation. She gives a history of abdominal cerclage in early pregnancy in view of a previous failed vaginal cerclage. Abdominal examination reveals an absence of uterine activity and an ultrasound examination reveals an absence of fetal heart activity.

19. A 28-year-old nulliparous woman presents to the early pregnancy assessment unit at 15 weeks' gestation with vaginal discharge. She was found to be 2 cm dilated. She gives a history of large loop excision of the transformation zone of the cervix 2 years ago. An ultrasound examination reveals the presence of fetal heart activity. A bicornuate uterus and a 2 cm dilated cervix with evidence of funnelling was also noted on the scan report.

Questions 20–24

Options for Questions 20–24

A Antibiotics
B Antenatal low molecular weight heparin (LMWH)
C Close surveillance and LMWH postnatally for 6 weeks
D Low dose aspirin only during first trimester
E Low dose aspirin plus steroids
F Low dose aspirin until 36 weeks' gestation
G Low dose aspirin antenatally plus LMWH postnatally for 7 days
H Low dose aspirin plus LMWH plus steroids
I Prophylactic antenatal LMWH plus postnatal for 6 weeks
J Prophylactic antenatal enoxaparin sodium plus postnatal enoxaparin sodium for 3–5 days
K Prophylactic LMWH in the first trimester
L Reassure the woman
M Therapeutic antenatal enoxaparin sodium plus prophylactic postnatal enoxaparin sodium
N Therapeutic antenatal enoxaparin sodium plus therapeutic postnatal enoxaparin sodium
O Varicose vein stripping

Instructions: For each scenario described below, choose the single most appropriate initial management from the list of options above. Each option may be used once, more than once, or not at all.

20. A 40-year-old nulliparous woman attends the maternal medicine clinic for a consultation at 13 weeks' gestation. A dating ultrasound scan at 12 weeks' gestation reveals a single viable intrauterine fetus. She gives a history of a single episode of deep venous thrombosis (DVT) following a road traffic accident 5 years ago. A recent thrombophilia screen prior to pregnancy is negative.

21. A 40-year-old nulliparous woman attends the early pregnancy assessment unit at 12 weeks' gestation with mild vaginal bleeding. A transvaginal scan reveals a viable dichorionic diamniotic twin pregnancy. Medical history reveals that she had an episode of DVT and a pulmonary embolism 2 years and 1 year ago respectively. A recent thrombophilia screen is negative.

22. A 40-year-old woman attends her antenatal appointment at 12 weeks' gestation. She gives history of three miscarriages (<10 weeks) with a single episode of a venous thromboembolism (VTE) following major surgery of the hip. Her blood test is positive for anticardiolipin antibody. A vaginal swab shows growth of group B *Streptococcus*.

23. A 40-year-old woman attends her antenatal appointment at 12 weeks' gestation. She gives a history of a stillbirth at 28 weeks' gestation and DVT 7 days following that delivery. Her blood test reveals an antithrombin III deficiency. She has been treated for toxoplasmosis in the past and her blood shows IgG antibodies for toxoplasmosis.

24. A 40-year-old Asian woman attends her antenatal clinic appointment at 12 weeks' gestation. She gives a history of eclampsia in her last pregnancy at 28 weeks' gestation and hence she had a Caesarean section. Now her blood pressure is 120/60 mmHg and her urine shows absence of protein.

Questions 25–29

Options for Questions 25–29

A   Evacuation of retained products of conception
B   Misoprostol
C   Misoprostol followed by mifepristone
D   Mifepristone followed by misoprostol
E   Methotrexate
F   Hysteroscopy
G   Hysterectomy
H   KCl injection to stop fetal heart activity
I   Laparoscopy
J   Laparotomy
K   Laparoscopic salpingectomy
L   Repeat ultrasound in 1 week
M   Repeat ultrasound scan by a senior member of staff
N   Reassure
O   Termination of pregnancy
P   Ultrasound scan by a fetal medicine consultant

Instructions: For each clinical scenario described below, choose the single most appropriate management from the list of options above. Each option may be used once, more than once, or not at all.

25. A 34-year-old woman attends the antenatal clinic for her booking (her first midwife appointment). She had a scan at 9 weeks following vaginal bleeding which showed a fetus with herniation of the gut through the umbilical area. The midwife comes to the registrar for advice as she is worried about the scan report.

26. A 32-year-old woman is referred to the early pregnancy assessment unit at 6 weeks' gestation with mild vaginal bleeding and suprapubic pain. Her urine shows 1 + leucocytes and no nitrates. A transvaginal scan reveals a viable intrauterine pregnancy with subchorionic bleeding.

27. A 28-year-old woman presents to the early pregnancy assessment unit with mild vaginal bleeding. A transvaginal ultrasound scan shows an intrauterine gestation sac of 14 × 15 × 14 mm with no fetal pole. She is unsure of the date of her last menstrual period.

28. A 34-year-old woman at 7 weeks' gestation is sent to the early pregnancy assessment unit by her GP. Her ultrasound scan confirms a missed miscarriage. She has multiple large fibroids.

29. A 28-year-old woman is referred to the early pregnancy assessment unit with a scan report of a missed miscarriage and she has been clearly informed by the ultrasonographer that the fetal heart beat is absent during the scan. The complete scan report reads as follows:

- patient's name and hospital number
- gestational age 10 weeks and 5 days
- fetal heart action present
- findings suggestive of missed miscarriage

Questions 30–34

Options for Questions 30–34

A	Vitamin A	I	Vitamin B12
B	Vitamin B1	J	Vitamin C
C	Vitamin B2	K	Vitamin D
D	Vitamin B3	L	Vitamin E
E	Folic acid	M	Vitamin K
F	Vitamin B5	N	Vitamin M
G	Vitamin B6	O	Vitamin I
H	Vitamin B7		

For each action described below, choose the single most appropriate vitamin from the list of options above. Each option may be used once, more than once, or not at all.

30. A water-soluble vitamin which is involved in myelin formation, synthesis of neurotransmitters, and also reduces total plasma homocysteine concentrations.

31. A lipid soluble vitamin acting on the lipid membrane and with synergistic interaction with vitamin C.

32. A vitamin photosynthesised by ultraviolet radiation in the epidermis.

33. A lipophilic vitamin important in post-translational modifications of proteins, particularly those involved in blood coagulation.

34. An essential water-soluble vitamin which has important roles in collagen synthesis, wound healing, absorption of non-haem iron and antioxidant action.

Answers: SBAs

1.   E One of the clinical presentations of a molar pregnancy is hypothyroidism

The typical signs and symptoms of a molar pregnancy are irregular vaginal bleeding, uterine enlargement disproportionate to gestational age and hyperemesis. Rare presentations include hyperthyroidism (not hypothyroidism), abdominal distension secondary to theca lutein ovarian cysts and early onset pre-eclampsia. More rare presentations include neurological symptoms such as seizures or respiratory symptoms. These are usually caused by metastatic deposits from invasive mole or choriocarcinoma rather than by the molar pregnancy itself.

2.   B She should wait another 5 months before trying to conceive

The follow-up plan for gestational trophoblastic disease is individualised. If the β-hCG concentration has returned to normal within 56 days of the pregnancy event (uterine surgical evacuation) follow-up should be for 6 months after the uterine surgical evacuation. If the β-hCG level has not returned to normal even after 56 days from the pregnancy event follow-up should be for up to 6 months from the normalisation of the serum β-hCG level.

With this patient, follow up should be for another 5 months, as a month has already passed and the β-hCG level normalised within 56 days. Women with a previous molar pregnancy are advised to contact the screening centre at the end of any future pregnancies regardless of outcome, to arrange a β-hCG blood test 6–8 weeks after the pregnancy to exclude recurrence of the disease.

3.   A Repeat the urinary pregnancy test in 2 weeks

This is likely to be a failed pregnancy of unknown location.

Al-Memar M, Kirk E, Bourne T. The role of ultrasonography in the diagnosis and management of early pregnancy complications. Obstet Gynaecol 2015; 17:173–181.

4.   D Repeat serum β-hCG measurement on day 7

This could be either a failed pregnancy of unknown location (PUL) or an ectopic pregnancy. PUL is not a diagnosis but a temporary classification until a final diagnosis has been made. If a PUL has been diagnosed, there is a 7–30% likelihood of ectopic pregnancy.

The management strategy for PUL described by Al-Memer et al (2015) is shown in **Table 15.1**.

Table 15.1 Management of pregnancy of unknown location		
β-hCG ratio (48 hours versus 0 hours)	Management	Likely diagnosis
>66% increase	Repeat the transvaginal scan on day 7	Likely intrauterine pregnancy
<66% increase	Repeat the transvaginal scan on day 7 or when the β-hCG level is likely to be >1000 IU/L	Possible ectopic pregnancy
>13% decrease	Perform a urinary pregnancy test in 2 weeks. If it is positive, measure β-hCG	Probably failed PUL
<13% decrease	Repeat β-hCG measurement on day 7	Either failed PUL or ectopic pregnancy
PUL, pregnancy of unknown location.		

Al-Memar M, Kirk E, Bourne T. The role of ultrasonography in the diagnosis and management of early pregnancy complications. Obstet Gynaecol 2015; 17:173–181.

5. A Abdominal ectopic pregnancies constitute 1% of all ectopic pregnancies

Abdominal pregnancies occur in 1/2200–1/10,200 of all pregnancies. The mortality rate is 7.7 times higher than for tubal pregnancies, and 89.8 times higher than for intrauterine pregnancies. An early abdominal pregnancy has been reported in a patient who underwent in vitro fertilisation for bilateral salpingectomy.

Agarwal N, Odejinmi F. Early abdominal ectopic pregnancy: challenges, update and review of current management. Obstet Gynaecol 2014; 16:193–198.

6. A 0.2/1000

The rate of ectopic pregnancy is 11/1000 and the mortality rate for women with an ectopic pregnancy is 0.2/1000. The women who die are usually vulnerable women who do not speak English, for example migrants, asylum seekers and refugees.

National Institute of Health and Care Excellence (NICE). Ectopic pregnancy and miscarriage: diagnosis and initial management [CG154]. London: NICE, 2012.

7. B Repeat scan in 7 days if the bleeding continues

The scan has revealed retained products of conception. Management is initially expectant for 7–14 days. Other options should be explored if there is a high risk of bleeding, a previous traumatic experience or evidence of infection. With expectant management, a repeat scan is only carried out in 7 days if the bleeding is continuing.

National Institute of Health and Care Excellence (NICE). Ectopic pregnancy and miscarriage: diagnosis and initial management [CG154]. London: NICE, 2012.

8. C In 14 days

When an early-pregnancy ultrasound is performed, the first finding to be noted is fetal heartbeat. If the heartbeat is not visible but there is a fetal pole, crown–rump length (CRL) is measured. If CRL is 7.0 mm or more on transvaginal ultrasound and no fetal heartbeat is seen, one should obtain a second opinion and/or rescan in 7 days. If no fetal heartbeat is seen when CRL is measured on a transabdominal ultrasound, the scan should be repeated in 14 days irrespective of the CRL measurement.

National Institute of Health and Care Excellence (NICE). Ectopic pregnancy and miscarriage: diagnosis and initial management [CG154]. London: NICE, 2012.

9. B Book a repeat scan for 7 days' time

If the gestational sac measures <25.0 mm on transvaginal ultrasound and there is no fetal pole, the scan should be repeated in 7 days. If the gestational sac measures >25.0 mm on a transvaginal ultrasound and there is no fetal pole, a second opinion should be sought and/or a second scan performed in 7 days. If the gestational sac has been measured transabdominally and there is no fetal pole, the scan should be repeated in 14 days.

National Institute of Health and Care Excellence (NICE). Ectopic pregnancy and miscarriage: diagnosis and initial management [CG154]. London: NICE, 2012.

10. A A single 800 μg dose of misoprostol

Mifepristone is not recommended for women with a missed or incomplete miscarriage. A single 800 μg dose of oral or vaginal misoprostol should be given. If there is no vaginal bleeding or products of conception are passed after 24 hours, the woman should contact the early pregnancy unit. Either 800 or 600 μg misoprostol, orally or vaginally, can be given for an incomplete miscarriage. A pregnancy test should be performed after 3 weeks of medical management. If it still positive, the woman should contact the early pregnancy unit.

National Institute of Health and Care Excellence (NICE). Ectopic pregnancy and miscarriage: diagnosis and initial management [CG154]. London: NICE, 2012.

11. D Methotrexate

This patient is an ideal candidate for methotrexate for the following reasons:

- Lack of an intrauterine pregnancy
- Small ectopic pregnancy <35 mm in size
- Lack of abdominal pain
- Serum β-hCG concentration <1500 IU/L

National Institute of Health and Care Excellence (NICE). Ectopic pregnancy and miscarriage: diagnosis and initial management [CG154]. London: NICE, 2012.

12. B Anti-D immunoglobulin prophylaxis should be offered to all rhesus-negative women who have had surgical management for an ectopic pregnancy or miscarriage

The dose of anti-D for women who are less than 20 weeks pregnant is 250 IU. It should only be given if there is a surgical procedure for a miscarriage or ectopic pregnancy. It is no longer recommended as part of medical management for a miscarriage or ectopic pregnancy, in threatened miscarriage or with a complete miscarriage or pregnancy of unknown location. A Kleihauer test should not be used to check for fetomaternal haemorrhage when there is miscarriage.

National Institute of Health and Care Excellence (NICE). Ectopic pregnancy and miscarriage: diagnosis and initial management [CG154]. London: NICE, 2012.

13. A Acupressure does not improve the symptoms of nausea and vomiting

Acupressure can help with symptoms of nausea and vomiting. Hyperemesis gravidarum is a diagnosis of exclusion and is made when there is nausea and vomiting, >5% pre-pregnancy weight loss, dehydration and electrolyte imbalance. Hypnotic therapies should not be used to treat it.

14. C Hold a multidisciplinary team meeting with a dietitian, nutritionist, pharmacist, endocrinologist, nurse, gastroenterologist and psychiatrist to discuss management

Assuming this patient lives in an area covered by the Abortion Act 1967, she may require a termination of pregnancy as the hyperemesis is compromising her health. At least 10% of women with severe hyperemesis gravidarum opt for termination of pregnancy, if offered it. All treatment options should be considered in a multidisciplinary setting before the decision to terminate is made. A psychiatric opinion should also be sought. Women should be offered thorough counselling before the decision to terminate is made.

Answers: EMQ

15. A Abdominal cerclage

A previous failed transvaginal cerclage is an indication of transabdominal cerclage. It can be done prior to pregnancy or during early pregnancy. However, women should be informed about the increased morbidity associated with it (infection bleeding and pregnancy loss).

16. D Cervical cerclage contraindicated

The contraindications for a cervical cerclage include:

- active pre-term labour
- clinical evidence of chorioamnionitis
- continuing vaginal bleeding
- pre-term premature rupture of membranes
- evidence of fetal compromise
- lethal fetal defect
- fetal death

17. N Suction evacuation through the suture

In this case, the woman is 8 weeks pregnant and can possibly get away with suction evacuation through the suture.

18. F Cut the suture through posterior colpotomy

Management decisions in cases of delayed miscarriage or fetal death in women with an abdominal cerclage can be difficult and should be made with senior involvement. An experienced doctor should carry out the procedure.

Suction evacuation through the suture up to 18 weeks has been described. Alternatively, the suture may be cut via posterior colpotomy. Failing this, a hysterotomy or Caesarean section may be necessary.

19. K Emergency cerclage not recommended

It is not recommended that an emergency history- or ultrasound-indicated cerclage is placed in women classified as high risk for preterm labour and birth. High risk women are those with Müllerian anomalies, previous cervical surgeries (cone biopsy, large loop excision of the transformation zone or a destructive operation such as laser ablation or diathermy) or multiple dilatation and evacuation.

National Institute for Clinical Excellence (NICE). Preterm labour and birth [NG25]. Manchester: NICE; 2015

20. I Prophylactic antenatal LMWH plus postnatal for 6 weeks

The RCOG classifies the risk assessment for women with a previous venous thromboembolism (VTE) in the categories recurrent or single VTE. The latter can be subclassified into:

- unprovoked VTE/idiopathic
- oestrogen-provoked (oestrogen-containing contraception or pregnancy) VTE
- thrombophilia (heritable or acquired) or family history-associated VTE (transient risk factor other than major surgery)
- Major surgery associated VTE

If a woman has a VTE which is unprovoked, oestrogen-related or if there is a transient risk factor other than major surgery, then LMWH should be offered throughout the antenatal period, and for 6 weeks postnatally. If the woman had a VTE which was provoked by major surgery, and has no other risk factors are identified then LMWH should be withheld until 28 weeks' gestation, and the patient should be assessed for new risk factors during pregnancy.

21. I Prophylactic antenatal LMWH plus postnatal for 6 weeks

Women with a recurrent VTE in the past, a previous unprovoked VTE, an oestrogen/pregnancy-related VTE or a previous VTE and a history of VTE in a first-degree relative (or a documented thrombophilia), or other risk factors should be offered thromboprophylaxis with LMWH antenatally and for 6 weeks postpartum.

22. I Prophylactic antenatal LMWH plus postnatal for 6 weeks

A previous VTE with a documented thrombophilia warrants antenatal plus postnatal LMWH for 6 weeks.

23. I Prophylactic antenatal LMWH plus postnatal for 6 weeks

Inherited thrombophilia in women who are asymptomatic and do not have other risk factors may be managed with close surveillance antenatally but should be considered for LMWH for at least 6 weeks postpartum if there is a high risk thrombophilia or a low risk thrombophilia with a family history. If there is a low risk thrombophilia, then 10 days LMWH should be considered in the postpartum period.

However, for women with antithrombin deficiency, more than 1 thrombophilic defect (including homozygous factor V Leiden, homozygous prothrombin G20210A and compound heterozygotes) or those with additional risk factors, advice of a local expert should be sought and antenatal prophylaxis considered. Any woman receiving antenatal thromboprophylaxis should receive postnatal thromboprophylaxis for 6 weeks.

24. F Low dose aspirin until 36 weeks' gestation

Women with previous pre-eclampsia should be started on low dose aspirin in the subsequent pregnancy. This should be done as soon as the pregnancy is confirmed and continued until 36 weeks' gestation.

Royal College of Obstetricians and Gynaecologists (RCOG). Reducing the risk of thrombosis and embolism during pregnancy and puerperium. Green-top guideline no. 37. London: RCOG Press; 2015. Calderwood CJ and Thanoon OI. Thromboembolism and thrombophilia in pregnancy. Obstet Gynecol Reprod Med 2009; 19:339–343.

25. N Reassure

Physiological gut herniation is a normal phenomenon that occurs during early pregnancy (it usually starts at 8 weeks and returns to the abdominal cavity before 12 weeks).

Physiology

Physiological herniation of the gut occurs as a result of the bowel growing faster than the abdominal cavity during the early gestational period. Subsequently, the intestine moves outside the embryonic abdomen, herniating into the base of the umbilical cord. This usually occurs at 8 weeks' gestation and is presumed to be due to the rapid growth of the cranial end of the midgut and the large size of the developing liver and kidneys. At approximately 10–12 weeks the abdomen enlarges and allows the intestines to return within the abdominal cavity (they should not be present beyond 13 weeks' gestation).

Ultrasound appearance

- herniation of the fetal gut out of the abdomen through the umbilical area
- usually seen in early pregnancy as mentioned above
- should not contain other organs, such as the liver
- the size of the herniation should be comparatively small (usually <10 mm)

If herniation of the gut is seen later in the pregnancy, one of the two differentials should be considered as listed below.

Omphalocele

- it is a defect in the abdominal wall in the midline at the umbilicus
- it occurs due to failure of the midgut to return back into the abdomen
- the bowel and abdominal content herniate through the base of the umbilical cord
- the bowel is covered by fine membranes
- it is usually associated with other defects and chromosomal anomalies, especially trisomy 13 and trisomy 18
- it is associated with a poor prognosis and outcome

Gastroschisis

- it is a defect in the abdominal wall, usually to the right of the umbilicus
- the bowel is freely floating in the amniotic fluid
- the bowel is not covered with any membranes
- the risk of chromosomal abnormality is low
- survival following surgery is 90%

26. N Reassure

Subchorionic bleeding during early pregnancy is not uncommon and usually resolves itself. This woman should be reassured and managed conservatively.

27. L Repeat ultrasound in 1 week

In known cases of intrauterine pregnancy, viability will be uncertain in approximately 10% of women at their first early pregnancy assessment unit (EPAU) visit.

Pregnancy of uncertain viability:

- Intrauterine sac (<25 mm mean diameter) with no obvious fetal pole
- <7 mm crown–rump length with no obvious fetal heart activity.

In order to confirm or refute viability, a repeat scan at a minimal interval of 1 week is necessary.

28. B Misoprostol

This woman has large uterine fibroids and should be managed by medical rather than surgical treatment unless emergency evaluation of retained products is necessary due to excessive bleeding. For the medical management of miscarriage mifepristone should not be offered; only misoprostol should be given either orally or vaginally. If the miscarriage is incomplete then 600 µg of misoprostol should be given. If it is a missed miscarriage then 800 µg should be given.

29. M Repeat ultrasound scan by a senior member of staff

There is a disparity in the scan report saying fetal heart action present but the final report implies missed miscarriage. Although the woman has been told clearly that the fetal heartbeat is absent, it is important to repeat the scan by seniors (ideally a consultant) just to confirm the viability again as otherwise this may lead to litigation.

National Institute for Health and Care Excellence (NICE). Ectopic pregnancy and miscarriage: diagnosis and initial management. London: NICE; 2012.
Buckett W and Regan L. Chapter 23: Sporadic and recurrent miscarriage. In: Shaw RW, Luesley D, Monga A (eds). Gynaecology (4th edn). Edinburgh: Churchill Livingstone, 2011.

30. G Vitamin B6

Vitamins are organic compounds essential for normal cell function, growth and development. The essential vitamins include vitamins A, C, D, E, K and the B series including B1 (thiamine), B2 (riboflavin), B3 (niacin), B5 (pantothenic acid), B6 (pyridoxine), B7 (biotin), B9 (folic acid) and B12 (cobalamin).

Vitamin B6 decreases in the third trimester of pregnancy (it is uncertain whether this is due to volume expansion or true deficiency). Vitamin B6 alleviates the severity of nausea but not vomiting in the first trimester. It is also associated with a statistically significant decrease in the risk of dental decay in pregnant women (of 16%), particularly when given in lozenge form, suggesting a local effect.

The effect of vitamin B6 supplementation on outcomes such as eclampsia, pre-eclampsia, low birth weight and breast milk production are inconclusive. Current evidence is not strong enough to support routine supplementation in pregnancy.

31. L Vitamin E

Vitamin E is an antioxidant. However, recent evidence (supplementation of vitamin E and vitamin C in pregnancy) showed no effect on pre-eclampsia, pre-term birth, small-for-gestational-age infants or any baby death. Current evidence does not support routine supplementation of these vitamins during pregnancy.

Duckworth S, Mistry HD, Chappell LC. Vitamin supplementation in pregnancy. Obstet Gynaecol 2012;14:175–178.

32. K Vitamin D

Vitamin D deficiency is more common in Asians than white people because the former require longer exposure to the sun to produce the same amounts of the vitamin. It is also more common in women who are fully covered and stay indoors.

In vitamin-D deficient mothers, a significant increase in infantile rickets is reported with decreased transfer of vitamin D to the fetus during pregnancy and breastfeeding. In the UK, approximately 15% of all adults may be deficient in vitamin D and the prevalence is said to increase to 90% in South Asian adults. Obesity before pregnancy is also associated with a significant increase in maternal and neonatal vitamin D deficiency independent of factors like ethnicity.

A systematic review showed that antenatal vitamin D supplementation is effective in improving the vitamin D status of Asian and white women and promotes growth in the first year of life in South Asian babies. The current NICE guidelines on antenatal care support the importance of maintaining adequate vitamin D stores in pregnancy, especially for those at highest risk of vitamin D deficiency (women of South Asian, African, Caribbean or Middle Eastern origin, women who have limited exposure to sunlight, women who eat a diet particularly low in vitamin D and women with a pre-pregnancy body mass index >30 kg/m^2). The recommended dose is 10 µg/day.

33. M Vitamin K

Vitamin K is required for the synthesis of coagulation factors II, VII, IX and X (synthesised in the liver). This can be deficient in women taking anticonvulsants (carbamazepine and phenytoin, which are liver enzyme inducers). Therefore, there is a potential risk of periventricular haemorrhage in babies born to these mothers. The current evidence suggests no significant decrease in periventricular haemorrhage with vitamin K supplementation during pregnancy and therefore the evidence to support routine supplementation is weak.

34. J Vitamin C

Vitamin C is an essential vitamin which is abundant in fruit and vegetables. It is important in wound healing and also promotes the absorption of non-haem iron in food. Multivitamin preparations for pregnancy generally contain low doses of vitamin C.

Royal College of Obstetricians and Gynaecologists (RCOG). Vitamin supplementation in pregnancy. Scientific Advisory Committee opinion paper 16. London: RCOG Press, 2009.
Walker SP, Permezel M, Berkovic SF. The management of epilepsy in pregnancy. BJOG 2009; 116:758–767.

Chapter 16

Gynaecological oncology

Questions: SBAs

For each question, select the single best answer from the five options listed.

1. A 50-year-old woman attended the rapid-access, 2-week wait gynaecological oncology clinic for postmenopausal bleeding. Her ultrasound showed thickened endometrium so a hysteroscopy and endometrial biopsy was undertaken. The consultant also performed a cervical smear because the previous smear had been 5 years previously. The woman is now being seen in the clinic 2 weeks later. The endometrial biopsy has shown inactive endometrium. The cervical smear has identified borderline nuclear changes in the squamous cells, and is negative for high-risk human papillomavirus.

   What is the appropriate next step in management?

   A Discharge to the care of her GP
   B Repeat the smear in 3 months
   C Repeat the smear in 6 months
   D Repeat the smear in 12 months
   E Referral to the colposcopy clinic

2. A 28-year-old woman has been referred to the colposcopy clinic. A cervical smear test revealed low-grade dyskaryosis with positivity for high-risk type 16 human papillomavirus. She smokes 15 cigarettes a day and has asthma. The colposcopy is satisfactory and normal (the entire squamocolumnar junction and margin of any visible lesion can be visualised with the colposcope).

   What is the management plan?

   A Discharge to GP care
   B Discharge to GP care with a plan of routine recall for a smear in 3 years' time
   C Discharge to GP care with a plan of routine recall for a smear in 3 years' time, and advice on smoking cessation
   D Follow-up in the colposcopy clinic in 6 months' time for a repeat smear and colposcopy
   E Follow-up in the colposcopy clinic in 1 year for a repeat smear and colposcopy

3. A 30-year-old parous woman has been referred to the colposcopy clinic with a cervical smear report of severe dyskaryosis. A colposcopy reveals dense acetowhite areas on both the anterior and posterior lips of the cervix, consistent with high-grade disease. The colposcopy is satisfactory and normal (the entire squamocolumnar junction and margin of any visible lesion can be visualised with the colposcope).

What is the plan for management?

A   Arrange for hysterectomy because she has completed her family
B   Take a cervical biopsy
C   Undertake cone biopsy under general anaesthesia
D   Discuss this at a multidisciplinary team meeting
E   Perform large loop excision of the transformation zone

4. A 28-year-old nulliparous woman is referred to the colposcopy clinic because of a cervical smear result of low-grade dyskaryosis and positivity for high-risk human papillomavirus. The colposcopy is satisfactory and normal (the entire squamocolumnar junction and margin of any visible lesion can be visualised with the colposcope).

What is the most appropriate plan of management?

A   Biopsy of the cervix
B   Discharge to the care of her GP
C   Discharge to GP care with a plan of routine recall for a smear in 3 years
D   Follow-up in the colposcopy clinic in 6 months for a repeat smear and colposcopy
E   Follow-up in the colposcopy clinic in 12 months for a repeat smear and colposcopy

5. A 16-year-old girl is referred by her GP as a gynaecological emergency with pain and abdominal distension. Clinical examination reveals a large abdomino-pelvic mass. CT reveals a large left-sided solid/cystic ovarian mass. Her CA-125 concentration is 100 U/mL. The blood results for tumour markers carcinoembryonic antigen, α-fetoprotein, β-hCG and lactate dehydrogenase levels are normal. Fertility-sparing surgery is undertaken. Histological examination of the excised tumour cells shows grade 1 glial tissue.

Which type of ovarian tumour is this most likely to be?

A   Brenner's tumour
B   Immature teratoma
C   Endodermal sinus tumour
D   Dysgerminoma
E   Embryonal carcinoma

6. A 55-year-old woman presents to her GP with abdominal bloating and pelvic pain. Tumour marker concentrations are CA-125 of 2890 unit/mL and carcinoembryonic antigen of 3.6 units/mL. She has been referred to the rapid-access gynaecologic clinic. She was then seen in the clinic and further investigation in the form of a CT scan is arranged. The scan reveals a large abdominal mass possibly filled with mucin. The findings are suggestive of mucinous carcinoma. During a staging laparotomy, the cyst ruptures. The histology is reported as mucinous carcinoma of the left ovary with rupture of cyst and normal right ovary, uterus, omentum and peritoneal biopsies.

What is the International Federation of Gynecology and Obstetrics (FIGO) stage in her case?

A   IB
B   IC1
C   IC2
D   IC3
E   IIA

7. A 62-year-old woman has been referred to the rapid-access, 2-week wait gynaecological oncology clinic for postmenopausal bleeding. An ultrasound reveals thickened endometrium. A hysteroscopy and an endometrial biopsy shows grade 1 endometrial cancer. MRI performed for staging indicates stage IA endometrial cancer.

What is the most appropriate management?

A   Insertion of a levonorgestrel-release intrauterine system (Mirena coil)
B   Transcervical resection of endometrium
C   Total abdominal hysterectomy with a bilateral salpingo-oophorectomy by longitudinal incision
D   Vaginal hysterectomy
E   Laparascopic hysterectomy and bilateral salpingo-oophorectomy

8. An 80-year-old woman presented to the rapid-access, 2-week wait gynaecologic clinic with vulval itching and soreness. Clobetasol propionate 0.05% prescribed by her GP for vulval application had had no effect. Examination revealed bilateral lichen sclerosis of the labia with midline labial fusion. Vulval adhesiolysis and vulval mapping biopsies were undertaken under general anaesthesia. Histology showed vulval squamous cell carcinoma of the left labia majora with a depth of invasion of >1 mm. MRI of the pelvis showed a thickened area on the left labia that measures <2 cm but no inguinal lymphadenopathy. After discussion in the multidisciplinary team meeting, she undergoes left-sided vulvectomy and left groin node dissection. The final histology report shows a 2 cm tumour with clear margins; 1 out of 5 nodes sampled from the left groin contains metastatic tumour.

What final International Federation of Gynecology and Obstetrics (FIGO) stage needs to be allocated after the definitive surgery for vulval cancer from histology results?

A   IA
B   IB
C   II
D   IIIA
E   IIIB

9. A 55-year-old woman is referred to rapid-access, 2-week wait gynaecologic clinic with a vulval lesion. Vulval examination reveals a 2.5 cm long left labial lesion. Biopsy of the lesion reveals squamous cell carcinoma of the vulva with >1 mm stromal invasion. Wide local excision and unilateral inguinal lymphadenectomy are undertaken.

    Non-clitoral lymphatic drainage typically first drains to which of the following set of lymph nodes?

    A   Cloquet or deep inguinal
    B   Internal iliac nodes
    C   External iliac nodes
    D   Superficial inguinal nodes
    E   Common iliac nodes

10. A 55-year-old woman is referred to rapid-access, 2-week wait gynaecologic clinic for postmenopausal bleeding. Pelvic ultrasound, which was organised by her GP, shows a thickened endometrium of 8 mm. Outpatient hysteroscopy and endometrial pipelle biopsy are carried out.

    What is the risk of endometrial cancer in a woman presenting with postmenopausal bleeding?

    A   1%
    B   5%
    C   10%
    D   20%
    E   25%

11. A 45-year-old woman is referred with menorrhagia and intermenstrual bleeding. The results of previous smears have been normal. Pelvic examination reveals a bulky uterus with no palpable adnexal masses. A transvaginal ultrasound scan shows a thickened endometrium of 20 mm and normal ovaries. Outpatient hysteroscopy and endometrial pipelle biopsy are carried out. The histology report indicates endometrial hyperplasia without atypia.

    What is the most appropriate first-line management?

    A   Cyclical progestogens on days 5–21 of the cycle
    B   High-dose oral progestogen
    C   Low-dose oral progestogen
    D   Levonorgestrel-releasing intrauterine system (Mirena coil)
    E   Progestogen-only pill

12. A 30-year-old woman has been referred to the genetic clinic for counseling. Her 36-year-old sister has been diagnosed with breast cancer, and genetic testing has reported a *BRCA1* gene mutation in this patient.

    What is her sister's lifetime risk of developing ovarian cancer?

    A   10–20%
    B   20–30%
    C   30–60%
    D   60–80%
    E   90%

13. A 30-year-old multiparous woman was referred to the colposcopy clinic on the basis of a cervical smear showing severe dyskaryosis. The colposcopy and biopsy revealed cervical intra-epithelial neoplasia grade 3 (CIN3). A large loop excision of the transformation zone was undertaken. The histology report indicated CIN2/3 with clear margins. Follow-up at 6 months involved colposcopy and another cervical smear. A colposcopy is normal, and the smear is reported to be normal and negative for high-risk human papillomavirus (HPV).

What is the best subsequent management?

A   Follow-up in 6 months for colposcopy, cervical smear and HPV testing
B   Follow-up in 12 months for colposcopy, cervical smear and HPV testing
C   Follow-up with the GP in 6 months for cervical smear
D   Follow-up with the GP in 12 months for cervical smear and HPV testing
E   Follow-up with the GP in 36 months for cervical smear and HPV testing

14. A 35-year-old woman has been referred to the colposcopy clinic with a referral smear reporting severe dyskaryosis. Colposcopy reveals frank invasive disease, which is confirmed by a cervical biopsy. A MRI of the pelvis shows a 3 cm cervical tumour with involvement of the vaginal fornices but no parametrial involvement. Examination under anaesthesia confirms these findings.

What is the International Federation of Gynecology and Obstetrics (FIGO) stage of the cancer?

A   I
B   Ib
C   IIa1
D   IIa2
E   IIB

15. A 49-year-old nulliparous woman is referred with perimenopausal bleeding. The results of previous smears have been normal. Pelvic examination reveals a bulky uterus with no palpable adnexal masses. Transvaginal ultrasound shows a thickened endometrium of 30 mm and normal ovaries. Outpatient hysteroscopy and endometrial pipelle biopsy are carried out. The histology report identifies endometrial hyperplasia with atypia.

What is the best plan of management?

A   Levonorgestrel-releasing intrauterine system (Mirena coil) and repeat hysteroscopy, with endometrial biopsy in 6 months
B   Levonorgestrel-releasing intrauterine system and repeat hysteroscopy, with endometrial biopsy at 6 and 12 months
C   Total abdominal hysterectomy
D   Total abdominal hysterectomy and bilateral salpingectomy
E   Total abdominal hysterectomy with bilateral salpingo-oophorectomy

Questions: EMQs

Questions 16–20

Options for Questions 16–20

A	Stage IA	G	Stage IIIA
B	Stage IB	H	Stage IIIB
C	Stage IC	I	Stage IIIC1
D	Stage II	J	Stage IIIC2
E	Stage IIA	K	Stage IVA
F	Stage IIB	L	Stage IVB

Instructions: For each scenario described below, choose the single most appropriate the International Federation of Gynecology and Obstetrics (FIGO) stage for endometrial cancer from the list of options above. Each option may be used once, more than once, or not at all.

16. A 60-year-old woman presents with postmenopausal bleeding (PMB) to the rapid-access gynaecologic clinic. An endometrial pipelle biopsy reveals an endometrioid adenocarcinoma. She is further investigated with a MRI scan which reveals uterine myometrial invasion of less than 50% and enlarged pelvic nodes. She subsequently undergoes a total abdominal hysterectomy, bilateral salpingo-oophorectomy and sentinel lymph node biopsy. You review her in the clinic at 2 weeks follow-up with a histology report of endometrial cancer with myometrial invasion of more than 50% and pelvic lymph node involvement.

17. A 44-year-old woman presents to the emergency department with heavy vaginal bleeding and intermenstrual bleeding for the last 6 months. Following a gynaecology review a hysteroscopy and endometrial biopsy were arranged. 2 weeks after her hysteroscopy she attends the rapid-access gynaecologic clinic and the histology reveals a papillary serous carcinoma. A CT scan of the chest is reported as normal while the MRI scan reveals a large uterine tumour infiltrating the serosal surface of the uterus and also involving the pelvic nodes. Subsequently, she undergoes a total abdominal hysterectomy, bilateral salpingo-oophorectomy and pelvic lymphadenectomy in an oncology centre. The final histology confirms the MRI findings.

18. An 82-year-old woman presents to the emergency department with postmenopausal heavy bleeding and her haemoglobin is 70 g/L. She receives 2 units of blood transfusion and undergoes hysteroscopy and an endometrial biopsy on an emergency basis, because she continued to bleed heavily. An endometrial biopsy reveals clear cell carcinoma. She subsequently undergoes a total abdominal hysterectomy, bilateral salpingo-oophorectomy and pelvic lymphadenectomy. The histology reveals clear cell carcinoma involving the uterine cervix and serosal surface.

19. A 55-year-old woman is referred to a rapid-access gynaecologic clinic with PMB. She returns to the clinic for her pipelle biopsy results which reveal endometrial cancer. She then undergoes a total abdominal hysterectomy and bilateral salpingo-oophorectomy. The final histology reveals tumour infiltration of less than 50% of the myometrium and involvement of the cervical stroma. Also, peritoneal washings are reported to be positive for malignant cells.

20. A 58-year-old woman attends the rapid-access gynaecologic clinic with PMB, following which she has outpatient hysteroscopy and endometrial biopsy. The histology revealed an endometrioid adenocarcinoma. She subsequently undergoes a total abdominal hysterectomy and bilateral salpingo-oophorectomy. The final histology is reported as endometrioid adenocarcinoma involving the endometrium and peritoneal washings were positive for malignant cells.

Questions 21–25

Options for Questions 21–25

A	Benign teratoma	G	Granulosa cell tumour
B	Choriocarcinoma	H	Gynandroblastoma
C	Dysgerminoma	I	Gonadoblastoma
D	Endodermal sinus tumour	J	Leydig cell tumour
E	Embryonal carcinoma	K	Malignant teratoma
F	Epithelial ovarian tumour	L	Sertoli cell tumour

Instructions: For each scenario described below, choose the single most appropriate tumour type from the list of options above. Each option may be used once, more than once, or not at all.

21. A 19-year-old girl is referred to the gynaecology clinic with a scan report of a bilateral ovarian mass. An MRI scan confirms a bilateral solid ovarian tumour. The blood test results show an increase in lactate dehydrogenase and placental alkaline phosphatase. She is referred to an oncology centre for further management, following which she undergoes staging for ovarian cancer and bilateral oophorectomy. Her final histology shows marked lymphocytic infiltration in the stroma surrounding the tumour cells.

22. A 20-year-old woman presents to the emergency department with abdominal distention and pain. Clinical examination reveals a palpable abdomino-pelvic mass and an ultrasound scan shows a unilateral solid ovarian mass on the right side. Her tumour marker α-fetoprotein is 300 U/mL and CA-125 concentration is 45 U/mL. She is then referred to the gynaecology oncology centre for further management. She had further imaging in the form of MRI and CT scans and undergoes staging laparotomy and right-sided oophorectomy. The histology reveals a Schiller–Duval body.

23. An 18-year-old girl presents to her GP with distention of the abdomen. An ultrasound scan reveals a unilateral solid/cystic mass on the left side. An MRI scan confirms that the ovarian tumour is confined to the left ovary and the right ovary looks normal. However, her tumour markers, β human chorionic gonadotropin

(β-hCG) and α-fetoprotein, are normal. She is then referred to the gynaecology oncology centre for further management, following which she undergoes staging laparotomy and left-sided oophorectomy. One of the components of the histology shows elements of glial tissue.

24. A 55-year-old menopausal woman presents to the emergency department with irregular vaginal bleeding. An abdominal scan shows a large pelvic mass on the right side and a thickened endometrium (20 mm). An MRI scan reveals similar findings. The blood test shows a raised a subunit of inhibin and CA-125 48 U/mL. She gives a family history of breast cancer and is currently on tamoxifen.

25. A 58-year-old woman presents to the emergency department with abdominal bloating and a decreased appetite. She had opened her bowels 2 days previously. Clinical examination reveals a distended abdomen with signs of subacute bowel obstruction. A CT scan of the abdomen and pelvis revealed a large complex pelvic mass (size 15 × 12 × 12 cm) with raised CA-125 (1000 U/mL) and normal carcinoembryonic antigen (CEA) (2 U/mL).

Questions 26–30

Options for Questions 26–30

A Cervical smear in 6 months
B Cervical smear in 12 months
C Cold coagulation of the cervix
D Diathermy to the cervix
E Discharge to GP and repeat smear in 6 months
F Discharge to GP and routine recall in 3 years' time
G Discharge to GP and routine recall in 5 years' time
H Knife cone biopsy
I Large loop excision of transformation zone (LLETZ)
J Punch biopsy of the cervix
K Repeat colposcopy in 6 months
L Repeat colposcopy in 12 months
M Radical hysterectomy
N Simple hysterectomy

Instructions: For each scenario below, chose the single most appropriated management option from the list of options. Each option may be used once, more than once or not at all.

26. A 28-year-old woman is referred to the colposcopy clinic by her GP. She is up to date with her smears, none of which have been abnormal apart from the current smear which is HPV 16 positive and shows mild dyskaryosis. Her colposcopy is satisfactory and normal.

27. A 49-year-old woman is referred to the colposcopy clinic by her GP. She is up to date with her smears, none of which have been abnormal apart from the current smear which is HP 16 and 18 positive and shows borderline changes in squamous cells. Her colposcopy is satisfactory and normal.

28. A 30-year-old woman is referred to the colposcopy clinic by her GP. She is up-to-date with her smears, none of which have abnormal apart from than the current smear which is high-risk HPV negative and shows mild dyskaryosis.

29. A 49-year-old woman is referred to the colposcopy clinic by her GP. She is up-to-date with her smears and never had any abnormal smears other than the current smear which is high-risk HPV negative and shows borderline changes in squamous cells.

30. A 38-year-old woman is referred to the colposcopy clinic by her GP. She is up to date with her smears, none of which have been abnormal apart from the current smear which shows severe dyskaryosis. Her colposcopy is satisfactory and reveals dense acetowhite areas at the 6 and 9 o'clock positions. She hates hospital and did not attend her previous two appointments.

Questions 31-35

Options for Questions 31-35

A Cervical smear in 12 months	zone
B Cervical smear in 24 months	I Need to be seen in the colposcopy
C Colposcopy and smear in 6 months for	clinic within 2 weeks of referral
test of cure	J Need to be seen in the colposcopy
D Discharge to the GP	clinic within 4 weeks of referral
E Discharge to the GP and carry out a	K Need to be seen in the colposcopy
routine recall in 3 years' time	clinic within 8 weeks of referral
F Discharge to the GP and carry out a	L Punch biopsy of the cervix
routine recall in 5 years' time	M Repeat colposcopy in 6 months
G Knife cone biopsy	N Repeat colposcopy in 12 months
H Large loop excision of transformation	

Instructions: For each scenario described below, choose the single most appropriate management from the list of options above. Each option may be used once, more than once, or not at all.

31. A 48-year-old woman with ten children is referred to the colposcopy clinic with a clinical impression of suspicious cervix. She is up to date with her smears, none of which have been abnormal. She has never had surgery before and is needle-phobic. She is social drinker and smokes 20 cigarettes per day. Her father has pancreatic cancer and her mother recently died of breast cancer.

32. A 35-year-old woman is referred to the colposcopy clinic with a smear report of glandular neoplasia. She suffers from contact dermatitis and is allergic to peanut oil. She does not have any support at home.

33. A 26-year-old woman is referred to the colposcopy clinic following a routine smear which was HPV 18 positive and revealed a borderline abnormality in the endocervical cells. She is terrified that she has cancer. She has been on ethinylestradiol with drospirenone (Yasmin) for the last 2 years and complains of some headache and tiredness. She also smokes 10 cigarettes per day. She does not have any abnormal vaginal bleeding. Colposcopy is satisfactory and normal.

34. A 40-year-old woman is referred to the colposcopy clinic by her GP with a referral cervical smear report of severe dyskaryosis. The colposcopy results are unsatisfactory and reveal severe acetowhite areas at the 3 o'clock and 5 o'clock positions with mosaicism. She is a chain smoker and gives a family history of strokes. She undergoes a large loop excision of transformation zone (LLETZ) under local anaesthesia.

35. A 39-year-old woman is referred to the colposcopy clinic by her GP with a referral cervical smear report of severe dyskaryosis. The colposcopy results are unsatisfactory and reveal a severe acetowhite area at the 3 o'clock and 5 o'clock positions with mosaicism. She is a chain smoker and gives a family history of stroke. She undergoes a LLETZ under local anaesthesia. The histology is reported as CIN3, completely excised. She has a colposcopy and a cervical smear at her 6-month follow up (called test-of-cure smear). The smear is normal and negative for high-risk HPV.

Questions 36–40

Options for Questions 36–40

A   Cervical smear in 12 months
B   Colposcopy and cervical smear in 12 months with high-risk HPV testing
C   Colposcopy and smear in 6 months for test of cure
D   Discharge to the GP
E   Discharge to the GP and routine recall in 3 years' time
F   Discharge to the GP and routine recall in 5 years' time
G   Knife cone biopsy
H   Large loop excision of transformation zone
I   Need to be seen in the colposcopy clinic within 2 weeks of referral
J   Need to be seen in the colposcopy clinic within 4 weeks of referral
K   Need to be seen in the colposcopy clinic within 8 weeks of referral
L   Referral to colposcopy
M   Routine recall in 3 years' time
N   Routine recall in 5 years' time

Instructions: For each scenario below, chose the single most appropriated management option from the list of options. Each option may be used once, more than once or not at all.

36. A 28-year-old woman was seen by her GP. She is up to date with her smears, none of which have been abnormal apart from her current smear which is shows glandular neoplasia. She is referred to the colposcopy clinic by her GP.

37. A 30-year-old woman is seen by her GP. She is up to date with her smears, none of which have been abnormal apart from her current smear which shows mild dyskaryosis and is HPV 16 positive.

38. A 51-year-old woman is seen by her GP. She is up to date with her smears, none of which have been abnormal apart from her current smear which shows borderline changes in squamous cells and is HPV 16 and 18 positive.

39. A 28-year-old woman is seen by her GP. She is up to date with her smears, none of which have been abnormal apart from her current smear which shows moderate dyskaryosis. She is seen in the colposcopy clinic, which reveals a high grade

abnormality. A large loop excision of transformation zone (LLETZ) is performed at the same appointment. A test-of-cure smear is performed at 6 months which shows normal cytology but is high-risk HPV positive.

40. A 28-year-old woman is seen by her GP. She is up to date with her smears, none of which have been abnormal apart from her current smear which shows low grade dyskaryosis. She is referred to colposcopy clinic. A colposcopy reveals a small area of low grade abnormality and a biopsy confirms cervical intraepithelial neoplasia 1 (CIN1).

Questions 41–45

Options for Questions 41–45

A	Measure CA-125 concentration	I	Repeat scan not necessary
B	Chemotherapy	J	Repeat the transabdominal ultrasound
C	CT		scan
D	MRI	K	Repeat the transvaginal scan (TVS)
E	Ovarian cyst aspiration	L	Refer to the colposcopy clinic
F	Ovarian cystectomy	M	Refer to the cancer centre
G	Oophorectomy	N	Refer to the gynaecology clinic
H	Ovarian transposition	O	Staging laparotomy

Instructions: For each scenario described below, choose the single most appropriate next step in the patient's management from the list of options above. Each option may be used once, more than once or not at all.

41. A 20-year-old woman attends the emergency department with acute abdominal pain. The surgeon suspects appendicitis and performs a diagnostic laparoscopy. You are the on-call registrar for that night and the surgeon calls you to give an opinion on an incidentally found large solid ovarian mass in the right adnexa with papillary projections on the surface. There is some free fluid in the pelvis and the other ovary appears normal.

42. A 58-year-old woman presents to her GP with gradual distension of the abdomen for the last 6 months. She is then referred to the gynaecology clinic for suspected ovarian cancer. An ultrasound scan of the pelvis reveals a large multilocular ovarian cyst on the right side. Her tumour markers are reported as: (a) CA-125 2000 U/mL, (b) CEA 1.2 ng/mL, and (c) CA-19.9 1 U/mL.

43. A 39-year-old woman is reviewed in the gynaecology clinic with symptoms of pelvic pain for the last 2 years. She was treated for endometriosis 5 years ago with laparoscopic laser ablation. Her ultrasound scan 2 months ago revealed a left-sided ovarian cyst (5.8 cm) with diffuse low-level internal echoes with one thin internal septae. Her CA-125 concentration is raised (61 U/mL).

44. A 28-year-old woman is referred to the gynaecology clinic with symptoms of menorrhagia with no intermenstrual and postcoital bleeding. Her pelvic examination is normal. However, an ultrasound scan of the pelvis shows an incidental finding of a simple ovarian cyst (size 3 × 3 × 3 cm) on the right side. Her serum CA-125 concentration is 15 U/mL. Her recent cervical smear was normal.

45. A 50-year-old woman is referred to the gynaecology clinic with two ultrasound scan reports: (a) a current one showing a simple left ovarian cyst of 3 × 4 cm in size, and (b) the previous one performed 4 months ago showing a simple left ovarian cyst of 5 × 4 cm in size. Her CA-125 concentration is 6 U/mL. She is otherwise asymptomatic and well.

Questions 46–50

Options for Questions 46–50

A	Arrhenoblastoma	I	Mucinous cystadenoma
B	Brenner tumour	J	Mucinous cystadenocarcinoma
C	Borderline serous ovarian tumour	K	Papillary serous carcinoma
D	Clear cell carcinoma	L	Serous cystadenoma
E	Endometrioid carcinoma	M	Serous cystadenocarcinoma
F	Dermoid cyst	N	Struma ovarii
G	Granulosa cell tumour	O	Thecoma
H	Krukenberg tumour		

Instructions: For each of the pathological findings described below, choose the single most appropriate tumour diagnosis from the list of options above. Each option may be used once, more than once, or not at all.

46. Signet ring cells on histology.

47. Transitional epithelium from Wolffian remnants.

48. Low malignant potential with no stroma invasion.

49. Müllerian origin with poor prognosis.

50. Usually seen in postmenopausal women and is associated with fibroma (Meigs' syndrome).

Questions 51–55

Options for Questions 51–55

A	Cervical biopsy	I	Thyroid function tests
B	Cervical smear	J	Pregnancy test
C	CT	K	Pelvic examination
D	Hysteroscopy and endometrial biopsy	L	Rectal examination
E	Diagnostic laparoscopy and proceed	M	Renal function tests
F	MRI	N	Saline hysterosonography
G	No further tests required	O	Speculum examination of cervix
H	Transvaginal scan (TVS) for endometrial thickness		

Instructions: For each case described below, choose the single most appropriate investigation in women with postmenopausal bleeding (PMB) from the above list of options. Each option may be used once, more than once or not at all.

51. A 48-year-old white woman is referred to the rapid-access gynaecologic clinic with PMB. Speculum examination reveals a stenosed cervical os and two failed attempts at endometrial pipelle biopsy. A transvaginal ultrasound shows an endometrial thickness of 6 mm. She claims to be fit and well.

52. A 48-year-old Asian woman presents to her GP with PMB. She had a left mastectomy and axillary node dissection for breast cancer 4 years ago. She is currently on two medications: tamoxifen and anastrozole. She has been up to date with her smears and all her previous smears, including the current one, are normal. A TVS performed in the clinic reveals 5 mm endometrial thickness and normal ovaries. A recent breast appointment shows no clinical evidence of recurrence of breast cancer.

53. A 48-year-old white woman visits the UK to see her daughter-in-law and her grandson. She is newly registered with a GP and presents with PMB for the last 2 weeks. She is up to date with her smears and has never had any abnormal smears. Pelvic examination is normal.

54. A 48-year-old Asian woman is referred to the rapid-access gynaecologic clinic for PMB which occurred 2 weeks ago. She did not have any further bleeding following that one episode. She is up to date with her smears which are normal, and a TVS reveals 3 mm endometrial thickness. Clinical examination reveals an atrophic cervix and vagina.

55. A 48-year-old white woman is referred to the rapid-access gynaecologic clinic for ongoing PMB for the last 3 weeks. So far all her previous smears have been normal and her endometrial thickness measures 4 mm on recent TVS. Clinical examination is normal.

Questions 56–60

Options for Questions 56–60

A	Adriamycin	H	Imiquimod
B	Carboplatin	I	Methotrexate
C	Cisplatin	J	Melphalan
D	Chlorambucil	K	Paclitaxel
E	Cyclophosphamide	L	Topotecan
F	Etoposide	M	Treosulfan
G	5–Fluorouracil	N	Vincristine

Instructions: For each side effect of chemotherapy described below, choose the single most appropriate drug from the list of options above. Each option may be used once, more than once or not at all.

56. A 49-year-old woman presents with haematuria. She has recently been diagnosed with ovarian cancer and has received two cycles of chemotherapy. Cystoscopy reveals haemorrhagic cystitis.

57. A 40-year-old woman presents with palpitations, numbness and tingling in the legs, and alopecia involving all body hair. She has recently been diagnosed with ovarian cancer and has received three cycles of chemotherapy. Clinical examination reveals pulse of 180 bpm and normal blood pressure. She is booked for debulking surgery in 10 days.

58. A 20-year-old woman is having treatment for a high-risk gestational trophoblastic disease. She has just finished her second cycle of chemotherapy. 1 week later she presents with feeling unwell with motor weakness, double vision and sore throat. Clinical examination reveals lower limb power of 3/5 and lateral rectus palsy of right eye, and blood results show myelosuppression.

59. A 40-year-old woman has recently been diagnosed with ovarian cancer and has received two cycles of chemotherapy. She presents with decreased urine output, tingling in the lower limbs and is hard of hearing following completion of the second cycle. Her blood results show high creatinine and low magnesium.

60. A 20-year-old woman had medical treatment for an ectopic pregnancy 15 days ago. She has been told not to get pregnant for at least 1 month following this injection because the drug has an antifolate action.

Answers: SBAs

1.   A Discharge to the care of her GP

Guidelines for the management of women with low grade cervical cytological abnormalities has been revised by the British Society for Colposcopy and Cervical Pathology (BSCCP). The NHS Cervical Screening Programme (NHSCSP) introduced HPV triage to differentiate between women at an increased risk of high grade CIN who should have colposcopy and women at low risk of CIN who can return to routine screening.

In the guideline it is recommended that women with borderline nuclear changes in squamous cells in their cervical smear and negative high-risk HPV can be discharged to their GP and return to routine cervical screening.

NHS Cancer Screening Programme. HPV triage and test of cure protocol: for women aged 25 to 64 years. London: NHS; 2010.
NHS Cervical Screening Programme. HPV Triage and test of cure implementation guide. NHSCSP good practice guide no. 3. London: NHS; 2011.

2.   B Discharge to her GP with a plan of routine recall for a smear in 3 years' time

As per the NHS Cervical Screening Programme (NHSCSP) policies, women with borderline or low grade cytological abnormality on cervical smear and high-risk HPV positive on testing should be referred to the colposcopy clinic for assessment. If the colposcopy is normal, then these women can be discharged to their GP and can return to routine recall for cervical smear. However, if the colposcopy and biopsy confirms CIN 1 then these women need a further follow up at one year in colposcopy clinic.

3.   E Perform large loop excision of transformation zone (LLETZ)

As per NHS Cervical Screening Programme (NHSCSP) policies, women with severe dyskaryosis should be referred to the colposcopy clinic urgently and need to be on the 2-week wait pathway. At colposcopy, if a high grade abnormality is confirmed then LLETZ needs to be offered and arranged. It can be done at the same setting (see and treat) or arranged at a later date. LLETZ has a success rate of 95%.

4.   E Follow up in the colposcopy clinic in 12 months for a repeat smear and colposcopy

As per NHS Cervical Screen Programme (NHSCSP) guidelines, women with borderline or a low grade cytological abnormality on their cervical smear and high risk HPV positive on testing should be referred to the colposcopy clinic for assessment. If the colposcopy is unsatisfactory (the entire squamo-columnar junction cannot be visualised), then these women need a further follow up in colposcopy clinic in a years' time.

5.   B Immature teratoma

Ovarian germ cells tumours can be benign or malignant. Although malignant germ cell ovarian tumours constitute around 15–20% of ovarian tumours, they represent only 2–5% of all ovarian cancers. They usually occur in the first 2 decades of life and are the most common tumours in this age group (60% of germ cell tumours occur in women under 21 years of age, and of these, one-third are malignant).

Teratomas are germ cell tumours and are classified as mature or immature. Mature teratomas are benign and arise from two or three germ cell layers. In 1–2% of cases, a mature teratoma undergoes malignant transformation (often to a squamous cell carcinoma).

Immature teratomas are malignant. They constitute 20% of germ cell tumours and 1% of all ovarian cancers. They are almost always unilateral (more than 90%). They are derived from ectoderm, endoderm and mesoderm, and contain both mature and immature elements (usually immature neural tissue). Neurotubules and rosettes can be seen histologically.

Immature teratoma is graded by the presence of glial or neural tissue, and prognosis depends on the glial tissue grading. Grade 1 represents a good prognosis, and grades 2 and 3 a poor prognosis. The treatment for germ cell tumours is fertility-sparing surgery followed by chemotherapy. Patients with malignant germ cell tumors will need the same staging surgery that is performed for epithelial ovarian cancer. If the patient wishes to preserve her fertility, the cancerous ovary and the fallopian tube on the same side are removed (unilateral salpingo-oophorectomy), but the uterus, ovary on the opposite side and the fallopian tube can be left behind. Adequately staged stage IA grade I immature teratomas will not require adjuvant chemotherapy. Grade 2 and grade 3 tumours are treated with adjuvant chemotherapy.

This patient's CA-125 concentration is mildly raised. CA-125 is a non-specific marker and can be raised in any disease causing inflammation of the peritoneum. Levels are raised in approximately 80% of all women with epithelial ovarian cancer (**Table 16.1**) but only 50% with International Federation of Gynecology and Obstetrics stage I disease. However, CA-125 has a low specificity in women less than 45 years of age because it can be elevated in several benign conditions. These include endometriosis, pelvic inflammatory disease, adenomyosis, fibroids, lymphoma, menstruation, ovarian hyperstimulation syndrome and pregnancy. It can also be raised with any other tumour causing peritoneal inflammation.

The prognostic factors for immature teratomas differs between children and adults. In children, the prognosis depends on the presence or absence of yolk sac components.

Table 16.1 Tumour markers in cancer	
Tumour marker	Cancer
Enzymes and proteins	
CA-125	Ovarian carcinoma (epithelial and primary peritoneal carcinoma)
CA-19.9	Colonic and pancreatic carcinoma
CA-15.3	Breast carcinoma
Lactate dehydrogenase, placental alkaline phosphatase 3% of dysgerminomas also produce β-hCG	Dysgerminomas
Oncofetal proteins	
Carcinoembryonic antigen	Upper gastrointestinal, colonic and pancreatic. It is also raised in mucinous ovarian tumours
α-Fetoprotein Half life 5–7 days	Endodermal sinus tumours, embryonal carcinomas, seminomas and hepatocellular carcinomas
α-Fetoprotein and β-hCG	Embryonal carcinoma (these can also produce oestradiol)
β-hCG Half life 16–48 hours	Gestational trophoblastic tumours, choriocarcinomas, non-gestational choriocarcinomas and embryonal carcinomas 3% of dysgerminomas produce hCG
Catecholamines and vanillylmandelic acid	Phaeochromocytoma
5-Hydroxytryptamine	Carcinoid tumour
Calcitonin	Medullary carcinoma of the thyroid
β-hCG, β-Human chorionic gonadotropin.	

Kumar B, Davies-Humphreys J. Tumour markers and ovarian cancer screening. Personal assessment in continuing education. In: Reviews, questions and answers, vol. 3. London: RCOG Press, 2003:51–53.

6.   B IC1

The International Federation of Gynecology and Obstetrics staging of ovarian cancer is shown in **Table 16.2**. Stage IC is either stage IA or IB with the tumour on the surface of one or both ovaries or surgical spill, or capsule rupture before surgery, or with ascites containing cancerous cells, or with positive peritoneal washings.

Stage IC is divided into IC1, IC2 and IC3. Surgical spill or rupture of a cyst during surgery is considered to be Stage IC1 ovarian cancer.

Surgical spill is important for staging purposes. Therefore it is important to document the findings and the operation clearly, including whether the rupture of cyst occurred prior to surgery or during surgery. This is also important for prognosis and survival (**Table 16.3**).

Table 16.2 International Federation of Gynecologic and Obstetrics classification of ovarian cancer

Stage	Characteristics
I	Growth limited to the ovaries
IA	Growth limited to 1 ovary. The ovarian capsule is intact without tumour on the external surface, and no malignant cells are present in washings or ascites
IB	Growth limited to both ovaries. The ovarian capsule is intact without tumour on the external surface, and no malignant cells are present in washings or ascites
IC	Either stage IA or IB but with tumour on the surface of 1 or both ovaries or surgical spill, or capsule rupture before surgery, or with ascites containing cancerous cells, or with positive peritoneal washings
IC1	Surgical spill
IC2	Tumour on the ovarian surface or capsule rupture before surgery
IC3	Positive peritoneal washings or ascites containing malignant cells
II	Growth involving 1 or both ovaries with spread to other pelvic organs (below the pelvic brim)
IIA	Metastasis to the uterus or tubes
IIB	Metastasis to other pelvic intraperitoneal organs
III	Growth involving 1 or both ovaries with histologically or cytologically confirmed peritoneal implants outside the pelvis and/or positive retroperitoneal lymph nodes or omentum
IIIA	Positive peritoneal spread confirmed microscopically or positive retroperitoneal lymph nodes
IIIA1	Positive retroperitoneal lymph nodes IIIA(i) – metastasis <10 mm in size IIIA(ii) – metastasis >10 mm in size
IIIA2	Microscopic peritoneal metastasis outside the pelvis ± positive retroperitoneal lymph nodes
IIIB	Macroscopic peritoneal metastasis <2 cm in size outside the pelvis ± positive retroperitoneal lymph nodes ± involvement of the liver and/or splenic capsule
IIIC	Macroscopic peritoneal metastasis >2 cm in size outside the pelvis ± positive retroperitoneal lymph nodes ± involvement of the liver and/or splenic capsule
IV	Distant metastasis excluding peritoneal metastasis
IVA	Analysis of pleural effusion showing malignant cells
IVB	Parenchymal liver and/or splenic metastasis and metastasis to extra-abdominal organs including inguinal lymph nodes and other lymph nodes outside the abdominal cavity

Table 16.3 5-year and overall survival rate for women with ovarian cancer

FIGO stage	5-year survival rate (%)
1	92
2	55
3	22
4	6
Overall survival for all stages	43
FIGO, International Federation of Gynecology and Obstetrics.	

Cancer Research UK. Ovarian cancer statistics. London: Cancer Research UK;2011.
International Federation of Gynecology and Obstetrics (FIGO). FIGO ovarian cancer staging. London: FIGO; 2014.

7. E Laparascopic hysterectomy and bilateral salpingo-oophorectomy

Endometrioid adenocarcinoma is the most common histological type of uterine cancer. The treatment for stage I disease is a total laparascopic hysterectomy and bilateral salpingo-oophorectomy. The risk of lymph node metastasis with grade 1 and stage 1 tumours is 1%. Because there is a risk of occult metastasis to adnexal tissues such as the tube and ovary, these organs should to be removed. The other reason for ovaries to be removed is that there may be an unrecognised oestrogen-secreting tumour.

Table 16.4 shows the International Federation of Gynecology and Obstetrics staging of endometrial cancer and Table 16.5 shows the survival rates for uterine cancer.

Table 16.4 International Federation of Obstetrics and Gynecology classification of endometrial cancer	
Stage	Description
I	Tumour confined to the uterus
IA	No invasion or invasion of less than half the depth of the myometrium
IB	Invasion equal to or more than half the depth of the myometrium
II	Tumour involving the cervical stroma but not extending outside the uterus
III	Local or regional spread of tumour outside the uterus
IIIA	Tumour involving the uterine serosa or adnexae
IIIB	Tumour involving the vagina or parametrium
IIIC	Metastases to the pelvic or para-aortic nodes
IIIC1	Metastases to the pelvic nodes
IIIC2	Metastases to the para-aortic nodes
IV	Tumour involving the bladder or bowel mucosa, or distant metastases
IVA	Tumour involving the bladder or bowel mucosa
IVB	Distant metastasis involving intra-abdominal metastases and/or inguinal lymph nodes

Endocervical gland involvement alone is no longer stage II disease. Positive cytology does not change the stage but is reported separately. Endometrioid carcinoma can be grade 1, 2 or 3.

Table 16.5 5-year and overall survival rate of women with uterine cancer	
FIGO stage	5-year survival rate (%)
I	95
II	77
III	39
IV	14
Overall survival for all stages	84.4

FIGO, International Federation of Gynecology and Obstetrics

National Cancer Institute. Endometrial cancer treatment – health professional version. Bethesda, Maryland: National Cancer Institute; 2017.

Cancer Research UK. Uterine cancer survival statistics. London: Cancer Research UK; 2011.

FIGO committee on Gynaecologic Oncology. FIGO staging for carcinoma of the vulva, cervix, and corpus uteri. Int J Gynaecol Obstet 2014; 125:97–98.

8.   D IIIA

The risk of cancer with lichen sclerosis is 2–4%, although 3–5% is sometimes quoted. If symptoms do not improve with local steroids, a mapping vulval biopsy is recommended to confirm the diagnosis.

Table 16.6 shows International Federation of Obstetrics and Gynecology staging of vulval cancer and **Table 16.7** shows survival rate for vulval cancer.

Table 16.6 International Federation of Gynecology and Obstetrics classification of vulval carcinoma

Stage	Characteristics
I	Tumour confined to the vulva or perineum with negative nodes
IA	Tumour confined to the vulva or perineum, ≤2 cm in size with stromal invasion of ≤1 mm, negative nodes
IB	Tumour confined to the vulva or perineum, >2 cm in size or with stromal invasion of >1 mm, negative nodes
II	Tumour of any size with adjacent spread (lowest third of the urethra/vagina/anus), negative nodes
IIIA	Tumour of any size with positive inguinofemoral lymph nodes (i) 1 lymph node metastasis of ≥5 mm (ii) 1–2 lymph node metastases of <5 mm
IIIB	(i) 2 or more lymph node metastases of ≥ 5 mm (ii) 3 or more lymph node metastases of <5 mm
IIIC	Positive node(s) with extracapsular spread
IVA	(i) Tumour invades other regional structures (upper two thirds of the urethra/vagina), bladder mucosa, rectal mucosa or fixed to pelvic bone (ii) Fixed or ulcerated inguinofemoral lymph nodes
IVB	Any distant metastasis, including pelvic lymph nodes

Table 16.7 5-year and overall survival rate for vulval cancer

FIGO stage	5-year survival rate (%)
I	80
II	60
III	40
IV	15

FIGO, International Federation of Obstetrics and Gynecology

Cancer Research UK. Survival statistics for vulval cancer. London: Cancer Research UK; 2011.

FIGO committee on Gynaecologic Oncology. FIGO staging for carcinoma of the vulva, cervix, and corpus uteri. Int J Gynaecol Obstet 2014; 125:97–98.

Homesley HD, Bundy BN, Sedlis A, et al. Assessment of current International Federation of Gynecology and Obstetrics staging of vulvar carcinoma relative to prognostic factors for survival (a Gynecologic Oncology Group study). Am J Obstet Gynecol 1991; 164:997–1003.

9. D Superficial inguinal nodes

Vulval lymphatics may cross the midline, and the pattern of lymphatic metastasis from midline tumours is slightly different from that of lateral tumours. The vulva generally drains into the superficial inguinal nodes, then into deep femoral nodes and finally to the external iliac lymph nodes. The deep femoral lymph nodes (around 3 to 5 nodes) are located medial to the femoral vein within the femoral triangle and under the cribriform fascia. The most superior node is called Cloquet's node. The clitoris and perineum have a bilateral lymph flow.

Unlike the rest of the vulva, the lymphatics from the clitoral region bypass the superficial inguinal nodes and pass directly into the deep femoral nodes. If the tumour lies in the midline, the deep femoral nodes can be involved without involvement of the superficial inguinal nodes. With lateral lesions, it is unlikely for the deep inguinal nodes to be involved if the superficial inguinal nodes are not.

10. C 10%

The majority of rapid-access 2-week wait gynaecologic clinic referrals are for women with postmenopausal bleeding (PMB). The risk of cancer in this group of women is around 10%. However, the risk of cancer if the endometrial thickness is <4 mm is <1%. Therefore, women who have had 1 episode of PMB but a normal pelvic examination and no abnormal findings on ultrasound can be discharged to GP care. The GP should be advised to refer the patient back again if there is a repeated episode of PMB.

National Institute for Health and Care Excellence (NICE). Gynaecological cancers – recognition and referral. London: NICE; 2015.

11. D Levonorgestrel-releasing intrauterine system (Mirena coil)

Management of women with endometrial hyperplasia without atypia:

- The majority regress spontaneously
- The risk of progressing to cancer is <5% over 20 years
- Risk factors should be modified – address obesity, stop hormone replacement therapy
- 10% of obese women harbour asymptomatic endometrial hyperplasia
- Treatment with progestogens produces a higher rate of disease regression (89–96%) than observation alone (74–81%)

Regarding first-line medical treatments of hyperplasia without atypia:

- Both continuous oral and local intrauterine [levonorgestrel-releasing intrauterine system (LNG-IUS)] progestogens are effective in achieving regression of endometrial hyperplasia without atypia
- The LNG-IUS should be the first-line medical treatment. This is because, compared with oral progestogens, it is associated with a higher disease regression rate and more favourable bleeding profile, while producing fewer adverse effects. Relapse is more common with oral progestogens

- An intrauterine system should be in place for a minimum of 6 months to obtain histological regression. It should be retained for 5 years in women who are at higher risk of relapse, e.g. if their BMI is >35 or if they are on oral progestogens. Endometrial biopsy at 6 and 12 months should be recommended and once two consecutive negative biosies are obtained, yearly follow with endometrial pipelle biopsies can be considered.
- Endometrial surveillance should be at 6-montly intervals – at least 2 consecutive negative biopsies are needed before the patient can be discharged
- Women who decline the LNG-IUS should be prescribed continuous progestogens (medroxyprogesterone 10–20 mg/day or norethisterone 10–15 mg/day)
- Cyclical progestogens should not be used because they are less effective in inducing regression of endometrial hyperplasia without atypia compared with continuous oral progestogens or the LNG-IUS.

Royal College of Obstetricians and Gynaecologists (RCOG) and British Society for Gynaecological Endoscopy. Management of endometrial hyperplasia. Green-top guideline No. 67. London: RCOG; 2016.

12. C 30–60%

The lifetime risk of breast cancer is 80% in a woman carrying the *BRCA1* mutation. 35–50% of the breast cancers are caused by mutations in the *BRCA1* gene on the long arm of chromosome 17. Men with the mutant gene do not usually develop breast cancer but transmit the gene to approximately 50% of their offspring.

Familial breast and ovarian cancer

Inherited genes play an important role in the development of breast, ovarian and colorectal cancers.

In the UK, the lifetime risk of developing breast cancer is 1 in 12, while for ovarian cancer it is 1 in 80. The incidence of breast cancer rises to 300/100,000 in women aged over 85 years compared with <10/100,000 in women under the age of 30 years. Breast cancer can occur in sporadic or hereditary forms. In cancers occurring in women under 35 years of age, up to 10% are inherited as dominant genes (**Table 16.8**).

About 1 in 800 women in the general population carry the *BRCA1* mutation and somewhat fewer than this the *BRCA2* mutation. Figures vary in terms of ethnic population and geographical location (e.g. about 1 in 50 of the Ashkenazi Jewish population carry these mutations). *BRCA1* and *BRCA2* equally increase the risk of developing breast cancer by 40–85% during a woman's lifetime, depending on the population. The risk of ovarian cancer is higher if *BRCA1* rather than *BRCA2* is present (**Table 16.9**).

Genetics: family history

- The relative risk of developing breast cancer is 1.1 for a mother, 3.8 for a sister and 6 for a daughter
- If there is 1 affected primary relative aged under 50 years, the lifetime risk is 5%
- If there are 2 affected primary relatives aged less than 50 years, the lifetime risk is 25%

- Around 5–10% of ovarian cancers are hereditary [e.g. show an association with *BRCA1* or *MLH1* (also known as *HNPCC*)]

BRCA1 and *BRCA2* mutations

- Overall these mutations occur in 3% of women with an ovarian tumour (5% aged less than 40 years) (see Table 16.8)
- Most epithelial ovarian cancers are sporadic, but 10% may be inherited with *BRCA1*, *BRCA2* and *HNPCC* gene mutations
- Mutations occurs in 80% of families with breast or ovarian cancer

Risk reduction measures for women who carry a *BRCA1* or *BRCA2* mutation

For breast cancer:

- Self-examination of the breasts
- Screening with mammography starting at the age of 30 years, carried out annually

Hormonal therapy

Tamoxifen is shown to reduce the risk of occurrences of hormone-receptor-positive, first-time breast cancer. The reduction is seen both in premenopausal and postmenopausal women who are high risk.

Surgical prophylaxis

Bilateral prophylactic mastectomy earlier on may reduce the risk of development of breast cancer in women by almost 95%.

For ovarian cancer:

- Yearly screening using transvaginal ultrasound and CA-125 concentration
- Combined oral contraceptive pill use, which reduces the risk of ovarian cancer by 40%. This is a good option in women who have not completed their family. The protective effect lasts for at least 10 years after stopping the pill
- Prophylactic oophorectomy once the family has been completed, although this does not prevent primary peritoneal cancers. It is recommended at age 40 years for women who carry a *BRCA1* gene mutation, and at age 45 years for women who carry a *BRCA2* gene mutation

Table 16.8 Genes associated with breast, ovarian and colorectal cancers	
Inherited genes	**Cancers**
ATM, BRCA1, BRCA2, CHEK2, RAD51, DIRAS3, ERBB2	Breast
BRCA1, BRCA2	Ovarian
MSH2 and *MSH6* on chromosome 2; *MLH1* on chromosome 3	Colorectal

Table 16.9 Lifetime cancer risk with *BRCA1* and *BRCA2*		
Lifetime risk	***BRCA1* (chromosome 17)**	***BRCA2* (chromosome 13)**
Breast cancer	60–80%	30–60%
Ovarian cancer	30–60%	20–30%

Morrison PJ, Hodgson SV, Haites NE (eds). Familial breast and ovarian cancer, genetics, screening and management. Cambridge: Cambridge University Press, 2002.

Royal College of Obstetricians and Gynaecologists. Ovarian cysts in postmenopausal women. Green-top Guideline no. 34. London: RCOG Press, 2003.

Shafi MI, Luesley DM, Jordan JA. Handbook of gynaecological oncology. Edinburgh: Churchill Livingstone, 2001.

13. E Follow-up with the GP in 36 months for cervical smear and human papillomavirus (HPV) testing

Test of cure (TOC) following large loop excision of the transformation zone [treatment of cervical intraepithelial neoplasia (CIN)]

The test-of-cure (TOC) policy is applied to all women who attend the clinic at their first follow-up appointment post treatment with LLETZ for cytology, irrespective of the fine histology grade of CIN. This also applies to women who were in the previous programme of 10-year surveillance and were followed up annually post treatment. Further management would be same in both groups as per the TOC results.

If the TOC results are normal, borderline or mild on cytology and the HR-HPV is negative, the patient will have further cytology in 3 years' time regardless of age. If the cytology is negative at 3 years' time, then women who are over 50 years of age will return to the normal recall pattern for that age which is a smear every 5 years.

Women with smears reported as showing moderate or severe dyskaryosis will be referred to colposcopy irrespective of their age.

Women will be referred to colposcopy if the TOC smear is reported as normal, borderline or mild dyskaryosis but HR-HPV is positive. If the colposcopy is satisfactory and negative then the first recall is in 3 years' time for any women.

Women who do not attend the colposcopy clinic after treatment (LLETZ) but go back to the GP before the first cytology follow up should still have the TOC.

National Health Service (NHS). National Health Service Cancer Screening Programme (NHSCSP): HPV triage and test of cure: implementation guide. NHSCSP Good Practice Guide No. 3. London: NHS; 2011.

National Health Service Cervical Screening Programme (NHSCSP). Colposcopy and Programme Management. Publication No. 20. London: NHSCSP; 2011.

Kelly RS, Patnick J, Kitchener HC, Moss SM, on behalf of the NHSCSP HPV Special Interest Group. HPV testing as a triage for borderline or mild dyskaryosis on cervical cytology: results from the Sentinel Sites study. Brit J Cancer 2011; 105:983–988.

14. C IIa1

The stage of the cancer describes the size of tumour as well as distant spread (**Table 16.10**).

Table 16.10 FIGO classification of cervical cancer	
Stage	**Characteristics**
I	Cancer is confined to the cervix (Extension to the uterus does not alter the stage of the disease)
IA	Microscopic diagnosis of invasive carcinoma with deepest invasion of ≥5 mm or more and horizontal extension of ≤7 mm
IA1	Microscopic diagnosis: stromal invasion ≤3 mm in depth and extension ≤7 mm
IA2	Microscopic diagnosis: stromal invasion >3 mm but <5 mm, and horizontal extension >7 mm
IB	Clinically visible cancer or preclinical cancer more than stage IA
IB1	Clinically visible cancer <4 cm
IB2	Clinically visible cancer >4 cm
II	Cervical carcinoma invades the parametrium but does not reach the lateral pelvic wall. Cervical carcinoma involves the upper two thirds of the vagina
IIA	No parametrial invasion but can involve up to the upper two thirds of the vagina
IIA1	Clinically visible cervical tumour <4 cm
IIA2	Clinically visible cervical tumour >4 cm
IIB	Obvious parametrial invasion but not up to the lateral pelvic wall
III	Cervical tumour extends to the pelvic wall and/or involves the lower third of the vagina and/or causes hydronephrosis or a non-functioning kidney
IIIA	Tumour involves the lower third of the vagina but there is no involvement up to the lateral pelvic wall
IIIB	Parametrial extension up to the lateral pelvic wall and/or hydronephrosis or a non-functioning kidney solely due to cervical tumour causing obstruction
IV	Cervical carcinoma extends beyond the true pelvis or has involved the adjacent organs (bladder mucosa and rectal mucosa). Bullous oedema does not alter the stage
IVA	Spread of cervical tumour to adjacent organs
IVB	Spread of cervical tumour to distant organs

Table 16.11 5-year survival rate for women with cervical cancer	
FIGO stage	**5-year survival rate (%)**
I	95
II	50
III	40
IV	05

Cancer Research UK. Survival statistics for cervical cancer. London: Cancer Research UK; 2011. International Federation of Gynecology and Obstetrics committee on Gynecologic Oncology. FIGO staging for carcinoma of the vulva, cervix, and corpus uteri. Int J Gynaecol Obstet 2014; 125:97–8

15. E Total abdominal hysterectomy with bilateral salpingo-oophorectomy

This woman is nearing menopausal age. There is a high risk of coexisting endometrial cancer with atypical hyperplasia, with an attendant small risk of occult metastasis to the ovary (in one study of 439 patients with stage I endometrial cancer, ovarian metastasis was found in 22 women or 5% of women). Therefore, it is better to offer salpingo-oophorectomy, after thorough counselling. Most NHS hospitals perform MRI to assess the disease before hysterectomy.

Endometrial hyperplasia with atypia and risk of cancer

- There is an 8% risk of progression to cancer in 4 years
- There is a 12% risk of progression to cancer after 9 years
- There is a 27.5% risk of progression to cancer after 19 years
- It is associated with coexisting carcinoma in up to 43% of women undergoing hysterectomy

Treatment of women with endometrial hyperplasia with atypia

- The risk of progression or persistence of cancer is high (30–50%) if there is atypical hyperplasia
- There is up to a 40% risk of endometrial cancer if there is complex atypical hyperplasia. Therefore a further hysteroscopy and thorough endometrial sampling should be considered despite the diagnosis of hyperplasia on endometrial pipelle biopsy
- If there is atypical hyperplasia, total hysterectomy should be undertaken because of the risk of underlying malignancy or progression to cancer
- Postmenopausal women with atypical hyperplasia should be offered bilateral salpingo-oophorectomy with the total hysterectomy
- In premenopausal women, the decision to remove the ovaries should be individualised. Bilateral salpingectomy should, however, be considered because it can reduce the risk of future ovarian malignancy

Takeshima N, Hirai Y, Yano K. Ovarian metastasis in endometrial carcinoma. Gynecol Oncol 1998; 70:183–187.

Answers: EMQs

16. I Stage IIIC1

Endometrial cancer is surgico-pathologically staged. In this case the final histology shows pelvic node involvement. Therefore, this woman has stage IIIC1 endometrial cancer.

17. I Stage IIIC1

In this scenario, the preoperative MRI scan suggests serosal and pelvic lymph node involvement. The final histology confirms the MRI scan findings. Therefore, this woman has stage IIIC1 endometrial cancer.

18. G Stage IIIA

Do not be misled by findings of cervical involvement in this scenario. The final histology also reveals serosal involvement. Therefore, this woman has stage IIIA endometrial cancer.

19. D Stage II

According to the revised FIGO classification uterine cancer involving cervical stroma is described as stage II. The classification of II into IIa and IIb has been removed from the current classification. Glandular involvement of the cervix is no longer classified as stage II.

20. A Stage 1A

According to the latest FIGO classification, the involvement of the endometrium and less than 50% of the myometrium is described as stage IA.

Positive peritoneal cytology no longer alters the stage of the disease according to the current FIGO classification.

The uterine tumours are surgico-pathologically staged.

The updated revised FIGO staging (2009) is as follows:

- Stage I: Tumour confined to the uterus
- Stage IA: Tumour confined to the endometrium or myometrial invasion of less than 50%
- Stage IB: Myometrial invasion of >50%
- Stage II: Invasion of the tumour into the cervical stroma but does not extend beyond the uterus
- Stage III: Local or regional spread of the tumour
- Stage IIIA: Tumour involves the serosa of the uterus, fallopian tubes or adnexae
- Stage IIIB: Vaginal or parametrial involvement

- Stage IIIC: Metastasis to pelvic or para-aortic lymph nodes
- Stage IIIC1: Metastasis to pelvic nodes
- Stage IIIC2: Metastasis to para-aortic nodes
- Stage IV: The tumour invades the bladder or bowel mucosa and/or distant metastasis
- Stage IVA: The tumour invades the bladder or bowel mucosa
- Stage IVB: Remote metastasis, including inguinal lymph nodes or intra-abdominal metastasis

Endocervical glandular involvement is no longer considered stage II.

Holland C. Endometrial cancer. Obstet Gynaecol Reprod Med 2010; 20:347–352.
Lewin SN. Revised FIGO staging system for endometrial cancer. Clin Obstet Gynecol 2011; 54:215–218.
FIGO committee on Gynaecologic Oncology. FIGO staging for carcinoma of the vulva, cervix, and corpus uteri. Int J Gynaecol Obstet 2014; 125:97–8

21. C Dysgerminoma

Germ cell tumours account for 10% of all ovarian tumours. They are derived from primitive germ cells of the embryonic gonad and usually occur in young women in their 20s. The major issue in managing these women is to be able to preserve fertility while not compromising the chances of a cure.

Dysgerminoma (the equivalent of seminomas in men) is the most common type of germ cell tumour. They are bilateral in 10–15% of the cases. The tumour cells resemble primordial germ cells and do not normally secrete hormones. However, raised β-hCG is seen in 3% of these tumours (β-hCG is elevated when trophoblastic elements are present, as is the case with choriocarcinomas and occasionally dysgerminomas when syncytiotrophoblastic giant cells are present). Lactate dehydrogenase and placental alkaline phosphatase can also be increased. Histologically, lymphocytic infiltration in the stroma is a hallmark of these tumours. The primary treatment is surgery followed by adjuvant chemotherapy in cases higher than stage IA. Fertility-sparing surgery needs to be considered in young women who wish to have children. The overall survival rate is 90%.

22. D Endodermal sinus tumour

The endodermal sinus tumour is the second most common tumour after dysgerminomas. The mean age of occurence is 18 years and one third can be pre-menarchal. They are usually large, fast-growing and unilateral in occurrence. Macroscopically, they are solid with areas of haemorrhage and necrosis. Microscopically, the characteristic feature is a Schiller–Duval body. The tumour marker α-fetoprotein is increased.

23. K Malignant teratoma

Mature teratomas are the same as dermoid cysts and are benign tumours. There is less than a 2% risk of developing cancer in a mature teratoma.

Immature teratoma is the same as malignant teratoma, it is usually unilateral and occurs before the 20s. They are derived from the ectoderm, endoderm and mesoderm. The degree of cellular immaturity decides the grade of the tumour and the element used is neural tissue. The treatment is surgery and chemotherapy.

Choriocarcinomas secrete β-hCG while embryonal carcinomas secrete both β-hCG and α-fetoprotein. Embryonal carcinomas constitute 5% of malignant granulosa cell tumours. These are one of the most aggressive tumours.

24. G Granulosa cell tumour

The granulosa cell tumour is the most common type of sex cord stromal tumour and can occur at any age. They usually secrete oestrogens and this may cause endometrial hyperplasia and endometrial cancer. Women in menopause can present with vaginal bleeding and young women may present with precocious puberty. The tumour marker is inhibin B, especially the a-subunit of inhibin. The main modality of treatment is surgery followed by chemotherapy in women with more than stage IA tumours. Long-term follow-up is necessary as these tumours have a tendency for late recurrence.

25. F Epithelial ovarian tumour

The incidence of ovarian cancer is 15 in 100,000 women per year in the UK and about 90% of these tumours are epithelial in origin. These can be serous, mucinous and other tumours. Serous cystadenocarcinoma is 3 times more common (accounting for 50% of all epithelial ovarian cancers) than mucinous cystadenocarcinoma. Mucinous and endometrioid cancers are the next most common tumours accounting for 10–15% each. Undifferentiated and clear cell carcinomas are uncommon.

CA-125 is raised above the normal cut-off level (>35 U/mL) in about 80% of all women with epithelial ovarian cancers, while it is raised in only 50% of FIGO stage 1 ovarian cancer.

Sanusi FA, Carter P, Barton DPJ. Non Epithelial Ovarian Cancers. Personal assessment in continuing education. Reviews, questions and answers. Volume 3. London: RCOG Press, 2003: 38–39.
Kumar B and Davies-Humphreys J. Tumour Markers and Ovarian Cancer Screening. Personal assessment in continuing education. Reviews, questions and answers. Volume 3. RCOG Press, 2003: 51–53.

26. F Discharge to GP and routine recall in 3 years' time

As per NHSCSP guidelines, women with borderline or low-grade cytological abnormalities on cervical smear and high-risk HPV positive on testing should be referred to colposcopy for assessment. If the colposcopy is normal, then these women can be discharged to their GP and can return to routine recall for cervical smear in 3 years' time.

27. G Discharge to GP and routine recall in 5 years' time

As per NHSCSP guidelines, women with borderline or low-grade cytological abnormality on cervical smear and high-risk HPV positive on testing should be referred to colposcopy for assessment. Because this woman's colposcopy is normal and she is 49 years old, she can be discharged to her GP and return to routine recall for a cervical smear in 5 years' time.

28. F Discharge to GP and routine recall in 3 years' time

The management of women with low grade cervical cytological abnormalities has been revised by the British Society for Colposcopy and Cervical Pathology. The NHS Cancer Screening Programme introduced HPV triage to differentiate between women at an increased risk of high grade CIN who should have colposcopy and women at low risk of CIN who can return to routine screening at 3 years or 5 years depending on the age of current cervical smear.

In the guideline it is recommended that women with borderline nuclear changes in squamous cells or low grade cervical smear and high risk HPV negative can be discharged to their GP and can return to routine cervical screening.

National Health Service Cancer Screening Programme (NHSCSP). HPV triage and test of cure protocol: for women aged 25 to 64 years. Sheffield: NHSCSP; 2011.

29. G Discharge to GP and routine recall in 5 years' time

All samples reported as borderline or low grade dyskaryosis are sent for HPV testing. If high-risk HPV is detected, referral to colposcopy is recommended. If high-risk HPV is not detected, the patient can return to normal screening intervals for age (3 or 5 yearly). On the other hand, women in whom high-risk HPV is not detected are very unlikely to develop cervical cancer.

30. I Large loop excision of transformation zone (LLETZ)

The chances of progression of moderate and severe dyskaryosis (amounting to CIN2 and CIN3) to invasive disease is much higher than mild dyskaryosis (amounting to CIN1), although it takes some time for progression. Therefore, the colposcopic finding of high grade abnormality warrants treatment. A LLETZ can be performed at the same visit (see and treat) if the follow-up will be compromised.

Public Health England. NHS cervical screening programme: colposcopy and programme management. Publication 20 (3rd Edn). London: Public Health England; 2016.

31. I Need to be seen in the colposcopy clinic within 2 weeks of referral

All women with an abnormal cervix or a cervix suspicious for cancer should be referred to the colposcopy clinic immediately. It is recommended that they should be seen within 2 weeks of referral.

32. I Need to be seen in the colposcopy clinic within 2 weeks of referral

The cervical screening programme is not designed to pick up glandular abnormalities. These are rare but associated with an underlying malignancy (adenocarcinoma) in 40% of cases and cervical intraepithelial neoplasia in almost 50% of cases. All women with 1 report of glandular neoplasia should be seen in a colposcopy clinic within 2 weeks of referral to colposcopy services.

33. E Discharge to GP and routine recall in 3 years' time

As per NHSCSP guidelines, women with borderline or low grade cytological abnormalities on cervical smear and are high-risk HPV positive on testing should be referred to colposcopy for assessment. If the colposcopy is normal, then these women can be discharged to their GP and can return to routine recall for cervical smear in 3 years' time.

34. C Colposcopy and smear in 6 months' time for test of cure

If the referral smear shows severe dyskaryosis and colposcopy reveals high grade abnormalities then the patient needs treatment with large loop excision of transformation zone (LLETZ). Following LLETZ, she would need the test-of-cure smear at 6 months.

National Health Service Cervical Screening Programme. (NHSCSP). Colposcopy and programme management. Publication 20 (3rd Edn). Sheffield: NHSCSP; 2016.

35. E Discharge to GP and routine recall in 3 years' time

Women treated for CIN are tested for high-risk HPV 6 months after treatment. If the cytology result is negative, low-grade dyskaryosis or borderline, the sample is tested for high-risk HPV. If high-risk HPV is not detected, the patient can return to a 3-year recall regardless of age (if the next test is negative, the patient can return to normal recall for age). If high-risk HPV is detected, the patient should be referred back to the colposcopy clinic.

Women with low-grade or negative post treatment cytology in whom high-risk HPV is not detected have a very low risk of residual disease. This avoids a 10-year follow up in the majority of women (around 85%). Women with high-risk HPV detected at test of cure will be further assessed for residual disease.

If moderate or severe dyskaryosis is detected on the cervical smear in a test of cure sample after treatment, the patient will referred back to colposcopy for further assessment. High-risk human papilloma virus testing is not performed on this sample.

National Health Service Cancer Screening Programme (NHSCSP). HPV triage and test of cure protocol: for women aged 25 to 64 years. London: NHSCSP; 2010.

36. I Need to be seen in the colposcopy clinic within 2 weeks of referral

As per NHSCSP guidelines, women with borderline or low grade cytological abnormality on a cervical smear and who are high-risk HPV positive on testing should be referred to colposcopy for assessment. If the colposcopy is normal, then these women can be discharged to their general practitioner and can return to routine recall for cervical smear in 3 or 5 years' time depending on the woman's age (<50 or >50 years respectively).

37. L Referral to colposcopy

In accordance with NHSCSP guidelines, women with borderline or low grade cytological abnormality on a cervical smear and high-risk HPV positive on testing should be referred to colposcopy for assessment. If the colposcopy is normal, then these women can be discharged to their general practitioner and can return to routine recall for cervical smear in 3 or 5 years' time depending on the womans' age (<50 or >50 years respectively).

38. L Referral to colposcopy

In accordance with NHSCSP guidelines, women with borderline or low grade cytological abnormality on a cervical smear and high-risk HPV positive on testing should be referred to colposcopy for assessment. If the colposcopy is normal, then these women can be discharged to their general practitioner and can return to routine recall for cervical smear in 3 or 5 years' time depending on the womans' age (<50 or >50 years respectively).

39. L Referral to colposcopy

When a woman has a test-of-cure smear following a LLETZ, and if the test-of-cure cervical smear is normal, borderline or low grade and positive for high-risk HPV, she needs to be referred back to colposcopy.

40. B Colposcopy and cervical smear in 12 months with high-risk HPV testing

In accordance with NHSCSP guidelines, women with borderline or low-grade cytological abnormalities on a cervical smear and are are high-risk HPV positive on testing should be referred to colposcopy for assessment. If the colposcopy is normal, then these women can be discharged to their general practitioner and can return to routine recall for cervical smears. However, if the colposcopy and biopsy confirms CIN 1 then these women need a further follow up at one year in the colposcopy clinic and a repeat smear, and high-risk HPV testing needs to be performed.

41. M Refer to the cancer centre

This was an emergency surgery for acute appendicitis. The ovarian cyst was an unexpected finding and the intraoperative findings are suspicious of malignancy. The patient has not been consented for complete staging operation for suspected ovarian malignancy and this needs to be done in the gynaecology oncology centre following full investigation [MRI scan of pelvis, staging CT scan of pelvis, abdomen and chest plus tumour markers (CA-125, CEA, HCG and AFP)]. She therefore needs urgent referral to the cancer centre.

42. M Refer to the cancer centre

The risk of malignancy index (RMI) in this case is >250. RMI >250 is considered high risk and the risk of cancer is 75%. She therefore needs referral to the cancer centre.

RMI is calculated by multiplying 3 parameters:

- Ultrasound (USG) features (U = 0 for a USG score of 0, U = 1 for a USG score of 1 and U = 3 for a USG score of 2–5)
- Menopausal status (use 3 for postmenopausal women and 1 for premenopausal women)
- CA-125 levels (actual value from the blood test)

The final number acquired after multiplication of the above factors is regarded as the RMI. This number determines the risk of ovarian cancer, e.g. <25 is considered low risk and the risk of cancer is <3%, RMI 25–250 is considered moderate risk and the risk of cancer is 20%, and RMI >250 is considered high risk for malignancy and the risk of cancer is 75%.

A RMI score of 200 is recommended to predict the likelihood of ovarian cancer (sensitivity of 78% and specificity of 87%). To plan further management, some centres utilise a threshold of 250 with a sensitivity of 70% and a specificity of 90%.

A CT scan of the abdomen and pelvis should be performed for all postmenopausal women with ovarian cysts who have a RMI score greater than or equal to 200, with onward referral to gynaecological oncology multidisciplinary team.

Royal College of Obstericians and Gynaecologists (RCOG). The management of ovarian cysts in postmenopausal women. Green-top guideline No. 34. London: RCOG; 2016.

43. D MRI

CA-125 is non-specific and can be raised in benign conditions such as endometriosis, fibroids, pelvic inflammatory disease and anything that causes irritation to the pelvic peritoneum. In this case, the cyst is likely to be an endometrioma because it has the typical appearance of an endometrioma on the ultrasound scan (a cyst with diffuse low-level internal echoes). However, in women with an intermediate risk (RMI of 61) an MRI scan should be arranged and her case referred to an MDT before proceeding to surgery.

44. I Repeat scan not necessary

Around 10% of women will have surgery in some form during their lifetime for an ovarian mass. The majority are benign in premenopausal women. The overall incidence of a symptomatic ovarian cyst in a premenopausal woman being malignant is approximately 1 in 1000 increasing to 3 in 1000 at the age of 50 years.

In premenopausal women, functional or simple ovarian cysts (thin-walled cysts without internal structures) which are <50 mm in maximum diameter usually resolve over two to three menstrual cycles without the need for intervention. A serum CA-125 assay does not need to be undertaken in all premenopausal women when an ultrasonographic diagnosis of a simple ovarian cyst has been made.

Aspiration of ovarian cysts, both vaginally or laparoscopically, is less effective and is associated with a high rate of recurrence.

The RMI in this case is 15. RMI <25 is considered to be low risk for malignancy. The risk of malignancy in such ovarian cysts is <1% and more than 50% of cases will resolve spontaneously within 3 months. Therefore, it is reasonable to manage them conservatively. Asymptomatic premenopausal women with such cysts (<50 mm diameter) generally do not require a follow-up because these cysts are very likely to be physiological and almost always resolve within three menstrual cycles.

Women with simple ovarian cysts between 50 and 70 mm in diameter should have yearly ultrasound follow-ups and those with larger simple cysts should be considered for either further imaging (MRI) or surgical intervention.

Lactate dehydrogenase (LDH), α-fetoprotein and β-hCG should be measured in all women under the age of 40 years with a complex ovarian mass because of the possibility of germ cell tumours.

45. K Repeat the transvaginal scan (TVS)

The risk of malignancy index in this case is 18 and is considered as low risk for malignancy. Hence, it can be followed by repeat scans and CA-125 levels every 3–4 months for 1 year when she can be discharged back to the GP. Ovarian cyst aspiration is no longer recommended.

Royal College of Obstetricians and Gynaecologists. Green-top Guideline No. 34. Ovarian cysts in postmenopausal women. London: RCOG Press, 2003.
Royal College of Obstetricians and Gynaecologists. Green-top Guideline No. 62. Management of suspected ovarian masses in premenopausal women. London: RCOG Press, 2011.
National Institute for Health and Clinical Excellence. Guidelines on ovarian cancer: the recognition and initial management (CT122). NICE, 2011.

46. H Krukenberg tumour

It is a metastatic tumour of the ovary which accounts for 1–2% of ovarian cancers. The primary tumour is usually from the gastrointestinal tract and also from the breast.

Macroscopically, both ovaries are often (80%) involved and may be symmetrically enlarged, which is consistent with its metastatic nature.

Microscopically, it is characterised by mucin-secreting signet ring cells in the ovarian tissue.

Immunohistochemical studies are positive for CEA and cytokeratin 20 (CK20) and negative for cytokeratin 7 (CK7) if the primary is from the colon.

The management is to identify and treat the primary tumour. If the metastasis is confined to the primary tumour, surgical removal may improve survival. If the metastasis is extensive, the treatment is usually palliative. However, the optimum treatment for such tumours is unclear.

47. B Brenner tumour

Transitional epithelium is the epithelium of the ureter, bladder and urethra. It can be seen in a Brenner tumour of the ovary.

48. C Borderline serious ovarian tumour

The hallmark of malignancy is stromal invasion. Ovarian tumours without stromal invasion and have malignant features rather than a benign appearance are referred to as borderline tumours.

49. D Clear cell carcinoma

Clear cell carcinoma is a poorly differentiated tumour and carries a poor prognosis.

50. O Thecoma

An ovarian mass (fibroma) when associated with right-sided pleural effusion is referred to as a fibroma (Meigs' syndrome).

Pathological classification of ovarian tumours

- Epithelial cell tumours
- Sex cord/stromal tumours
- Germ cell tumours
- Embryonic tumours
- Miscellaneous
- Metastatic

Epithelial tumours

- 80% of ovarian tumours
- 90% of all primary malignant tumours

Types

- Serous cystadenoma
- Serous cystadenocarcinoma
- Serous borderline tumour
- Mucinous cystadenoma
- Mucinous cystadenocarcinoma
- Mucinous borderline tumour
- Brenner tumour
- Endometrioid tumour
- Clear cell tumour

Serous tumours

- Most common epithelial tumour
- Cystadenoma – usually uniocular or bilocular
- Cystadenocarcinoma – partly cystic/solid
- Increased CA-125

Mucinous tumours

- Cystadenoma – multilocular
- Rupture may cause pseudomyxoma peritonei and small bowel obstruction
- Cystadenocarcinoma – usually solid
- Can be associated with appendicular cancer
- Increased CEA and CA-125

Clear cell carcinoma

- Müllerian origin
- Poor prognosis
- 10% bilateral
- 15% associated with primary in the uterus
- Highly malignant

Brenner tumours

- Transitional epithelium from Wolffian remnants
- Fibrous elements
- Usually benign (99%)
- If malignant, may be associated with bladder tumour

Borderline tumours

- Low malignant potential
- No stromal invasion
- May have extra ovarian spread in 20% of cases
- Serous – 50% bilateral
- Mucinous – 5% bilateral
- 5-year survival: stage I = 97% and stage III = 85%

Endometrioid carcinoma

- May be secondary from endometrial carcinoma
- Can arise in endometriosis

Sex cord/stromal tumours

- Thecoma
- Granulose cell tumour
- Androblastoma

Granulosa cell tumours

- Solid and 75% have endocrine function
- Usually occur in women >60 years of age but also can occur before puberty
- Can present with PMB, irregular cycle and bleeding and precocious pseudo puberty
- Juvenile – 5% are malignant and aggressive
- Treatment is chemotherapy

Androblastoma (arrhenoblastoma)

- Sertoli – most common, usually benign

- 70% oestrogenic, 20% androgenic and 10% no secretion
- Leydig cell and mixed Sertoli–Leydig tumours – very rare

Germ cell tumours

- Most common type in woman aged <30 years
- Malignant: 2–3%; 30% in women aged <20 years
- Categorised by the degree of cellular differentiation

Dysgerminoma

- 50% of malignant germ cell tumours
- Usually in women aged <30 years
- Bilateral: 10–15%
- Not associated with hirsutism
- Secretes lactate dehydrogenase and placental alkaline phosphatase
- Secretes β-hCG in 3% of the cases
- Has lymphoid infiltration of the stroma on histological examination
- Radio and chemo sensitive
- Chemotherapy preserves ovarian function

Embryonic tumours

- Mature cystic teratoma (dermoid) is a benign tumour and is usually seen in women of childbearing age. They are unilocular and bilateral in 10–15% of cases. In 1% of cases, malignant change can occur
- Immature teratomas are common in the first 2 decades of life and are malignant. They are unilateral and frequently contain neural tissue. Occasionally, they may secrete thyroid hormones (struma ovarii) and serotonin (carcinoid)
- Embryonal carcinoma – secrete β-hCG and α-fetoprotein

Extra embryonic differentiation

- Yolk sac or endodermal sinus tumour – secrete α-fetoprotein
- Present at 14–20 years of age
- Unilateral, chemosensitive
- Malignant ovarian choriocarcinoma – secrete β-hCG
- May present with precocious puberty
- Poor prognosis and poor response to chemotherapy

Miscellaneous

- Gonadoblastoma – benign
- Streak ovary or testis
- Leydig cell tumours
- Small cell carcinoma

Metastatic tumours

- Constitute up to 10% of tumours
- Most common from stomach, breast and colon
- Krukenberg tumour – mucin secreting tumour
- Bilateral and solid
- Signet ring cells on histology

Sanusi FA, Carter P, Barton DPJ. Non epithelial ovarian cancers. Personal assessment in continuing education. Reviews, questions and answers. RCOG Press, 2003; 3:38–39.
Kumar B and Davies-Humphreys J. Tumour markers and ovarian cancer screening. Personal assessment in continuing education. Reviews, questions and answers. RCOG Press, 2003; 3:51–53.
Shafi MI, Luesley DM, Jordan JA. Handbook of Gynaecological Oncology. Edinburgh: Churchill Livingstone; 2001.

51. D Hysteroscopy and endometrial biopsy

Due to an oestrogen deficiency, the endometrial thickness in postmenopausal women is much thinner compared to premenopausal women. The probability of endometrial cancer increases with increasing endometrial thickness. A thickness of >5 mm increases the likelihood of endometrial cancer in postmenopausal women and thus warrants investigation in the form of endometrial pipelle sampling or hysteroscopy plus endometrial biopsy. A thickness of <5 mm has a negative predictive value of 98%. A meta-analysis also found that endometrial thickness of 5 mm or less reduced the risk of endometrial pathology by 84%.

The differential diagnosis of postmenopausal bleeding (PMB) includes:

- Genital atrophy (88% of PMB)
- Atrophic endometritis, atrophic vaginitis
- Endometrial cancer (8% of PMB)
- Endometrial hyperplasia (up to 10% of PMB)
- Endometrial polyp (5–9% of PMB)
- Cervical polyp and cervical cancer
- Ovarian tumours (2% of PMB)

The majority (80%) of women with endometrial cancer present with PMB. The second most common malignancy is cervical cancer and the third most common is ovarian cancer. Malignancies arising from the vagina, vulva and fallopian tube are rare.

Extragenital causes of bleeding should be ruled out in women with recurrent PMB or PMB following hysterectomy (bleeding may be from bladder cancer or urethral polyps, caruncle or prolapsed urethral mucosa).

52. D Hysteroscopy and endometrial biopsy

Postmenopausal bleeding refers to any vaginal bleeding that occurs in menopausal women (absence of menstrual period for 1 year) other than the expected cyclical bleeding that occurs in women taking a sequential regimen of hormone replacement therapy. Until proven otherwise, this bleeding warrants investigation to rule out cancer and therefore needs referral to the gynaecology oncology clinic as a target patient. All patients should be seen in the clinic within 2 weeks of referral. However, the diagnosis can be made by 31 days once the patient is seen and if it is cancer the treatment should be initiated by 62 days from the time seen, or 30 days from the time of diagnosis.

Tamoxifen is an oestrogen antagonist in breast tissue and an agonist in endometrial tissue. It is used in the treatment of breast cancer following surgery in women with receptor positive breast cancer. The duration used is usually 5 years because there is no evidence to show benefit after this period (the risks outweigh benefits).

There is a slightly increased risk of endometrial cancer in such women and there are no associated specific ultrasound findings. The only way forward is endometrial biopsy in women with abnormal vaginal bleeding. By agonist action, tamoxifen causes endometrial thickening and it is difficult to define a cut-off value of endometrial thickness on ultrasonography for initiating investigation although some articles suggest 12 mm. However, women on tamoxifen presenting with PMB need urgent hysteroscopy and endometrial biopsy to rule out endometrial cancer.

53. H TVS for endometrial thickness

All women presenting with postmenopausal bleeding need urgent TVS if clinical findings are normal. This helps the clinician to decide the necessity of an endometrial biopsy in such women. However, in women with normal endometrial thickness, one should take an individual approach in deciding the need for endometrial biopsy and this may depend on the risk factors in such women. If the endometrial thickness is > 5 mm, an endometrial biopsy should be done in the form of an endometrial pipelle biopsy or hysteroscopy and endometrial biopsy.

54. G No further tests required

The most common cause of postmenopausal bleeding is atrophic endometritis or vaginitis (88%). If the endometrial thickness is normal and the clinical findings are suggestive of atrophy, reassure women. However, if these women continue to bleed, they would need a hysteroscopy and endometrial biopsy.

55. D Hysteroscopy and endometrial biopsy

Any woman with ongoing postmenopausal bleeding will need an endometrial biopsy despite normal endometrial thickness on the TVS.

National Institute of Health and Clinical Excellence (NICE). Referral for suspected cancer (CG27). NICE, 2011.

Rogerson L and Jones S. The investigation of women with postmenopausal bleeding. Pace review No. 98/07. London: RCOG Press, 2003: 10–13.

Gupta JK, Chien PF, Voit D, Clark TJ, Khan KS. Ultrasonographic endometrial thickness for diagnosing endometrial pathology in women with postmenopausal bleeding: a meta-analysis. Acta Obstet Gynecol Scand 2002; 81:799–816.

Franchi M, Ghezzi F, Donadello N, Zanaboni F, Beretta P, Bolis P. Endometrial thickness in tamoxifen-treated patients: an independent predictor of endometrial disease. Obstet Gynecol 1999; 93:1004–1008.

Smith-Bindman R, Weiss E, Feldstein V. How thick is too thick? When endometrial thickness should prompt biopsy in postmenopausal women without vaginal bleeding. Ultrasound Obstet Gynecol 2004; 24:558–565.

Sahdev A. Imaging the endometrium in postmenopausal bleeding. BMJ 2007; 334:635–636.

56. E Cyclophosphamide

Alkylating agents bind covalently to DNA side chains and cause cross-linkage and strand breaks. They act on multiple phases of the cell cycle (therefore they kill both slowly and rapidly proliferating cells). Alkylating drugs include melphalan, chlorambucil, cyclophosphamide, ifosfamide and treosulfan. Cyclophosphamide is an alkylating agent which is inactive in itself and has to be converted to an active drug (4-hydroxy cyclophosphamide) in the liver. It then decomposes within the cells to form phosphoramide mustard and acrolein (this is excreted in the urine and is toxic to bladder epithelium). It is less myelotoxic than other alkylating agents (melphalan causes leukaemia in the long run).

It causes haemorrhagic cystitis (ifosfamide also causes this side effect) which can be neutralised by administering acetylcysteine or mesna (it neutralises the effects of acrolein). It can also cause alopecia. It is not currently used as first line treatment for ovarian cancer.

57. K Paclitaxel

Paclitaxel belongs to the taxane group of drugs and acts by binding to microtubules (it prevents depolymerisation into tubulin dimers), thereby disrupting mitosis. When administered intravenously, it is 95% protein bound and is metabolised in the liver by the cytochrome P450 enzyme system. However, 5–10% is excreted in the kidneys.

Side effects include neutropaenia, arrhythmias, sensory peripheral neuropathy and alopecia. It is also associated with hypersensitivity reactions which can be reduced by the administration of glucocorticoids and H1 and H2 antagonists prior to infusion.

58. N Vincristine

Vincristine belongs to the vinca alkaloids and acts by binding to tubulin (it prevents polymerisation), thus causing mitotic arrest in the G2 and M phases of the cell cycle. It is highly protein bound (like paclitaxel) and is metabolised in the liver. Side effects include neurotoxicity (paraesthesia, motor weakness and cranial nerve palsy) and myelosuppression.

59. C Cisplatin

Cisplatin and carboplatin belong to the platinum group of drugs (they act by cross-linking with DNA strands). Conventionally, cisplatin was used as a first line treatment alone or in combination therapy for the treatment of ovarian cancer.

Cisplatin is administered intravenously and is 90% protein bound. It is mainly excreted by the kidneys and is highly nephrotoxic (dose limiting toxicity). This can be reduced to some extent by forced diuresis. The newer drug carboplatin is much less nephrotoxic than cisplatin and has therefore replaced it in modern chemotherapy for ovarian cancer. Cisplatin also causes peripheral neuropathy and is toxic to the middle ear causing high frequency hearing loss and tinnitus.

60. I Methotrexate

Methotrexate is an antimetabolite and acts by inhibiting dihydrofolate reductase. It is excreted mainly in the kidneys. It is used in the treatment of gestational trophoblastic disease and also ectopic pregnancy. Side effects include mucositis, nausea, vomiting, photosensitivity, nephrotoxicity and hepatotoxicity.

Shafi MI, Luesley DM, Jordan JA. Handbook of Gynaecological Oncology. Edinburgh: Churchill Livingstone, 2001.

Chapter 17

Urogynaecology and pelvic floor problems

Questions: SBAs

For each question, select the single best answer from the five options listed.

1. A 45-year-old woman with four children attends the urogynaecology clinic with urgency, and incontinence when coughing or sneezing and during intercourse. There is no significant past medical history and she is not taking any medication. Her body mass index is 35 kg/m² and she drinks three cups of tea every day.

    What is your initial management plan?

    A Conservative management
    B Ask the patient to keep a bladder diary and employ conservative measures and pelvic floor exercises for 6 months
    C Ask the patient to keep a bladder diary and employ conservative measures and pelvic floor exercises for 3 months
    D Pad tests
    E Urodynamic studies

2. A 66-year-old multiparous woman attends the general gynaecology clinic complaining of occasional incontinence when coughing and sneezing. She also says there is 'something coming down the vagina' that is causing a 'dragging' sensation. On examination, there is procidentia.

    How will you manage her?

    A Pelvic floor exercises
    B Reassurance and discharge
    C Referral to a specialist in urogynaecology
    D Insertion of a ring pessary
    E Insertion of a shelf pessary

3. A 45-year-old woman has been referred to the urogynaecology clinic with recurrent urinary tract infections over the last 3 months. Despite repeated courses of antibiotics, frequency and dysuria have continued. Today's urinary dipstick test is positive for leucocytes.

    What is the next step in management?

    A   Ask the patient to keep a bladder diary
    B   Give antibiotics
    C   Measure the post-voiding residual urine
    D   Repeat the urinary dipstick test
    E   Send a midstream urine sample to the laboratory for microscopy and sensitivity

4. A 45-year-old woman attends the general gynaecology clinic with complaints of urgency, frequency and urge incontinence. There is no significant past medical history and she is not taking any medication. She also reports faecal incontinence.

    How will you manage her?

    A   Bladder training
    B   Desmopressin
    C   Oxytocin
    D   Pelvic floor exercises
    E   Referral to a specialist service

5. A foundation year 1 (FY1) doctor is taking a history from a woman who has been referred to the urogynaecology clinic. She is 50 years old and is complaining of nocturia, urgency and frequency, with occasional incontinence when she coughs. The doctor is not sure whether this woman needs a urodynamics test.

    In which of the following circumstances should urodynamic tests be performed?

    A   Before surgery in women who have symptoms of posterior compartment prolapse
    B   Before surgery in women who have symptoms of voiding dysfunction
    C   Before surgery in women who have symptoms of an underactive bladder
    D   Before surgery in women who have symptoms of stress incontinence
    E   Prior to starting conservative management

6. A 46-year-old woman with a body mass index of 25 kg/m^2 attends the urogynaecology clinic, complaining of an inability to stop herself from urinating when she first feels the desire to micturate. She has never had any children. She does not drink tea or coffee but drinks 1.5 L of water during the day. There is no significant past medical history and she is not taking any medication. A urine dipstick test is negative for leucocytes and nitrites.

    What is the correct treatment to offer?

    A   Advise her to drink less water
    B   Bladder training for 6 weeks
    C   Bladder training for 8 weeks
    D   Bladder training for 12 weeks
    E   Pelvic floor exercises for 3 months

7. A 47-year-old multiparous woman is seen at a 6-month follow-up in the urogynaecology clinic. She gives a history of arthritis, for which she is taking medication. She is still complaining of frequency, urgency and urge incontinence. Medical treatment with oxybutynin and tolterodine has not improved the symptoms. She is really unhappy about this and wants to know what can be done to improve her symptoms.

    What is the next management option?

    A   Continued anticholinergics
    B   Percutaneous sacral nerve stimulation
    C   Percutaneous posterior tibial nerve stimulation
    D   Transcutaneous sacral nerve stimulation
    E   Transcutaneous posterior tibial nerve stimulation

8. A 60-year-old woman diagnosed with overactive bladder was prescribed oral oxybutynin to be taken daily. You see her 4 weeks after she started the medication. When you review her symptoms in the clinic, she says they have not improved on this medication.

    How should she be managed next?

    A   Oxybutynin for another 4 weeks
    B   Bladder training
    C   Urodynamic studies
    D   Reassurance
    E   Replacement of the oxybutynin with darifenacin

9. A 47-year-old woman attends the urogynaecology clinic with symptoms of urgency, urge incontinence, frequency and nocturia. Conservative and medical treatment has not improved them. Urodynamic studies suggest an overactive bladder. There is no significant past medical history and she is not taking any medication.

    What is the appropriate management?

    A   Multidisciplinary team review and injection of 100 units of botulinum A toxin
    B   Multidisciplinary team review and injection of 200 units of botulinum A toxin
    C   Multidisciplinary team review and injection of 400 units of botulinum A toxin
    D   Percutaneous sacral nerve stimulation
    E   Transcutaneous posterior tibial nerve stimulation

10. A 47-year-old multiparous woman is referred to the urogynaecology clinic because for the last 6 months she has been experiencing incontinence when she coughs and sneezes. She has tried conservative management with pelvic floor exercises, but this has not worked.

    How should she be managed?

    A   Botulinum toxin A
    B   Continued pelvic floor exercises
    C   Desmopressin
    D   Hysterectomy
    E   Synthetic mid-urethral tape

11. A 52-year-old woman attends the gynaecology clinic with a history of a 'heaviness/dragging' sensation in her vagina. She had a hysterectomy 10 years ago overseas and does not know the reason for it. She is otherwise healthy and well. She is not currently taking any medication. Examination reveals stage 1 post-hysterectomy vaginal vault prolapse.

How should she be managed?

A   Insertion of a ring pessary
B   Insertion of a shelf pessary
C   Open abdominal sacrocolpopexy
D   Pelvic floor training
E   Sacrospinous fixation

12. You are the registrar in theatre and are about to perform a vaginal hysterectomy for menorrhagia. The patient has a body mass index of 24 kg/m² and has not had any previous surgeries. The consultant asks what additional measure can be taken to reduce the chances of a post-hysterectomy vaginal vault prolapse while performing vaginal hysterecomy.

What procedure can be used to reduce the chances of a vaginal vault prolapse?

A   McCall culdoplasty
B   Open abdominal sacrocolpopexy
C   Subtotal hysterectomy
D   Sacrospinous fixation
E   None of the above

13. A 77-year-old woman attends the gynaecology clinic accompanied by her daughter. Her husband died 10 years ago and her daughter is her carer. The patient gives a 1-year history of feeling uncomfortable when she sits down. She has diabetes, hypertension and mild chronic obstructive pulmonary disease. On examination, she is frail, and procidentia is found. She has tried two ring pessaries but these were not successful in managing her symptoms.

What is the correct management?

A   Colpocleisis
B   Sacrocolpoplexy
C   Insertion of a shelf pessary
D   Pelvic floor training
E   Vaginal hysterectomy

14. Which one of the following is a risk factor for pelvic organ prolapse?

A   Afro-Caribbean ethnicity
B   Having bouts of diarrhoea
C   Heavy lifting
D   Smoking cigarettes
E   A previous vaginal delivery

15. A 25-year-old nulliparous woman is seen in the antenatal clinic at 30 weeks' gestation. The pregnancy has been low risk but she would like an elective Caesarean section because she is anxious about future pelvic organ prolapse.

What will you tell her regarding an elective Caesarean section?

A   A Caesearean section prevents prolapse
B   A Caesarean section does not prevent prolapse
C   A Caesearean section prevents prolapse when performed by a consultant
D   It is unclear whether a Caesarean section prevents prolapse
E   A vaginal birth prevents prolapse

Questions: EMQs

Questions 16–20

Options for Questions 16–20

A	Amitryptyline	I	Trospium chloride
B	Botulinum toxin	J	Propiverine HCl
C	Darifenacin	K	Dobutamine
D	Desmopressin	L	Drospirenone
E	Duloxetine	M	Desogestrel
F	Fesoterodine	N	Digoxin
G	Oxybutynin	O	Fexofenadine
H	Tolterodine		

Instructions: For each mechanism of action described below, choose the single most appropriate drug from the list of options above. Each option may be used once, more than once, or not at all.

16. Selective serotonin and noradrenergic reuptake inhibitor

17. Anticholinergic plus musculotrophic plus local anaesthetic

18. Anticholinergic plus calcium channel blocker

19. Competitive muscarinic receptor antagonist which is a prodrug

20. Uroselective, M3 muscarinic acetylcholine receptor antagonist

Answers: SBAs

1. **C Ask the patient to keep a bladder diary and employ conservative measures and pelvic floor exercises for 3 months**

   Mixed incontinence is treated in terms of the predominant symptom. Conservative management is the first choice, including 3 months of pelvic floor exercises. Pelvic floor training should consist of eight contractions carried out 3 times a day. Electromyography as biofeedback should not be routinely used with pelvic floor training. The exercises should be continued if an improvement is seen.

2. **C Referral to a specialist in urogynaecology**

   Women who have a symptomatic prolapse that is visible at or below the introitus should be referred to a specialist.

3. **C Measure the post-voiding residual urine**

   If recurrent urinary tract infections are occurring, the post-void residual volume should be measured by a bladder scan or catheterisation.

4. **E Referral to a specialist service**

   A patient should be referred to a specialist service if there is:

   - Bladder or urethral pain
   - A benign pelvic mass
   - Associated faecal incontinence
   - Suspected neurological disease
   - Suspected urogenital fistulas
   - Previous surgery for incontinence
   - Previous pelvic cancer surgery or pelvic radiation therapy

5. **B Before surgery in women who have symptoms of voiding dysfunction**

   Videourodynamics and ambulatory urodynamics should not be performed before starting conservative treatment. Urodynamic studies should be performed:

   - Before surgery in women who have symptoms of anterior compartment prolapse
   - Before surgery in women who have symptoms of voiding dysfunction
   - Before surgery in women who have symptoms of overactive bladder
   - In patients who have had prior surgery for stress incontinence

   They should not be performed if the history suggests pure stress urinary incontinence.

6.   B Bladder training for 6 weeks

First-line management for urgency or mixed urinary incontinence is bladder training for 6 weeks.

7.   B Percutaneous sacral nerve stimulation

Discussion of such patients in a multidisciplinary team (MDT) meeting helps to manage patients better. Patients who have not responded to medical treatment can be offered percutaneous sacral nerve stimulation but this decision must be made only in a MDT setting. Moreover, such treatment may be used for women who cannot perform intermittent catheterisation, and such woman therefore cannot be treated with botulinum toxin A.

Transcutaneous posterior tibial nerve stimulation should not be offered as there is insufficient evidence to recommend its use. In occasions where both conservative and medical treatments have failed and the woman declines botulinum toxin A or percutaneous sacral nerve stimulation, transcutaneous posterior tibial nerve stimulation can be considered but the decision has to pass through the MDT.

8.   E Replacement of the oxybutynin with darifenacin

Oxybutynin (immediate release), tolterodine (immediate release) or darifenacin (once daily preparation) should be offered for an overactive bladder. If the first medication does not improve the symptoms, the dose should be changed or another drug offered. A telephone interview or face-to-face consultation should be offered to all patients 4 weeks after starting a new medication, but if the side effects are intolerable, an earlier appointment should be offered from the start of the medical therapy.

9.   B Multidisciplinary team review and injection of 200 units of botulinum A toxin

If overactive bladder syndrome has been proved by urodynamic studies and the patient has not responded to conservative or medical treatment, she should be discussed in the multidisciplinary team meeting and then be given 200 units of botulinum toxin A, injected into the bladder wall.

She should be informed of the risk of urinary retention with botulinum toxin A injection and the potential need for clean intermittent catheterisation, and it should be confirmed that the patient is willing to catheterise herself because otherwise botulinum toxin A injections cannot be given. If botulinum toxin A is effective, follow-up should be offered at 6 months, or sooner if the symptoms return.

10.   E Synthetic mid-urethral tape

If conservative measures fail, one of the following should be offered:

- Synthetic mid-urethral tape
- Open colposuspension
- Autologous rectus fascial sling

A synthetic tape should be safe and of the highest quality. It should be made of type 1 macroporous polypropylene. Coloured tape allows for better visibility, easier insertion and revision of the procedure if necessary. If a transobturator approach is used, the woman should be informed that there are no long-term data on outcome.

Currently, there is some controversy about the use of mesh devices because they are now known to cause long-term complications. This answer is correct at the time of going to press, but modifications of guidelines are anticipated by 2019 at the latest. The RCOG website has up-to-date information.

11. D Pelvic floor training

Pelvic floor muscle training is advised for stage 1 and 2 vaginal prolapse, including post-hysterectomy vaginal prolapse. A vaginal pessary should be used for stage 3 and 4 post-hysterectomy vaginal prolapse.

12. A McCall culdoplasty

A McCall culdoplasty or suture of the cardinal and uterosacral ligaments to the vaginal cuff at the time of hysterectomy can prevent a post-hysterectomy vaginal prolapse. Sacrospinous fixation at the time of hysterectomy should be considered if the vault descends to the introitus during closure. Subtotal hysterectomy does not prevent a post-hysterectomy vaginal vault prolapse.

13. A Colpocleisis

Colpoclesis is a procedure that is suitable for frail elderly women who are not sexually active.

14. C Heaving lifting

The risk factors for pelvic organ prolapse are:

- White ethnic origin
- Older age
- Constipation
- Heavy lifting
- Two children or more
- Genetic predisposition

15. D It is unclear whether a Caesarean section prevents prolapse

The role of Caesarean section in the prevention of incontinence and symptomatic prolapse is unclear. In theory, it may be assumed that it does prevent pelvic organ prolapse because the woman does not go into labour and a vaginal delivery is associated with utero-vaginal prolapse. However, it is not easy to predict which women are more prone to develop pelvic organ prolapse. A perineal massage and the application of hot packs in the second stage of labour have shown to reduce the risk of a perineal tear but not the risk of prolapse.

Answers: EMQs

16. E Duloxetine

Duloxetine is a selective serotonin and noradrenergic reuptake inhibitor, which increases the contraction of the rhabdosphincter. It is used in the treatment of stress incontinence. The dose is 40 mg twice daily and can be reduced to 20 mg daily after reassessment in 2 weeks. The side effects include nausea, vomiting, constipation, diarrhoea, dry mouth, insomnia, drowsiness, headache, dizziness, anorexia and blurred vision. The contraindications to its use include liver disease, pregnancy and breastfeeding.

17. G Oxybutynin

Oxybutynin is anticholinergic, musculotropic and also has local anaesthetic effect. The dose is 2.5 mg 3 times daily to 5 mg 4 times daily. It causes more dryness of mouth than selective anticholinergic drugs and is used in the treatment of detrusor instability.

18. J Propiverine HCl

Propiverine HCl is an anticholinergic and a calcium channel blocker. It antagonises muscarinic receptors and directly relaxes the muscle. The side effects are dry mouth and blurring of vision. The dose is 15–30 mg twice daily.

19. F Fesoterodine

Fesoterodine is a newer anticholinergic drug used in the treatment of detrusor instability. It is a competitive, non-uroselective muscarinic receptor antagonist and is a prodrug. The dose is 4–8 mg once daily. The side effects include insomnia, less often nasal dryness, pharyngo-laryngeal pain, cough and vertigo.

20. C Darifenacin

Darifenacin is a M3 muscarinic acetylcholine receptor antagonist and is uroselective. The daily dose is 7.5–15 mg once daily. It is not recommended for women with severe hepatic impairment.

Solifenacin has similar actions to darifenacin and is not recommended in women a with severe hepatic impairment.

Other drugs

Trospium chloride is a non-selective, anticholinergic drug and a competitive muscarinic receptor antagonist. The dose is 20 mg twice daily. It causes less dry mouth compared to oxybutynin. It is used in the treatment of detrusor instability.

Tolterodine is a competitive, non-uroselective muscarinic antagonist (M1, 2, 3, 4 and 5), which causes less dryness of the mouth than oxybutynin. The dose is 2–4 mg once daily.

Desmopressin enhances the reabsorption of water in the kidneys by increasing cellular permeability of the collecting ducts and is highly effective for women with nocturia. The dose is 200–400 µg once daily at night-time.

Abboudi H, Fynes MF, Doumouchtsis SK. Contemporary therapy for the overactive bladder. Obstet Gynaecol 2011; 13:98–105.